A RAPID ACTION GUIDE

When seconds count

● Every emergency demands urgent action.
But sometimes the urgency is so pressing
that seconds can mean the difference between
minor and major damage or injury — in some
cases, between life and death.

● This "Rapid action" section is a guide to
help you to cope with emergencies of the
specially urgent kind that can occur in and
around the home.

● The instructions give only the essential
information needed for taking immediate
action. Additional details about all of the
emergencies dealt with here are given in
the main sections of the book.

Someone who has stopped breathing will probably suffer brain damage after about four minutes and die within ten minutes. Mouth-to-mouth resuscitation puts air into the lungs until the victim can breathe again.

ARTIFICIAL RESPIRATION

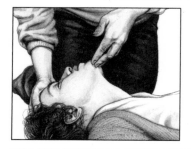

1 With one hand on the forehead and the fingers of the other hand under the chin, tilt the head backward to open the airway.

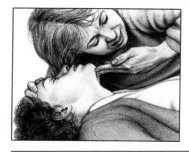

2 Look at the chest for movement. Listen for sounds of breathing. Feel for exhaled breath on your cheek. If none of these signs is present, the victim is not breathing and needs artificial respiration.

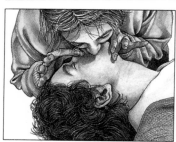

3 Pinch the nose closed with your fingers and blow two full breaths into his mouth, pausing in between to take a breath yourself. (For infants, cover both nose and mouth, and breathe gently.)

4 Look, listen and feel for air exchange. Check the neck pulse. If there is a pulse but no breathing, continue giving one breath every five seconds. (Give one every four seconds to a child; one every three seconds to an infant.)

5 When breathing begins, put the victim into the recovery position like this (see page 31).

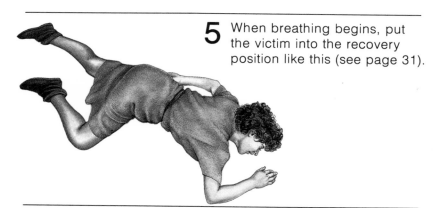

BLEEDING

Even if you cannot stop the bleeding altogether, reducing the flow of blood may be enough to save life.

Large foreign body in skin ▶

Bleeding that will not stop ▶

Bleeding from nose, ear or mouth ▶

If a deep cut causes blood to flow

1 Lay the victim down. Remove clothing from around the wound if you can do so without wasting time.

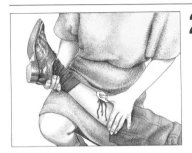

2 If there is no large foreign object in the wound, press down hard on it with any clean, absorbent material, or even your bare hands. If possible, raise the wound above the level of the heart to slow the flow of blood.

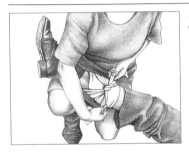

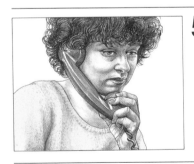

3 Maintain the pressure until the bleeding stops. While doing so, place an absorbent pad, such as the inside of a clean folded handkerchief or pillowcase, over the wound and bandage it firmly in place with a scarf or piece of clean linen.

4 If blood seeps through the dressing, do not remove it. Put another on top.

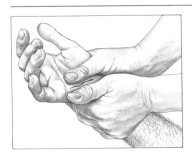

5 Take the victim to the emergency department of your local hospital. If you need an ambulance, call 911, or call the ambulance directly if your area is not yet served by this toll-free emergency number. For telephone assistance in a crisis, simply dial zero.

If the wound is large

Squeeze the sides of the wound together gently but firmly, and maintain the pressure until the bleeding stops. If possible, raise the wound above the level of the heart. Continue as for a deep cut (step 3 above).

If there is a large foreign body in the skin

1 If bleeding is profuse, squeeze the edges of the wound together around the object.

- *DO NOT TRY TO REMOVE IT, AS IT MAY BE PLUGGING THE WOUND.*

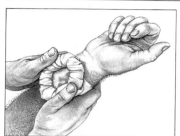

2 Put a piece of clean cloth over the wound. Then put a thick circular pad of clean material around the wound, preferably higher than the object, to prevent pressure on it (see page 58).

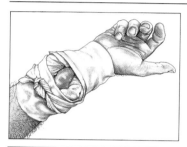

3 Bandage it with diagonally applied strips of material that do not go over the foreign body.

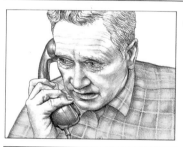

4 Call 911 and ask for an ambulance, or take the victim to the emergency department of your local hospital.

If the bleeding will not stop

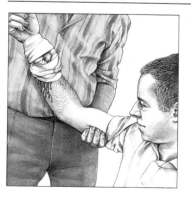

1 **A severely bleeding arm**
As a last resort, press your fingers between the muscles on the underside of the upper arm. This will compress the brachial artery, which roughly follows the seam of the sleeve. Press up and in, pushing the artery against the bone.

- *DO NOT MAINTAIN MAXIMUM PRESSURE FOR LONGER THAN 5 MINUTES LEST YOU CAUSE IRREPARABLE DAMAGE TO THE LIMB.*
- *DO NOT APPLY A TOURNIQUET.*

SEE NEXT PAGE

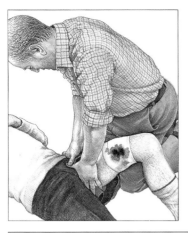

A severely bleeding leg

As a last resort, lay the victim down with the injured leg bent. Press down in the center of the fold of the groin with both thumbs, one on top of the other, against the rim of the pelvis. This will compress the femoral artery.

- *DO NOT MAINTAIN MAXIMUM PRESSURE FOR LONGER THAN 5 MINUTES LEST YOU DAMAGE THE LIMB IRREPARABLY.*
- *DO NOT APPLY A TOURNIQUET.*

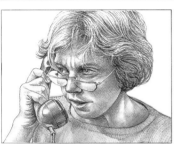

2 Tell someone to call 911 or your local ambulance service.

If an injured person bleeds from nose, ear or mouth

1 This can indicate severe injury to head or chest. Put the victim in a half-sitting position, with the head inclined toward the injured side, to allow the blood to drain.

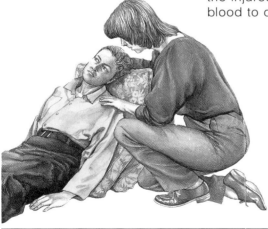

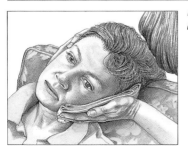

2 Cover the bleeding point, but do not apply pressure.

SEE NEXT PAGE

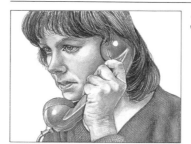

3 Call 911 and ask for an ambulance. If your area is not yet served by this toll-free emergency number, dial zero and ask the operator to get help for you.

4 If the person becomes unconscious, put her in the recovery position like this (see page 31).

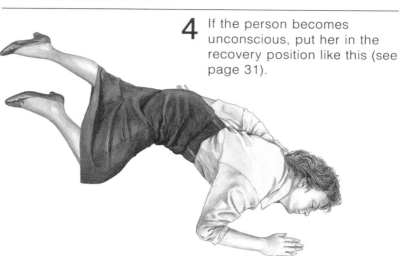

BURNS AND SCALDS

Many burns need medical attention because of the risk of infection and shock. A young child or a sick or old person should always be taken to a doctor.

If the burn or scald is smaller than a 25¢ piece

Large burns and
scalds ▶

1 If possible, remove rings, watch or constricting clothing before the area starts to swell.

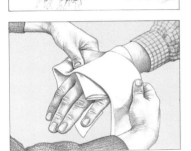

2 **Is it very painful?**
If so, the burn is probably superficial. Put it under slow-running cold water for ten minutes, or longer if pain continues.
Cover the burn with clean, non-fluffy material. A sterile dressing is best, but the inside of a folded handkerchief, bound on with cloth, will do.

Is it peeling or charred?
If the skin looks gray, and is peeling or charred and not very painful, the burn may be deep and serious. Cover it (see above) and go to the doctor or to the emergency department of a hospital.

- *DO NOT USE ADHESIVE DRESSINGS.*
- *DO NOT APPLY FAT, OINTMENT OR LOTION.*
- *DO NOT BREAK A BLISTER OR TOUCH A BURN.*

If the burn or scald is larger than a 25¢ piece

1 If possible, remove rings, watch or constricting clothing before the area starts to swell.

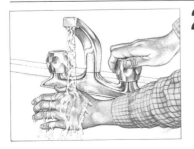

2 Cool the burn by holding it under cold, running water for at least ten minutes, or longer if the pain continues. Cool a large area with a damp, clean cloth, but do not waste time before getting medical help.

SEE NEXT PAGE

7

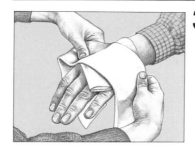

3 Cover the burn with clean, non-fluffy material. A sterile dressing is best, but the inside of a clean folded handkerchief, bound on with a scarf or other cloth, will do.

4 See your doctor or go to the emergency department of your local hospital.

- *DO NOT USE ADHESIVE DRESSINGS.*
- *DO NOT APPLY FAT, OINTMENT OR LOTION.*
- *DO NOT BREAK BLISTERS OR TOUCH THE BURN.*

If the burn or scald covers a large area of the body

A person who receives burns over a large area of the body, such as an arm, thigh, lower leg or chest, is likely to suffer shock, and needs urgent hospital treatment.

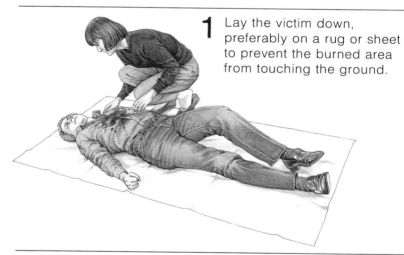

1 Lay the victim down, preferably on a rug or sheet to prevent the burned area from touching the ground.

2 If possible, remove any rings, watch, shoes or constrictive clothing before the area begins to swell.

Remove clothing soaked in boiling liquid when it has begun to cool.

- *DO NOT REMOVE ANYTHING THAT IS STICKING TO THE BURN.*

SEE NEXT PAGE

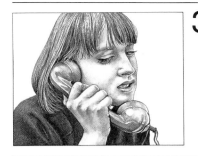

3 Call 911 and ask for an ambulance, or arrange to take the victim to the emergency department of your local hospital.

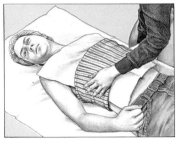

4 Cover the burn with clean, non-fluffy material, such as a freshly washed pillowcase. Fix it in place with a scarf or a piece of clean cloth.

- *DO NOT APPLY FAT, OINTMENT OR LOTION.*
- *DO NOT TOUCH THE BURN.*

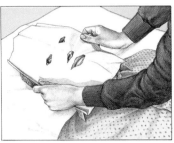

For burns to the face, make a mask from a clean pillowcase by cutting holes for nose, mouth and eyes.

- *DO NOT APPLY FAT, OINTMENT OR LOTION.*
- *DO NOT TOUCH THE BURN.*

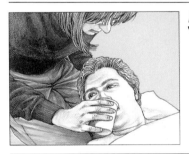

5 If the victim is conscious, give frequent sips of cold water to replace lost fluid.

6 If a person with burns on the front becomes unconscious, put him in this recovery position. Turn the head to one side and tilt it back to open the airway. Raise the opposite side of the body by supporting it on a large cushion.

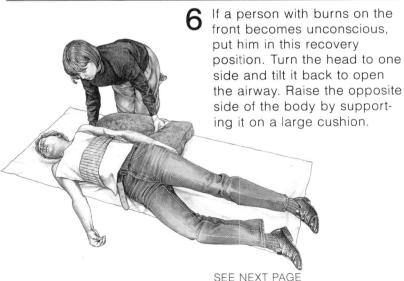

SEE NEXT PAGE

BURNS AND SCALDS

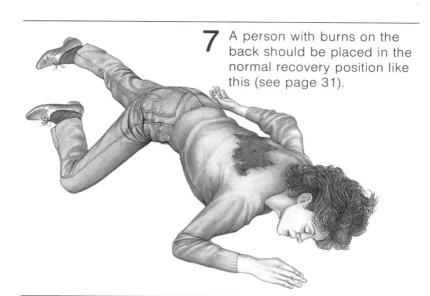

7 A person with burns on the back should be placed in the normal recovery position like this (see page 31).

BURNS AND SCALDS

BURST PIPE OR LEAKING TANK

When water pours through a ceiling, it is probably coming from a burst pipe.

If water pours through the ceiling

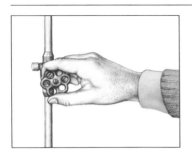

1 Close the main shutoff valve. It is usually in the basement near the water meter, or on the supply pipe from the well in a well system.

Leaking tank ▶

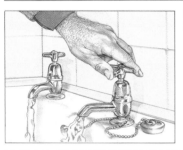

2 Open a faucet in the lowest part of the house to drain the water from the pipes. When the water stops flowing from the faucet, the flow from the leak will have stopped also.

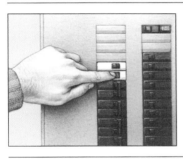

3 If water is running down a light fixture, switch off the light and cut the power to that circuit by tripping a breaker or removing a fuse at the main control panel or fuse box.

- *DO NOT TURN THE CIRCUIT BACK ON UNTIL IT HAS BEEN CHECKED BY AN ELECTRICIAN.*

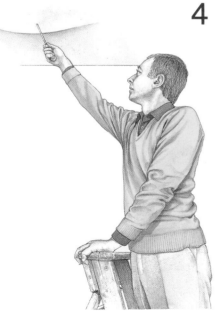

4 If the ceiling plaster is bulging, put a large bowl or bucket beneath the bulge and pierce the plaster with a screwdriver or chisel. Stand out of the way, and have spare buckets ready. This will limit damage to your ceiling to one area.

   Call a plumber as soon as these four steps are completed.

If your hot water tank is leaking

1 Switch off the heat source, whether electricity, gas or oil.

2 Shut off the cold water supply to the tank.

3 Call a plumber.

BURST PIPE OR LEAKING TANK

CHOKING

Anything that goes down a person's windpipe, rather than the food passage, must be brought up again as soon as possible.

If the victim is conscious

1 Do not interfere with a person who is choking, as long as he can cough forcefully. Encourage him to cough. It may be all that is needed to dislodge the blockage.

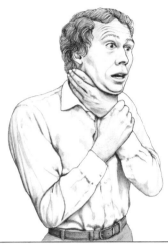

2 If this fails, and the victim is coughing or breathing with extreme difficulty, or he can no longer cough or breathe, quickly ask him if he is choking. If he is unable to speak or nods his head "yes," have someone call for medical aid and begin the Heimlich maneuver. (Immediate intervention is in order, too, if the victim clutches his throat – an instinctive sign of choking – or turns blue.)

Treating children ▶

Treating infants ▶

Unconscious victim ▶

CHOKING

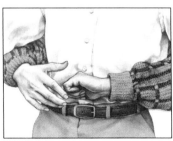

3 Stand behind him and, with your arms around him, clench your fist and thrust it, thumb knuckle inward, at a spot well below the breastbone, slightly above the navel, and well away from either side of the rib cage.

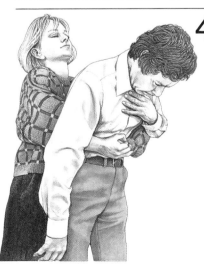

4 Hold your fist with the other hand and pull both hands toward you with a quick upward-and-inward thrust from the elbows. You are trying to elevate the diaphragm so that the air thus forced out of the lungs may dislodge the blockage. Repeat continuously until the blockage is dislodged or the victim becomes unconscious.

Treating children

1 Encourage the child to cough. Do not interfere as long as she is coughing forcefully.

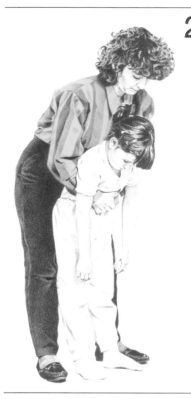

2 If the child ceases to cough and is making a high-pitched sound when inhaling, perform the Heimlich maneuver (steps 2 to 4 on the previous page).

Treating infants

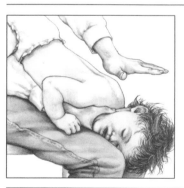

1 If a choking infant can no longer breathe or make sounds, support him face down on your forearm, which should be resting on your thigh. With the heel of your other hand, give him four rapid but light blows between the shoulder blades.

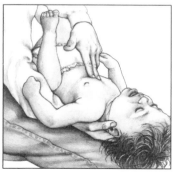

2 If this fails, turn the infant on his back so that his head is lower than his torso. Imagine a line drawn between his nipples, and place two fingers in the center of his chest about one finger's width below that line. (Make sure you do not touch the tip of the sternum.) Press inward rapidly four times.

If the victim becomes unconscious

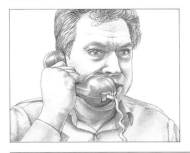

1 If a third person is present, tell him to call 911 and ask for an ambulance. If you are on your own, continue to help the victim.

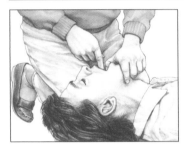

2 Place the victim on his back and open his mouth. Insert your index finger into his mouth and use a hooking action to dislodge food or any other thing along his cheek that might be blocking his airway. (You never perform blind finger sweeps on a child or infant.)

- *BE CAREFUL NOT TO FORCE AN OBJECT DEEPER INTO THE AIRWAY.*

3 If this fails, put one hand on the victim's forehead and the other under his chin to tilt his head, thus opening his airway.

4 Pinch his nose closed and blow two full breaths into his mouth, pausing in between to take a breath yourself.

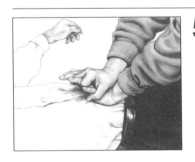

5 If artificial respiration does not restore breathing, straddle the victim's thighs and perform the Heimlich maneuver. Position the heel of one hand in the center of his abdomen, well below the breastbone, slightly above the navel, and well away from either side of the rib cage. Cover that hand with the other hand, fingers interlaced.

SEE NEXT PAGE

CHOKING

6 Without bending your elbows, press the abdomen inward and upward rapidly six to ten times.

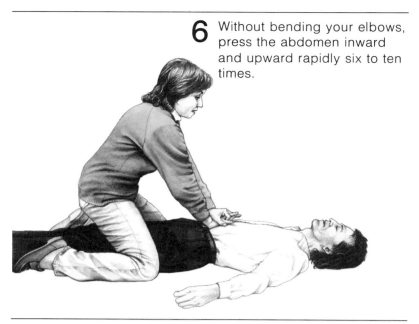

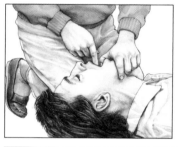

7 Perform the finger sweep again to see if the blockage has been dislodged. If it has, hook it out with a finger. If not, repeat steps 4 to 7 for as long as necessary.

DRUG OVERDOSE

An overdose of any drug (either an addictive drug or an ordinary medicine) is serious and requires urgent medical treatment. Symptoms include abnormal dilation or contraction of the pupils of the eyes, vomiting, difficulty in breathing, unconsciousness, sweating and hallucinations.

If a person takes a deliberate or accidental overdose

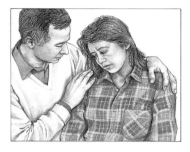

1 Ask the victim what has happened. Obtain any information about the drug that you can as soon as possible. The victim may become unconscious at any time.

- *DO NOT TRY TO INDUCE VOMITING. IT WASTES TIME AND MAY BE HARMFUL.*

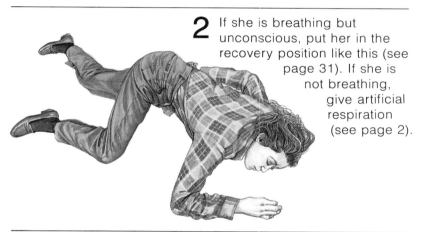

2 If she is breathing but unconscious, put her in the recovery position like this (see page 31). If she is not breathing, give artificial respiration (see page 2).

Alcohol poisoning ▶

DRUG OVERDOSE

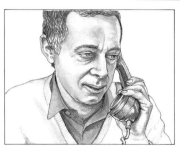

3 Call your poison control center; the number is listed in the front of your telephone directory. The medical personnel on the line will give you step-by-step instructions.

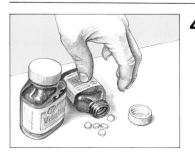

4 The poison control center will need information on any bottles or pill containers found near the victim. Send these and a sample of vomit in the ambulance if the patient is being hospitalized. These will help doctors determine the most appropriate treatment.

If a person becomes unconscious from alcohol poisoning

1 Put him in the recovery position like this, so that he does not choke on his own vomit (see page 31).

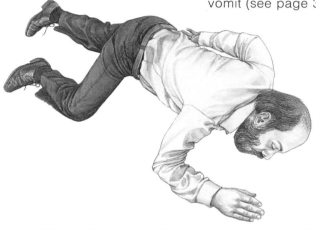

2 Call your poison control center. The center's staff will give you step-by-step instructions.

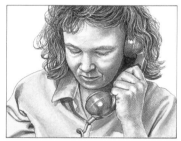

DRUG OVERDOSE

ELECTRIC SHOCK

If someone receives an electric shock at home or at work, break the victim's contact with the current in the quickest, safest way possible.

How to deal with situations involving an electrical injury

1 Stop the current by pulling out the plug. If for some reason you cannot reach the plug, switch off the power at the main fuse box.

- *DO NOT USE THE SWITCH ON THE APPLIANCE. A FAULTY SWITCH MAY BE THE CAUSE OF THE ACCIDENT.*

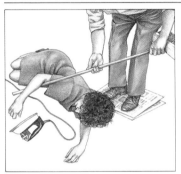

2 If there is no way to switch off, stand on dry insulating material, such as a thick layer of newspaper, a rubber mat or a wooden box, and push the victim's limbs away from the source with a broom or wooden chair.

- *DO NOT USE ANYTHING THAT IS DAMP OR MADE OF METAL.*

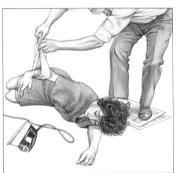

Alternatively, loop a rope, a pair of pantyhose or any dry fabric around the victim's feet or under the arms, and pull her free.

- *DO NOT TOUCH THE VICTIM WITH YOUR HANDS.*
- *DO NOT USE ANYTHING WET, SUCH AS A DAMP TOWEL.*

3 Once the victim is freed, tilt the head backward to open the airway. Check if she is breathing by looking for the rise and fall of her chest, by listening for breaths, and by feeling their movement against your cheek. If these signs are absent, have someone call 911, and begin artificial respiration immediately (see page 2).

SEE NEXT PAGE

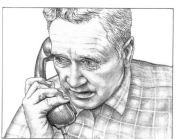

4 Even if the victim seems unharmed, call 911 and ask for an ambulance, or drive her to the emergency department of your local hospital. Tell the hospital how long she was in contact with the electricity.

ELECTRIC SHOCK

FIRE

When fire has taken hold in a house, get out quickly. Smoke, especially from plastic foam upholstery, can be deadly.

If a frying pan or a deep fryer catches fire

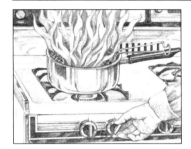

1 Turn off the heat on the stove. However, you should cover or extinguish the flames first (see 2 below) if the controls are at the back of the stove.

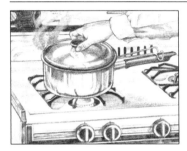

2 Cover the pan with its own lid, or use an extinguisher labeled B or ABC (see page 150) on the flames. If the fire is not out in 15 seconds, get everyone out of the house, close the kitchen door and call 911 or the fire department.

- *DO NOT MOVE THE PAN.*
- *DO NOT THROW WATER ON IT.*
- *DO NOT LIFT THE LID OFF A DEEP FRYER FOR HALF AN HOUR, EVEN IF THE FLAMES SEEM TO HAVE DIED DOWN.*

If an electrical appliance or plug catches fire

1 Get everyone out of the house. Then call 911 or the fire department.

2 If you can do so safely, try putting out the fire with an extinguisher labeled C or ABC (see page 150), while waiting for the fire department.

- *NEVER THROW WATER ON AN ELECTRICAL FIRE.*
- *DO NOT TOUCH ANY SWITCH ON A BURNING APPLIANCE OR PLUG.*

TV set on fire ▶

Oil heater on fire ▶

Foam furniture on fire ▶

Clothing on fire ▶

Smell of burning at night ▶

Trapped on upper floor ▶

FIRE

If a TV or computer catches fire

1 Get everyone out of the house. Then call 911 or the fire department.

2 Meantime, try to put out the fire with an extinguisher labeled C or ABC (see page 150), but only if you can do so safely. If you are not successful, get out of the house. Close the room door as you leave.

  • *DO NOT USE WATER, BECAUSE RESIDUAL ELECTRICITY MAY REMAIN IN THE SET, EVEN AFTER THE CURRENT IS SHUT OFF.*

If an oil heater catches fire

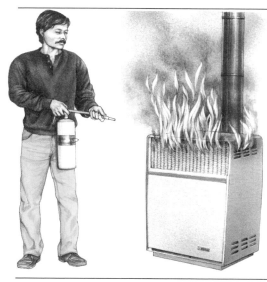

Follow steps 1 and 2 above with one important exception. Use only extinguishers labeled B or ABC. Never throw water on an oil fire.

FIRE

If a foam sofa or armchair catches fire

Burning plastic foam gives off choking black smoke that can overcome you very quickly. Do not try to put out the fire.

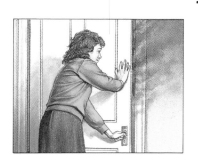

1 If you simply dropped a cigarette on the sofa, you would likely douse the fire right away by drenching the sofa with water. But once a fire has taken hold, get out of the room and close the door to prevent the smoke from spreading.

SEE NEXT PAGE

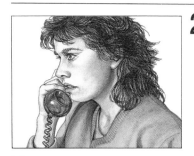

2 Get everyone out of the house and call 911 or the fire department, preferably from a neighbor's house.

If a person's clothes catch fire

1 Prevent the victim from rushing about in a panic; the movement will fan the flames.

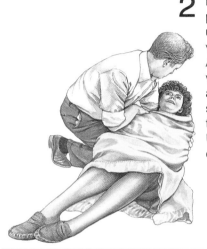

2 Lay the victim down to prevent the flames from rising up to the head, and roll the victim along the ground. Alternatively, you can use water to douse the flames, or a blanket, coat or drapes to smother them, but only after the person is on the ground. Use these methods only if you can do so without delay.

3 Treat the victim according to the extent of the burns (see pages 7, 8, 9 and 10).

Trapped on upper floor ▶

FIRE

If you smell burning at night

1 Alert everyone in the house.

2 Get everyone outside and count heads at a predetermined meeting place.

- *SMOKE DETECTORS ARE YOUR BEST BET AGAINST LOSS OF LIFE AND PROPERTY THROUGH FIRE. A DETECTOR WILL HAVE SENSED THE FIRE AND AWAKENED YOU LONG BEFORE YOU CAN SMELL THE SMOKE.*

SEE NEXT PAGE

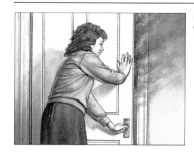

3 Shut all doors behind you to restrict the spread of flames and smoke.

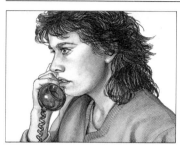

4 Go to the nearest telephone and call 911 or the fire department.

- *DO NOT GO BACK INSIDE.*

If you are trapped on an upper floor

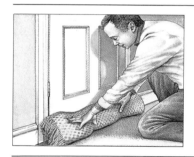

1 Go to a room at the front of the house, close the door and block up cracks with bedding or clothes.

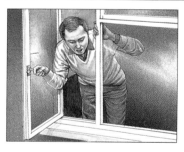

2 Open the window and call for help. Throw or hang something out the window to attract attention.

- *DO NOT JUMP OUT THE WINDOW, EXCEPT AS A LAST RESORT.*

FIRE

GAS LEAK

Your first priority is to get everyone out of the area.

If you smell gas indoors

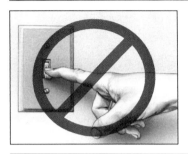

1 Avoid anything that might produce a spark or flame — a cigarette lighter, electric switch, lamp, flashlight, or telephone.

  • *DO NOT SWITCH OFF ANY LIGHT OR OTHER APPLIANCE ALREADY IN OPERATION.*

2 Get everyone out of the house. Leave the doors open as you go out so that the area gets ventilated.

3 Once in the open air, put any unconscious persons in the recovery position (see page 31).

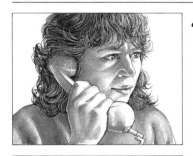

4 Call 911 or your gas company from a neighbor's house. Call for an ambulance if someone had become unconscious.

  • *DO NOT RETURN TO THE HOUSE UNTIL GAS OFFICIALS HAVE DECLARED THAT THE AREA IS SAFE.*

GAS OFFICE

Tel. ....

If you smell gas outside

1 Examine your surroundings for signs of excavation or construction. Gas leaks sometimes occur as a result of pipeline damage during such activities.

GAS LEAK

SEE NEXT PAGE

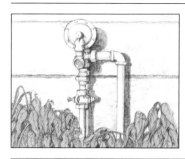

2 A ring of dead or wilting vegetation may also be a sign of gas leaking from an underground pipeline. Weather, too, can be a factor: underground gas leaks often bubble to the surface after rain.

3 Put out cigarettes; extinguish any naked flames; do not start up your car.

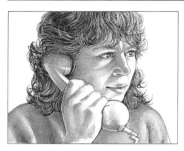

4 Get away from the gas odor. Once you are out of the area, call 911 or the gas company, and mention anything that may help the gas company pinpoint the leak.

GAS OFFICE

Tel. ....

GAS LEAK

POISONING

A house contains many substances, such as bleach, insecticides and paint stripper, that are highly dangerous to children. Get medical help quickly if a child swallows one.

If a child swallows a harmful household product

1 If the victim is conscious, try to discover what has been swallowed. Remember that he may become unconscious at any time.

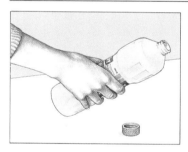

2 Call 911 or the poison control center. The center's medical staff will give you step-by-step instructions.

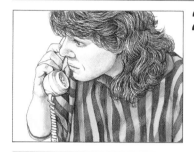

3 Have the container in your hand when you make the call, so that you can describe the contents accurately. If the victim has to go to hospital, bring the container and a sample of vomit with you. Such evidence can help doctors prescribe the appropriate antidote.

4 You will find instructions on the recovery position on page 31. You may be told to put an unconscious victim in this position while waiting for an ambulance, say.

Plant poisoning ▶

POISONING

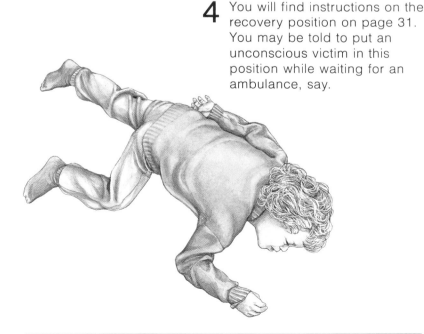

If a child eats a poisonous plant

The most common poisonous plants are azaleas, mistletoe, dieffenbachia, rhododendrons, jimsonweed, daffodil bulbs and mushrooms. Symptoms of poisoning include vomiting, diarrhea and stomach pains.

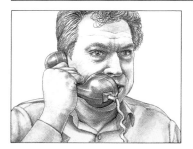

Call the poison control center. If you are directed to the nearest hospital, bring a sample of the plant, or give it to the ambulance attendants.

POISONING

STROKE OR HEART ATTACK

STROKE SYMPTOMS There may be headache, paralysis on one or both sides of the body, or difficulty swallowing and speaking. Possibly confusion and loss of consciousness.

HEART ATTACK SYMPTOMS Sudden crushing pain in the chest, often spreading to arms, neck and jaw. Possibly breathlessness.

Dealing with a possible stroke or heart attack

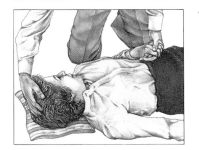

1 **Suspected stroke**
If the patient is conscious, put her in the recovery position, or lay her down with head and shoulders slightly raised and supported with a pillow. Place the head on one side to allow saliva to drain from the mouth.

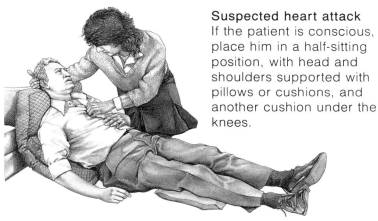

Suspected heart attack
If the patient is conscious, place him in a half-sitting position, with head and shoulders supported with pillows or cushions, and another cushion under the knees.

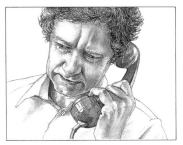

2 Call 911 or an ambulance immediately.

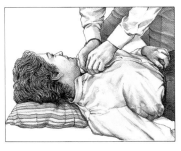

3 Loosen clothing around neck, chest and waist to help circulation and breathing.
- *DO NOT GIVE THE PATIENT ANYTHING TO EAT OR DRINK.*
- *DO NOT ALLOW A HEART ATTACK PATIENT TO MOVE UNNECESSARILY: IT WILL PUT EXTRA STRAIN ON THE HEART.*

STROKE OR HEART ATTACK

SEE NEXT PAGE

4 If the patient becomes unconscious, place her in the recovery position like this (see page opposite).

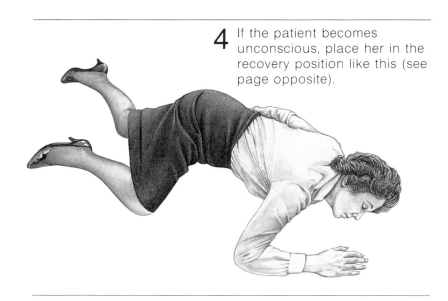

**STROKE OR
HEART ATTACK**

UNCONSCIOUS PERSON

Unless you suspect a fracture of the spine or neck, turn an unconscious, but breathing, victim to the recovery position. This will prevent blood, saliva or the tongue from blocking the windpipe. The recovery position is a priority treatment.

Putting an unconscious victim in the recovery position

1 Kneel beside the victim, about 9 in. (23 cm) away. Turn the head toward you, and tilt it back to open the airway.

2 Lay the nearer arm along the victim's side, slightly tucking it under the body and keeping it straight. Put the other arm across the chest. Place the far ankle over the near ankle.

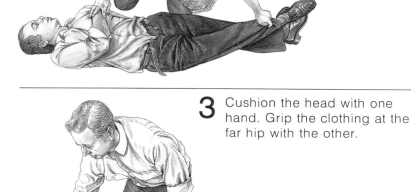

3 Cushion the head with one hand. Grip the clothing at the far hip with the other.

4 Turn the victim onto his side by pulling quickly toward you, supporting him with your knees.

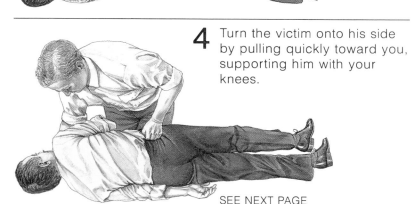

SEE NEXT PAGE

Turning a heavy person ▶

If an arm or leg is broken ▶

UNCONSCIOUS PERSON

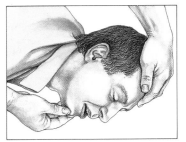

5 Tilt the head back to straighten the throat. This keeps the airway open, allowing the victim to breathe freely.

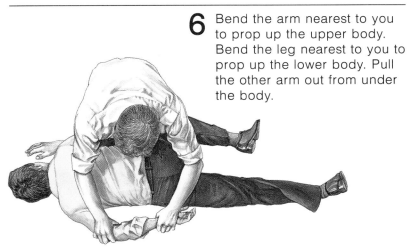

6 Bend the arm nearest to you to prop up the upper body. Bend the leg nearest to you to prop up the lower body. Pull the other arm out from under the body.

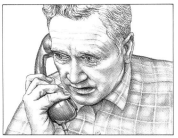

7 Call 911 and ask for an ambulance.

If the victim is heavy

Grip the clothing at the hip with both hands and roll the body against your knees. If possible, get a second person to support the head while you turn the body.

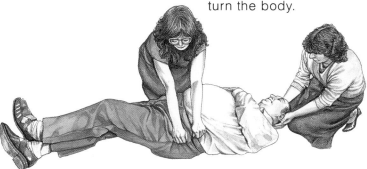

Alternatively, the helper can kneel facing you and push the victim while you pull.

If an arm or a leg is broken

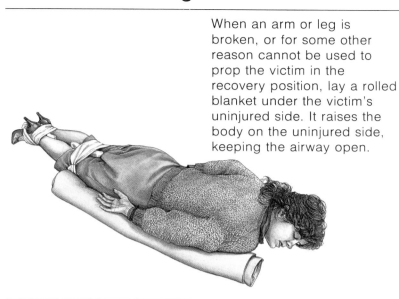

When an arm or leg is broken, or for some other reason cannot be used to prop the victim in the recovery position, lay a rolled blanket under the victim's uninjured side. It raises the body on the uninjured side, keeping the airway open.

EMERGENCY:
READER'S DIGEST ACTION GUIDE

The credits that appear on page 354 are hereby
made a part of this copyright page.

Based on *What to Do in an Emergency*, published
by The Reader's Digest Association Limited,
London. Published in Canada as *Action Guide:
What to Do in an Emergency.*

Library of Congress Cataloging in Publication Data
Emergency: Reader's digest action guide.
    Based on: What to do in an emergency.
    Includes index.
1. Medical emergencies — Handbooks, manuals, etc.
2. First aid in illness and injury — Handbooks, manuals,
etc. I. Reader's Digest Association. II. What to do in
an emergency.
RC86.8.E54   1988   616.02′52   88-18537
ISBN 0-89577-319-8

Printed in Belgium

READER'S DIGEST
ACTION GUIDE

WHAT
TO DO
IN AN EMERGENCY

EMERGENCY

THE READER'S DIGEST ASSOCIATION, INC.
PLEASANTVILLE, NEW YORK · MONTREAL

Acknowledgments

STAFF

Editors: Andrew Byers,
  Philomena Rutherford
Art supervisor:
  John McGuffie
Designer: Michel Rousseau
Research: Wadad Bashour
Text preparation:
  Joseph Marchetti
Coordination: Susan Wong

CONTRIBUTORS

Writers
Dr. George Birdwood
Ted Clements
Frank Eaglestone
Fred Fearnley
Dr. Max M. Glatt
Anthony Greenbank
Marcus Jacobson
Dr. Harvey Marcovitch
Dr. Frank Preston
Tom Sanders
Major Bertram Seymour
Mike Stockman
Superintendent Brian Turner

Researchers
Martha Plaine
Paul Poirier

Artists
Andrew Aloof
Dick Bonson
Charles Chambers
Brian Delf
Jennifer Eachus
Colin Emberson
Grose/Thurston
Nicholas H.T. Hall
Haywood and Martin
Rosalind Hewitt
Ivan Lapper
Gordon Lawson
Malcolm McGregor
David Nockels
Tim Pearce
Stephen Pointer
A.W.K.A. Popkiewicz
Bill Prosser
Elaine Sears
Lyne Young

Photographers
Andra Nelki
David Sheppard
Maurice Vezinet

Consultants
William Anderson
Dr. Basil Booth
Malcolm Conway
Dr. James Cox
Eric Franklin
Brian Garland
Yvan Gélinas
Geoff Good
Dr. Mark Harries
Pippa Isbell
Angela Large
Walter LeStrange
Bob McDowell
Dr. W. Donald Mackenzie
Malcolm Parsons
Leonard A. Sipes, Jr.
Gillian Smedley
Roger Smith
Inspector Philip Snoad
Sidney Swallow
John Sworder
Chris Vecchi
Richard Whitehouse
Tony Wilkins
Jim Williams
Professor Michael Zander

**The editors thank the
following organizations
for their assistance:**
Addiction Research Foundation,
  Toronto
Alberta Avalanche Safety
  Association, Edmonton
Alliance of Canadian Travel
  Associations, Ottawa
American Academy of
  Ophthalmology, San
  Francisco
American Association of Poison
  Control Centers, San Diego
American College of Nurse-
  Midwives, Washington
American College of
  Obstetricians and
  Gynecologists, Washington

American Diabetes Association,
  Alexandria, Va.
American Gas Association,
  Arlington, Va.
American Heart Association,
  Dallas
American Horse Council,
  Washington
American Humane Society,
  Denver
American Medical Association,
  Chicago
American National Red Cross,
  Washington
American Public Power
  Association, Washington
American Society of Travel
  Agents, Washington
AMTRACK, Washington
ASPCA, New York
Association for the Care of
  Asthma, Philadelphia
Bell Canada, Montreal
Boy Scouts of Canada, Montreal
Canada Housing and Mortgage
  and Housing Corporation,
  Ottawa
Canada Safety Council, Ottawa
Canadian Association of Fire
  Chiefs, Ottawa
Canadian Coast Guard, Ottawa
Canadian Conference for Motor
  Transport Administrators,
  Ottawa
Canadian Federation of Humane
  Societies, Ottawa
Canadian Heart Foundation,
  Ottawa
Canadian Medic Alert
  Foundation, Toronto
Canadian National, Montreal
Canadian Orienteering
  Federation, Vanier, Ont.
Canadian Recreational
  Canoeing Association, Ottawa
Canadian Red Cross (Ontario
  Division), Toronto
Canadian Standards
  Association, Rexdale, Ont.

Canadian Stroke Recovery Association, Don Mills, Ont.
Canadian Yachting Association, Ottawa
Center for Disease Control, Atlanta
Consumer and Corporate Affairs Canada, Ottawa
Consumers' Association of Canada, Ottawa
Earthquake Engineering Institute, El Cerrito, Cal.
Emergency Care Institute, Bellevue Hospital, New York
Emergency Preparedness Canada, Ottawa
Environment Canada (Atmospheric Environment Service), Ottawa
Epilepsy Foundation of America, Landover, Md.
Federal Emergency Management Agency, San Francisco
Federal Highway Administration (Bureau of Motor Carrier Safety), New York
Fire Prevention Canada Association, Ottawa
Gaz Métropolitain, Montreal
Health and Welfare Canada (Bureau of Hazardous Chemicals, Laboratory Center for Disease Control, Pesticide Division), Ottawa
Hôtel-Dieu Hospital (Burn Center), Montreal
Hydro-Québec, Montreal
Insurance Bureau of Canada, Toronto
International Association of Chiefs of Police, Washington
International Association for Medical Assistance to Travelers, Guelph, Ont., and Lewiston, N.Y.
International Institute of Ammonia Refrigeration, Chicago

Jewish General Hospital, Montreal
Johnson and Johnson (Canada), Montreal
Johnson and Son, Ltd., Brantford, Ont.
McGill University (Department of Meteorology), Montreal
Massachusetts Poison Control Center, Boston
Montreal Poison Control Center
National Association of Community Health Workers, Washington
National Association of Home Builders of the United States, Washington
National Association of Social Workers, Silverspring, Md.
National Cave Rescue Commission, Bloomington, Ind.
National Clearing House of Alcohol Information, Rockville, Md.
National Council on Alcoholism, New York
National Crime Prevention Council, Washington
National Electronic Injury Surveillance System, Washington
National Fire Protection Association, Quincy, Mass.
National Institute on Drug Abuse, Ann Arbor, Mich.
National Research Council of Canada (National Committee on Earthquake Construction), Ottawa
National Sheriffs Association (National Neighborhood Watch), Alexandria, Va.
National Speleological Society, Huntsville, Ala.
National Water Safety Congress, Warrenton, Va.
New York State Police, Albany, N.Y.
Ontario Hydro (Safety Measures Division), Toronto
Ontario Ministry of Health, Toronto
Ontario Provincial Police (Traffic and Marine Division), Toronto

Ontario Safety League, Toronto
Parks Canada (Locks and Canals Division), Ottawa
Public Works Canada (Fire Commissioner of Canada), Ottawa
Quebec Safety League, Montreal
Royal Canadian Mounted Police (Drug Squad), Toronto
Royal Life Saving Society (Ontario Branch), Toronto
St. John Ambulance, Ottawa
St. Lawrence Seaway Authority, Montreal
Smith and Nephew Ltd., Montreal
SPCA, Montreal
Standards Council of Canada, Ottawa
Stroke Control Club International, Galveston, Tex.
Transport Canada (Traffic Accident Statistics Department), Ottawa
Underwriters Laboratories, Northbrook, Ill.
United States Army Corps of Engineers, Washington
United States Coast Guard (Boating Safety Education), Washington
United States Consumer Product Safety Commission, Washington
United States Geological Survey, Reston, Va.
United States National Center for Health Statistics, Washington
VIA Rail, Montreal
Victorian Order of Nurses, Ottawa
Woods Hole Oceanographic Institute, Woods Hole, Mass.

Contents

1 WHEN SECONDS
   COUNT
   a rapid action guide

40 When emergency
    strikes

42 FIRST AID AND
    MEDICAL
    EMERGENCIES

140 IN THE HOME
     AND AT WORK

190 EMERGENCIES
     ON THE ROAD

218 EMERGENCIES
     IN THE WATER

266 EMERGENCIES ON VACATION AND IN THE COUNTRY

302 NATURAL DISASTERS

312 CRIME

326 ALCOHOL AND DRUGS

344 INDEX

354 CREDITS

When emergency strikes

BE PREPARED

The time to read this book is *before* an emergency strikes, so that, forewarned, you know what to do as soon as danger threatens. Just as the middle of a darkening forest is no place to begin learning how to use a map and compass, the middle of a crisis is no time to begin discovering how to deal with it.

Safety experts also stress that, in any crisis, thinking is as crucial as doing. First assess the situation quickly, they say – then act. The experts identify three major rules to bear in mind: do not panic; improvise; and weigh the risks.

How this book is organized

This book aims to cover all the crises that you are likely to run into. The first two sections – *When seconds count* and *First aid and medical emergencies* – are arranged alphabetically. In other sections, the information is arranged thematically: crises affecting swimmers, for example, are grouped separately from boating crises in the section called *Emergencies in the water.*

Within each section, there are also reassuring tips on ways of staying out of trouble, and real-life stories about people who have survived the most terrifying dangers by using their knowledge and their wits.

DO NOT PANIC

In any crisis, staying calm is the most important rule of all. Panic can turn a problem into a tragedy; and staying calm can do more than any other single factor to save a life – yours or someone else's.

A swimmer caught in weeds underwater can untangle himself with his hands if he keeps his head. If, in panic, he lunges blindly for the surface, he may pull the weeds tighter – and drown. Panic destroys judgment and paralyzes the muscles.

Knowledge is one antidote to it. The best cure, though, is an unshakable determination not to give way to it. Keep telling yourself that panic will only make things worse.

IMPROVISE

No emergency is quite like any other. Treating a bad cut at home when you have a first aid kit at hand and an ambulance only a telephone call away is very different from trying to cope with the same problem when you are out camping far from help.

In any situation, if you do not have exactly what you need, be prepared to make do with whatever is at hand. Look around for possible substitutes. Keep looking until you find one.

A life preserver and rope, for example, are the best equipment for helping someone who has fallen into water. But if there is no life preserver nearby, a child's rubber ring, a couple of towels knotted together or even a pair of trousers can save a life, too.

WEIGH THE RISKS

Sometimes in a crisis there is no absolutely safe way out. There may be no choice but to take one risk in order to avoid a greater one. If your brakes fail on the highway, for instance, you may have to drive deliberately into a guardrail – and risk wrecking your car – in order to avoid risking your life in an uncontrollable crash.

This action guide provides immediate information to help you cope with an emergency. Safety experts in many fields attest to the appropriateness of the procedures recommended in this guide. But in a specific emergency, only you, the person on the spot, can weigh the risks of each possible procedure against the advantages and pick the best. To do so effectively requires clear understanding and a cool head. This action guide will help to give you both.

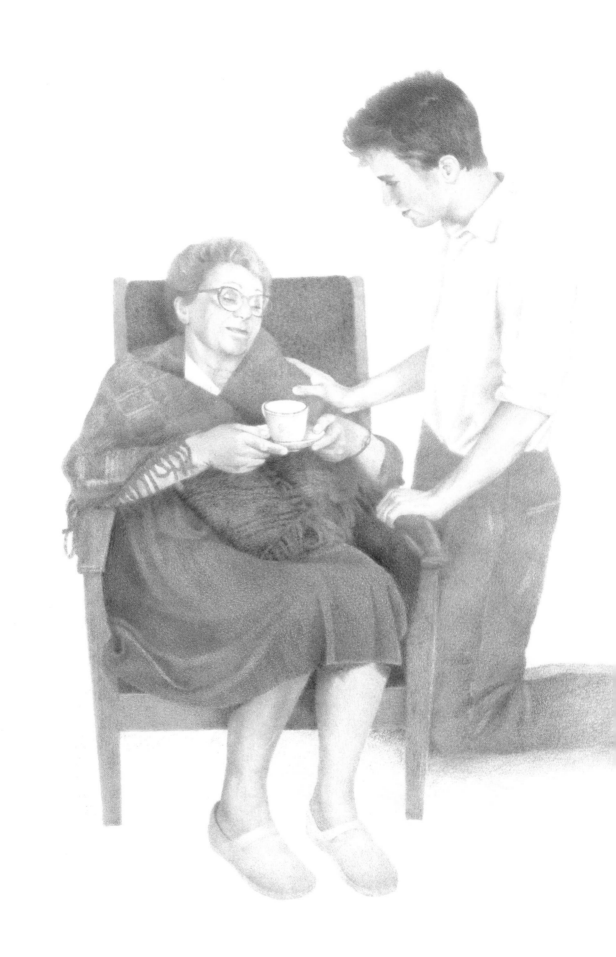

First aid and medical emergencies

44	What you need in a first aid kit
46	Abdominal injuries
48	Amputation
48	Animal bites
49	Ankle injuries
49	Appendicitis
50	Artificial respiration: mouth-to-mouth resuscitation
52	Artificial respiration and chest compression (CPR)
54	Asphyxiation
54	Asthmatic attack
55	Back or neck injuries
56	Bandages
59	Black eye
60	Bleeding
63	Blindness
64	Blisters
64	Boils
65	Bruises
66	Burns and scalds
68	Chest injuries
71	Chest pain
71	Chicken pox
72	Childbirth
76	Childhood illnesses
82	Choking
86	Concussion
86	Cramp
87	Crush injuries
88	Crying baby
89	Cuts
90	Diabetic coma
90	Dislocated joints
91	Drowning
92	Drug overdose
92	Ear injuries
93	Electric shock
94	Epileptic seizure
94	Eye injuries
96	Fainting
97	Flu
97	Food poisoning
98	Fractures
99	Frostbite
100	Gas poisoning
101	German measles
101	Grazes
102	Gunshot wounds
102	Head and face injuries
105	Heart attack
106	Heat exhaustion and heatstroke
108	Hiccups
108	Hypothermia
109	Hysteria
110	Insect stings and bites
111	Measles
111	Miscarriage
112	Moving an injured person
116	Mumps
116	Nose injuries
117	Poisoning
118	Pulse and breathing
119	Rabies
120	Rib fractures
120	Shock
121	Slings
124	Slipped disc
124	Smoke inhalation
125	Snakebite
126	Splinters
127	Splints
130	Sports injuries
132	Sprains and strains
133	Stab wounds
134	Stroke
135	Sunburn
135	Tooth injuries
136	Unconsciousness
139	Vertigo
139	Whooping cough

What you need in a first aid kit

A home first aid kit is mainly intended for minor injuries that you can treat yourself, but it should also be equipped to deal with more serious injuries until the victim gets professional medical help. It should be kept in a well-sealed box. Keep the box in a locked medicine cabinet in your bathroom, or put it on the top shelf of the hall closet, where it will be out of the reach of children. Do not keep first aid materials in unsealed containers in the bathroom or kitchen; they may deteriorate in the damp air. When you go on family vacations, take the kit with you.

Write the addresses and telephone numbers of your doctor and the emergency department of your local hospital on a piece of paper and fix it to the inside of the first aid box. Tape it to the underside of the lid, for instance.

Do not keep old medicines left over from a previous illness. Flush them down the toilet.

First aid kits can be bought ready-made from most drugstores, but you can make up your own from the items shown here, and at the same time become familiar with what your kit contains.

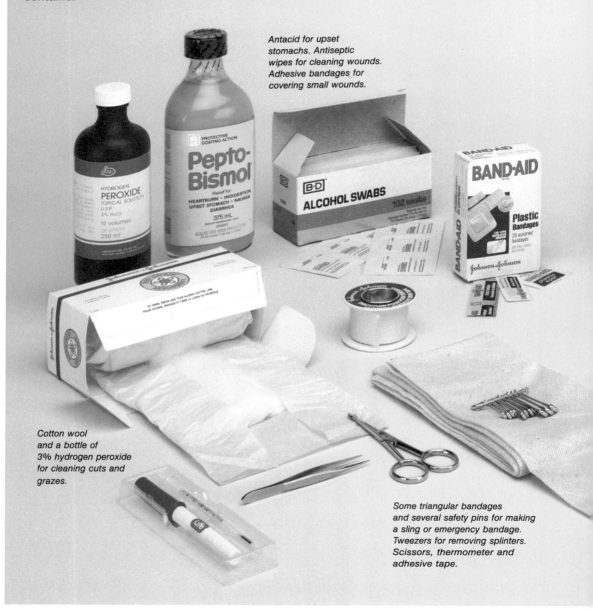

Antacid for upset stomachs. Antiseptic wipes for cleaning wounds. Adhesive bandages for covering small wounds.

Cotton wool and a bottle of 3% hydrogen peroxide for cleaning cuts and grazes.

Some triangular bandages and several safety pins for making a sling or emergency bandage. Tweezers for removing splinters. Scissors, thermometer and adhesive tape.

A kit for hikers

On outings – particularly in remote areas – take a small first aid kit which includes a survival blanket (also called a space blanket). The blanket can be wrapped around an injured person to preserve warmth in freezing temperatures.

The kit should also contain a triangular bandage, an elastic bandage for ankle injuries, some sterile dressings, adhesive bandages and a packet of antiseptic wipes for cleaning a wound when no water is available. Store the kit in a small plastic box.

How to improvise a dressing

If you have to treat a wound when no first aid kit is available, you can improvise dressings and bandages from a range of materials.

• For a dressing, take a clean handkerchief and fold it inside out so that the side that was protected from dirt can be placed on the wound. For a larger dressing, use a clean pillowcase or towel in the same way.

• Another way is to strip the wrapping off a packet of paper handkerchiefs and put the pad on the wound. Alternatively, discard the first few sheets of a toilet roll, then make a pad.

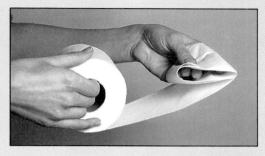

MAKING A TOILET PAPER DRESSING *Wind toilet paper round your fingers to make a pad. Put its bottom, untouched side on the wound.*

• Do not put fluffy material such as absorbent cotton directly onto a wound because the fibers will become embedded in it.

• Whatever you make the dressing from, avoid touching the surface that will be in contact with the wound. Otherwise, dirt on your fingers could introduce infection.

• An improvised dressing can be bandaged on with any piece of reasonably clean material, such as a scarf, tie or old linen.

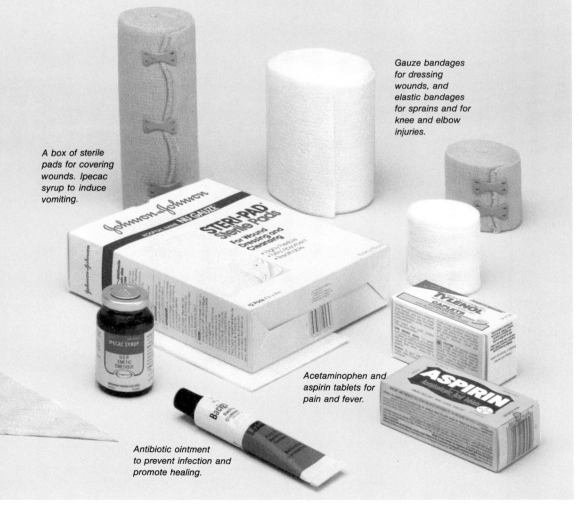

Gauze bandages for dressing wounds, and elastic bandages for sprains and for knee and elbow injuries.

A box of sterile pads for covering wounds. Ipecac syrup to induce vomiting.

Acetaminophen and aspirin tablets for pain and fever.

Antibiotic ointment to prevent infection and promote healing.

Abdominal injuries

A car accident, a fall or a stab wound can cause serious injuries to vital organs inside the abdomen – the lower two-thirds of the trunk.

The abdomen contains organs such as the bladder, intestines and uterus which are richly supplied with blood. An injury which damages the blood vessels can be as dangerous as one that affects the organs themselves.

Often the wound is clearly visible, and sometimes an organ may even be protruding.

If the wound runs lengthwise on the body, lay the victim flat on the back with the feet slightly raised on a cushion or folded jacket.

If the wound runs across the body, lay the victim on the back with the knees bent and the head and shoulders raised on a folded jacket or cushion. These two positions will help to hold the wound closed.

Treating the wound
Gently remove the clothing from around the wound, taking care not to cough, sneeze or even breathe on it, as it may become infected.

Put a dressing or a folded piece of clean linen over the wound to staunch the bleeding, and tie it in place with a bandage or scarf.

Cover the victim with a coat or blanket, leaving the arms outside. Call for an ambulance, but do not leave the victim alone.

Loosen any tight clothing – at the neck and

VICTIM WITH A WOUND LENGTHWISE TO THE BODY

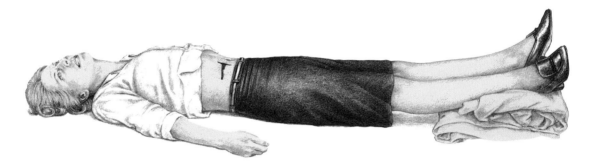

If the wound is running lengthwise to the body, lay the victim flat on her back with the feet slightly raised on a folded blanket, jacket or other convenient support. Do not raise the head off the ground. This position tenses the muscles of the abdomen and helps to close the wound.

VICTIM WITH A WOUND ACROSS THE BODY

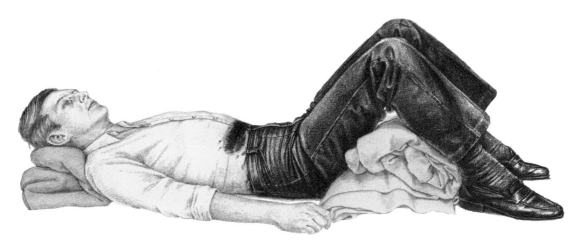

If the wound runs across the abdomen, lay the victim on his back, with folded coats or blankets under the shoulders. Bend the knees and support them, too, with anything at hand. This position relaxes the abdominal muscles and helps to keep the wound closed.

waist, for example – to assist breathing and help blood circulation.

Do not offer anything to eat or drink, as the victim may need a general anesthetic at the hospital. If he complains of thirst, moisten his lips with water.

If the victim becomes unconscious, carefully support the abdomen and gently turn him into the recovery position (see page 136).

If the victim coughs or vomits, support the wound by pressing gently on the dressing to prevent internal organs from protruding.

If internal organs are already protruding from the wound, do not try to push them back or touch them.

Internal injuries of the abdomen

In some accidents there may be no external signs of injury, but the victim may be bleeding internally.

All suspected cases of internal bleeding should be examined by a doctor as soon as possible. The warning signs are:

- Pain and tenderness in the abdomen.
- Tightening of the abdomen.
- Bruises and abrasions.
- Nausea and vomiting.
- Muscular spasms.
- Paleness, cold clammy skin and sometimes sweat on the forehead.
- Faintness.

HOW TO BANDAGE AN ABDOMINAL WOUND

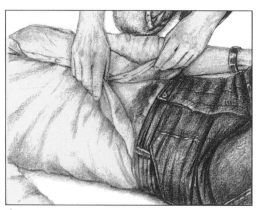

1 Gently remove the victim's clothing from around the wound to expose it for treatment. Do not cough, sneeze or breathe on the wound, as that may cause it to become infected. Do not touch the wound with your hands.

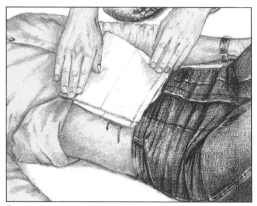

2 Cover the wound and any protruding organs lightly with a large dressing, ideally a sterile dressing from a sealed wrapper. Alternatively, use a piece of clean linen refolded so that the unexposed side faces the wound.

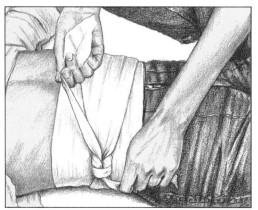

3 Fix the dressing in place with a bandage, so that it covers, but does not press down on, the wound. Tie the knot away from the wound so that it does not press on the injury, either. If you cannot get a bandage under the victim's back, secure the dressing with adhesive tape.

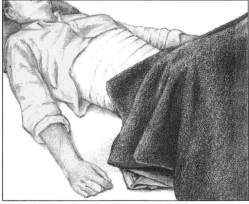

4 Keep the victim warm by covering him with a blanket or coat, leaving his arms outside so that you can check his pulse without disturbing him. Make sure that a doctor or an ambulance has been called, but do not leave the victim alone. Reassure him that help is on its way.

Amputation

A finger, a toe or even a major limb which has been severed in an accident can sometimes be sewed back on by microsurgery.

But do not waste time preserving the limb until you have taken care of the victim, whose life is the first priority.

Do not try to restore the severed limb yourself – by binding it in place with surgical tape, for example. You will only cause the victim great pain, and damage the tissues, which will make surgery more difficult.

What you should do
• Lay the victim down and put a pad of gauze or clean linen, such as the inside of a clean, folded handkerchief, on the stump, and fix it in place with a bandage. A scarf will do.
• Immobilize an injured arm by bandaging it to the chest. If a leg is injured, bandage it to the other leg.
• If possible, raise the injured limb above the level of the heart to reduce bleeding.
• Reassure the injured person and encourage him to keep still, then call 911 or your local ambulance service.
• Once you have dealt with the victim, try to find the severed limb. Wrap it in a clean cloth, such as a handkerchief or a pillowcase, and put it in a plastic bag.
• Keep it cool, if possible by packing ice around the plastic bag. Do not let the ice come in direct contact with the limb.
• Give the limb to the ambulance crew, or doctor, to go to hospital with the victim.

Animal bites

Bites from animals can introduce germs from the animal's mouth into the wound, possibly causing infection (see *Rabies*, page 119). There is a similar risk with human bites.

The area of any bite should be thoroughly washed, and if the skin has been broken the victim should see a doctor. Serious wounds should be treated at the emergency department of a hospital.

Report dog bites to your local animal control agency. Most municipalities have laws that require owners to control their dogs.

CLEANING AND DRESSING A BITE

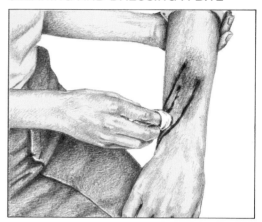

1 *Wash the area thoroughly with soap and warm water, or a mild antiseptic. Dry gently, wiping down and away from the wound. Cover with a clean dressing.*

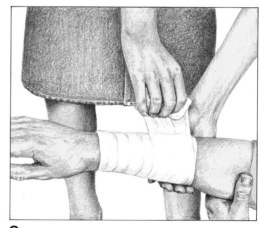

2 *Hold the dressing in place with a clean bandage or adhesive tape. Take the victim to a doctor, because injections against tetanus or a course of antibiotics may be required.*

Ankle injuries

The ankle is the joint that most often suffers sprains – the stretching or tearing of a ligament linking the bones.

A sprain may be caused by twisting the foot as you walk or run. It causes pain in the joint, which becomes worse if it is moved, and the joint swells up.

The injury may take up to 14 days to heal, depending on the severity. For treatment, see *Sprains and strains*, page 132.

A serious sprain can be hard to distinguish from a fracture. So if there is any doubt, and the victim cannot support himself on the ankle, assume that a bone is broken.

Treating a fractured ankle

A fracture of the ankle can follow a fall or a stumble that makes the ankle bend excessively, or it can be caused by falling on the foot from a height. The warning signs are:
• Immediate pain, which is often severe.
• The ankle soon becomes swollen or bruised.
• Pain when moving the ankle.
• It may be difficult or impossible to stand on the injured leg.

If you suspect a fractured ankle, apply a cold compress to limit the swelling, and see a doctor as soon as possible.

Make the cold compress by soaking a small towel or other material in cold water, wringing it out and wrapping it around the ankle. Or tie up some ice cubes in a plastic bag, wrap them in a cloth and crush them with a hammer. Then apply the compress to the ankle.

Appendicitis

Spasms of pain in the abdomen may be the first sign of appendicitis. The pain is caused by inflammation of the appendix, a short tube, closed at one end, that projects from the junction of the small and large intestines.

Appendicitis can occur if the open end of the appendix is blocked by fragments of hard waste matter, or if the appendix becomes kinked. As a result, infection sets in and the walls of the appendix become inflamed and swollen.

If the condition is left untreated, it may subside, only to recur – a condition known as chronic appendicitis.

If the condition is acute, however, the pain increases until the appendix finally bursts, spreading the infection through the area immediately around it, or throughout the intestine. This is a surgical emergency, requiring prompt treatment. For this reason, a doctor should be seen as early as possible in cases of suspected appendicitis, especially in children or old people.

The symptoms can take between 4 and 48 hours to develop. Because symptoms are extremely variable, the condition can be difficult to diagnose. Call the doctor immediately if the pain gets worse, becomes continuous, or keeps the sufferer awake — and call him in any case if the pain lasts longer than four hours.

The danger signs
• Recurring spasms of pain. At first they may be felt near the navel, but sometimes in the lower right side of the abdomen.
• After a few hours, there is a constant severe aching in the lower right side of the abdomen.
• The lower right side of the abdomen is tender to the touch. The pain becomes more severe if the sufferer moves; it may interfere with sleep.
• The sufferer feels sick and may vomit. Often there is constipation, although the bowels may move normally, or even be loose.
• Food and drink are usually refused.
• It may hurt to walk, or to pass urine.
• The breath may smell foul.
• Body temperature generally rises to 102°F (39°C) in adults, and can be even higher in children. But sometimes it is only slightly raised.

What you can do to help
• Keep the sufferer lying still with a hot-water bottle wrapped in a towel on the abdomen.
• Rinse the mouth with sips of water, but do not give food or drink.
• Do not administer laxatives.

First aid and medical emergencies

Artificial respiration: mouth-to-mouth resuscitation

A person who has stopped breathing will die within minutes, maybe as few as six. After as little as three minutes without oxygen the brain can suffer irreversible damage. So it is urgent to get air into the lungs as quickly as possible.

Sometimes it is difficult to know if someone's breathing has stopped. You should kneel down, put your ear beside the victim's mouth and nose and look along the chest. If the person is breathing, you should be able to hear and feel it, and to see the chest rising and falling with each breath.

When breathing stops, the lips, cheeks and ear lobes take on a bluish-gray tinge. Breathing may stop merely because the airway has become blocked for one of three reasons: the head may have fallen forward, making the airway narrower; the tongue may have slipped back in the throat, covering the airway; vomit or saliva may have collected at the back of the throat, blocking the airway.

• Your first step is to ask someone to call 911 or an ambulance. Once that is taken care of, you must set about opening the victim's airway. Lay him on his back on a firm surface and tilt his head backward with one hand, while you lift his chin with the other hand.

• Keeping your hand on the forehead to maintain the tilt, use the fingers of your other hand to clear any obstruction in the mouth.

• Simply opening the airway may be enough to cause breathing to start spontaneously. Once breathing has stabilized, put the victim in the recovery position (see page 136) until the ambulance arrives.

Breathing for a victim

• If the victim does not begin to breathe when the airway is opened, begin mouth-to-mouth respiration immediately. This is a simple but most effective way of getting air into the lungs of someone who has stopped breathing, or whose breathing is very weak or labored.

• Pinch the nose shut, and seal your lips around the open mouth.

• Blow two full breaths into the victim's mouth, making the chest rise and fall each time, and gulping a big breath of air yourself between each ventilation. If there is no chest movement, reposition the victim's head by the head-tilt chin-lift method described above, and give two more breaths. If there is still no chest movement, suspect an obstruction (see *Choking*, page 15).

• If there is chest movement, check the neck, or carotid, pulse with your index and middle fingers. If there is no pulse, start external chest compressions (see pages 52-53).

• If there is a pulse, but the victim is not yet breathing, continue artificial respiration, giving one vigorous breath every five seconds. Remove your mouth to allow the victim to exhale and turn your head to watch for the rise and fall of the chest. Continue until the victim breathes by himself, or help arrives.

CLEARING THE AIRWAY

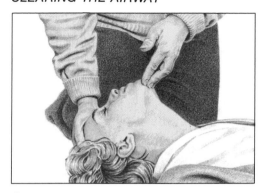

1 *Tilt the head back by lifting the chin with one hand and pressing down on the forehead with the other. This opens the airway.*

MOUTH-TO-MOUTH RESPIRATION

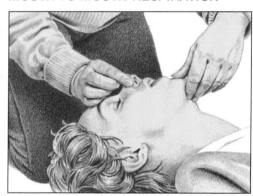

1 *Pinch the nose shut with your finger and thumb and deliver two quick full breaths. Check the neck pulse (see* Has the heart stopped beating? *page 52) and watch the chest fall.*

Babies and small children

• When resuscitating a baby or small child, seal your lips around both mouth and nose, because the area is so small.

• Give two gentle puffs of air, then feel the pulse: check inside the upper arm in infants.

• If there is a pulse, continue giving gentle puffs of air – one every three seconds for an infant, one every four seconds for a child.

If mouth-to-mouth is impossible

• Occasionally it is not possible to use a victim's mouth for artificial respiration – perhaps because there are injuries to the mouth. In such a case breathe into the nose, holding the mouth shut as you do so.

First aid and
medical emergencies

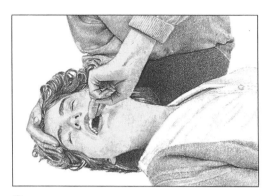

2 *If the victim does not begin breathing, turn her head to the side and, with your fingers, clear her mouth of any foreign matter.*

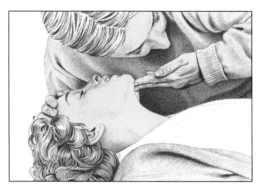

3 *Listen for breathing. See if the chest rises and falls. Place your ear close to her nose and mouth and feel for exhaled air.*

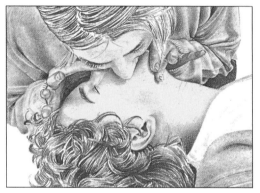

2 *If there is a pulse and chest movement but no breathing, replace your mouth and continue giving one breath every five seconds. Keep going until the victim starts breathing again.*

MOUTH-TO-NOSE RESPIRATION

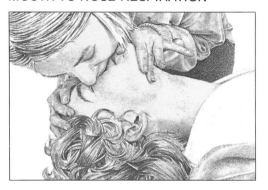

With the head tilted, and holding the mouth shut with one hand, seal your lips around the nose, and breathe into the victim in the same way as for mouth-to-mouth respiration.

GIVING ARTIFICIAL RESPIRATION TO A BABY
Put the baby on a firm surface and clear the airway. Then cover both nose and mouth with your mouth and puff in gently twice, making the chest rise. Remove your mouth and check the pulse on the infant's upper arm as you watch the chest fall. Then continue the puffs, slightly faster than you would normally breathe yourself – about one every three seconds.

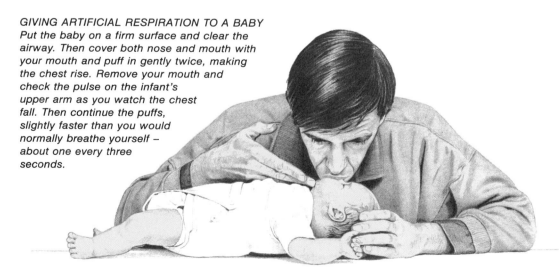

51

Artificial respiration and chest compression (CPR)

WARNING – CARDIOPULMONARY RESUSCITATION (CPR) REQUIRES TRAINING, SKILL AND PRACTICE. THE UNTRAINED COULD CAUSE SERIOUS DAMAGE.

If a person's heart stops beating, blood will no longer be pumped to the brain, and mouth-to-mouth respiration will be useless by itself. Brain damage will begin within minutes.

Compressing the victim's chest will force the blood through the circulatory system. If the brain continues to receive blood, the heart may spontaneously resume beating.

External chest compression is always used with mouth-to-mouth respiration to provide the blood with oxygen. But chest compression can be a dangerous technique. The heart is sensitive, and if it is compressed while still beating faintly it may stop completely.

Compression should be used only by a person trained in first aid – and only after he or she has established conclusively that the victim's heartbeat has stopped. The technique should never be practiced on a healthy person.

Consequently this information is intended only as a memory aid for trained people. They will know that chest compressions are preceded by artificial respiration (see pages 50-51) and are given only when the heart has stopped beating (see box, this page).

Compressing the victim's chest
Compression is carried out on the lower half of the breastbone. The heel of the hand should be centered on a point two finger-widths up from the bottom of the breastbone.

• With your second hand on top of the first, depress the chest of an adult by 1½ in. (4 cm), and repeat at the rate of 80 to 100 per minute. Do 15 compressions, then inflate the lungs twice by mouth-to-mouth respiration. Repeat this cycle four times, then check the pulse.

HAS THE HEART STOPPED BEATING?

The only reliable way to discover if the heart has stopped beating is to feel the pulse of one of the carotid arteries in the victim's neck to either side of the Adam's apple. The pulse on the wrist is not a reliable indication.

Feel the neck pulse after giving the first two breaths in mouth-to-mouth respiration. If there is no pulse, have someone call 911, or an ambulance, and begin external chest compression.

Check the pulse again after one minute, and then after every three minutes. If the pulse returns, it means that the heart has started beating again.

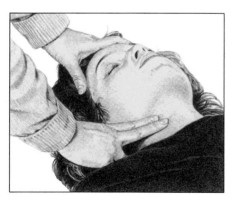

To feel the pulse of the carotid artery, place your fingers gently in the hollow of the neck between the Adam's apple and the muscle at the side.

CHEST COMPRESSION ON AN ADULT

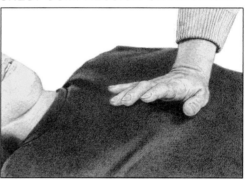

1 Kneeling beside the victim, place the heel of one hand on her chest, two finger-widths up from the bottom of the breastbone. Keep your thumb and fingers raised, so that they do not press on the ribs.

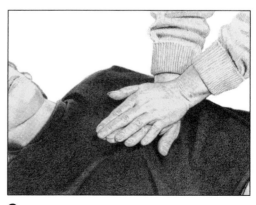

2 With your second hand over the first, apply pressure with the heel of your hand. Press down 1½ in. (4 cm), keeping your thumbs and fingers raised. Let the chest rise again.

• When you detect a neck pulse, stop compression, but continue mouth-to-mouth respiration until breathing starts. Keep checking the pulse. If it stops, restart compression.

Treating children
• Use one hand only to compress the chest of a child one to eight years of age.
• The depth of the compression should be 1 to 1½ in. (2.5–4 cm) and the speed should be 80 to 100 times a minute.
• Give one small breath after five compressions. Continue this cycle of one breath, five compressions, until the pulse returns.

Treating infants
• Give chest compression to a baby using two fingers only, the index and middle finger of one hand. The depth of compression must be no more than 1 in. (2.5 cm), and the speed 100 times a minute.

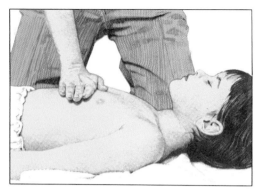

COMPRESSION ON A YOUNG CHILD
Using only the heel of one hand, press down the lower breastbone 1–1½ in. (2.5–4 cm) at a rate of 80 to 100 presses per minute. Give five presses, then one breath, using mouth-to-mouth respiration.

COMPRESSION ON A BABY

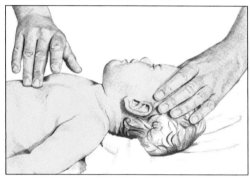

1 *Put the baby on a firm surface, or hold it on your arm, cradling the head in your hand. Put your index finger on the breastbone at the level of the nipples. A finger-width below this point — between the middle and the ring fingers — is the area of chest compression.*

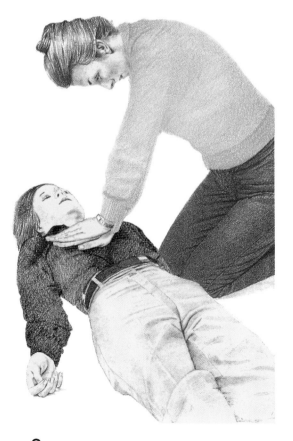

3 *Give 15 presses at normal pulse rate, then inflate the lungs twice by mouth-to-mouth respiration. Repeat the sequence four times a minute. Check the carotid pulse after one minute, then every three minutes.*

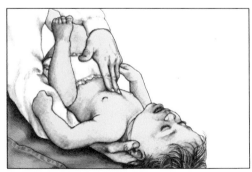

2 *Using two fingers, press down about 1 in. (2.5 cm). Give 100 compressions per minute, pausing to ventilate the baby after each five compressions. Give 15 presses, then two lung inflations.*

Asphyxiation

A person suffering from asphyxiation (lack of oxygen in the blood) may die unless first aid is given promptly. Nerve cells in the brain can die after only three minutes without oxygen.

Common causes of asphyxiation
• Blockage of the airway by food, blood, vomit or broken teeth, or by the tongue falling to the back of the throat. Such blockages can occur with an unconscious person.
• Compression of the chest or damage to the lungs – possibly in a road accident.
• Gas poisoning – possibly from carbon monoxide given off by a car exhaust in a confined space.
• Electrical accidents.
• Suffocation – possibly from a plastic bag being placed over the head.
• Strangulation – possibly from attempted suicide by hanging.
• A severe attack of asthma or bronchitis.

Warning signs
• Breathing is difficult, and may become noisy and eventually stop altogether.
• The face turns blue, and the veins on the head and neck are swollen.
• The victim gradually loses consciousness and may have convulsions.

What you should do
• If a person is suffocating because his mouth and nose have become blocked, remove the cause. If, for example, a plastic bag covers his head, tear it.
• Check for danger to yourself and to the victim. If there is a continuing threat — from escaping gas, for example — stop it at the source or drag the victim clear.
• If the victim has been strangled, quickly cut or untie the cord or other material around the neck. If possible, keep the knot intact as possible evidence for the police.
• Check that the victim is breathing. If not, clear the airway (see page 50).
• If breathing does not start, give mouth-to-mouth respiration (see page 50).
• If you suspect that the airway is blocked by food, treat for choking (see page 82).
• Once breathing is normal, turn the victim into the recovery position (see page 136).
• Call for an ambulance but do not leave the victim alone. Keep a careful watch on breathing, and give artificial respiration again if it falters.

Asthmatic attack

Most asthma attacks, while distressing, do not threaten life. However, a few particularly serious attacks are fatal each year.

During an asthmatic attack the muscles around the air tubes go into a spasm, impeding breathing. At the same time, the walls of the air tubes swell, and the tubes are further blocked by thick, tenacious mucus.

Warning signs of a severe attack
• Noisy, wheezy breathing.
• Pale or bluish-gray complexion.
• Beads of sweat on the forehead.
• An anxious expression.
• In a prolonged attack, mental confusion because of lack of oxygen.
• The victim struggles for breath, and is often

HOW TO HELP DURING AN ATTACK

1 *If possible, sit an asthma sufferer in an upright chair drawn close to a table or the back of another chair on which he can rest his forearms. His back should be fairly straight, and his elbows spread out.*

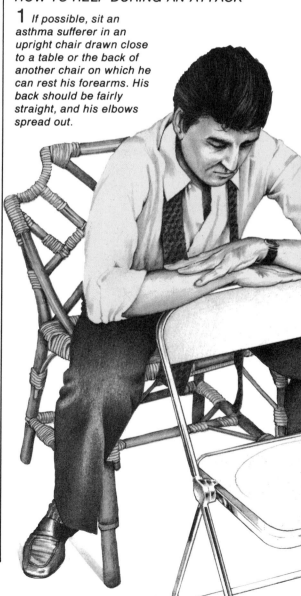

found sitting hunched up grasping the chair arms, a tabletop or other support.

What you can do
• Most asthmatic attacks occur at night, often when the sufferer is in bed. In this case, open the window to provide fresh air and prop up the sufferer in bed with pillows. Even though the window is open, keep the room warm.
• If the patient has taken his medication but the attack persists, call his doctor or take him to the hospital. Reassure the sufferer, telling him that expert help is on the way.
• If you have to take a victim to hospital, transport him sitting up in the front passenger seat rather than lying down in the back.

Causes of asthma attacks
• Respiratory infection may cause inflammation of the air tubes.
• Allergy to various substances, including house-dust mites, animal fur or feathers, pollen and some foods.
• Nighttime attacks in children are often associated with house-dust mites, down pillows or pets sleeping in the bedroom.
• Anxiety or excitement seems to bring on attacks in some people.

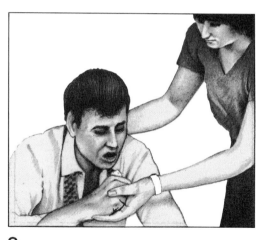

2 *If the sufferer has an inhaler, help him to use it.*

Back or neck injuries

Mishandling a person whose back or neck is broken can cause permanent paralysis or even death.

A victim with a suspected broken back or neck should be moved only if he is in immediate danger — in a burning building, for example. Otherwise leave him where he is. Any moving should be left to ambulance attendants who will have the right equipment.

Before you even touch an injured person, look for possible clues. For example, if he is lying at the foot of a ladder or a flight of stairs, it is possible he has suffered a back or neck injury.

Warning signs
• Loss of feeling and movement below the injured area, or a sensation of having been cut in half.
• Pain at the site of injury.
• A tingling sensation or pins and needles in the hands and feet (denotes neck injury).
• Inability to move fingers, wrists, toes or ankles when asked to do so, with no symptoms of a broken arm or leg.
• Inability to feel pain when the skin is gently nipped.
• Difficulty in breathing.

What you should do
• Tell the victim to lie still.
• Cover him with a blanket and comfort him as much as possible. Do not raise the head or try to rest it on anything. Call for an ambulance.
• If the victim is unconscious, and lying on his back, do not turn him over into the recovery position. Leave him face up and, with your fingers, clear his mouth of any obstructions to breathing.
• Watch his breathing carefully. If it stops, begin mouth-to-mouth respiration (see page 50) immediately, even though tilting the head risks further damage to the spine. Be as careful and gentle as you can.

First aid and medical emergencies

Bandages

In medical emergencies, bandages have three different uses. They keep a dressing in place over a wound, preventing dirt and germs from entering; they maintain pressure on a wound, controlling and absorbing bleeding; and they can be used to support or immobilize an injured part of the body (see *Slings*, page 121, and *Splints*, page 127).

Bandages are usually made of gauze or muslin, but in an emergency they can be improvised readily from sheets, pillowcases, stockings, scarves, shirts, dresses, or any other suitable material.

If no bandage is available, a dressing can be secured with strips of adhesive tape.

Dressings, which are used to absorb blood and prevent infection, are usually a pad of cotton wool covered with gauze. Fluffy material such as absorbent cotton should not go directly on a wound because the fibers will stick.

In an emergency, a dressing can be made from a pad of any clean, dry, absorbent material. The inside of a folded handkerchief, a towel or pillowcase – even a pad of paper tissues or toilet paper – can all be used (see *How to improvise a dressing*, page 45).

Sterile dressings sealed in protective wrapping can be bought from any drugstore. These sterile pads will keep indefinitely in a family medicine cabinet.

Bandages, some gauze, some elastic, come in varying widths of 1 to 6 in. (2.5 to 15 cm). Triangular bandages for making slings can be up to 3 ft. (1 m) long.

APPLYING THE BANDAGE TO A WOUND

1 *Start by putting the end of the bandage on the limb and making a firm turn to hold it in place. Apply the outer surface to the skin so that you can unroll it easily. Bandage a limb in the position in which it is to remain.*

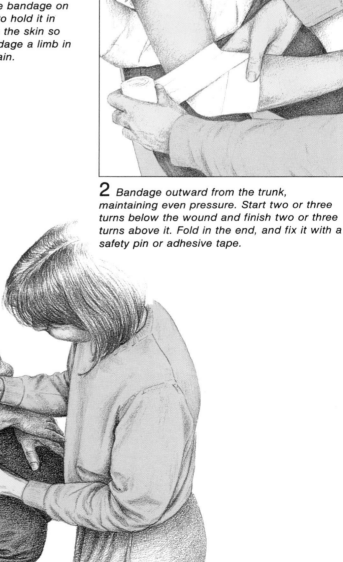

2 *Bandage outward from the trunk, maintaining even pressure. Start two or three turns below the wound and finish two or three turns above it. Fold in the end, and fix it with a safety pin or adhesive tape.*

How to use a bandage

Traditional bandages come in rolls of non-stretch, open-weave gauze and, without practice, can be difficult to apply. Crepe or elastic bandages are easier to put on, and because they follow the contours of the body the pressure they exert on the wound is more evenly distributed.

Rolled bandages can be bought in different widths for different purposes: a 1 in. (2.5 cm) bandage for fingers and toes; 2 in. (5 cm) for hands; 3 in. (7.5 cm) for arms and legs; and 4 or 6 in. (10 or 15 cm) for the trunk.

Is the bandage too tight?

It is easy to bind a bandage so tightly that it interferes with the victim's nerves or blood circulation. After applying a bandage, and again ten minutes later, check for the following warning signals.

• The patient has a tingling feeling in the fingers or toes, or loses feeling altogether.

• The fingers or toes are very cold.

• The patient is unable to move the fingers or toes.

• The beds of the fingernails or toenails are unusually pale or blue.

• The pulse of an injured arm is weak compared to the other arm, or completely absent.

If any of these danger signs occurs, remove the bandage and apply it again more loosely.

Other types of bandage

Triangular bandages can be bought from most drugstores or they can be made by cutting a

FINISHING OFF A BANDAGE WITH A KNOT

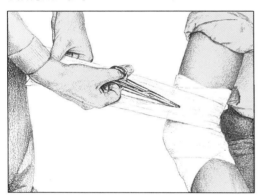

1 *If you do not have a safety pin or adhesive tape, leave a piece of bandage free. The length will depend on the thickness of the area being bandaged. Cut the end of the bandage in half lengthways.*

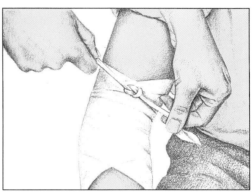

3 *Take the two ends around the limb again and tie them off, preferably with a reef knot (right end over left end, then left end over right). Once again, make sure that the knot does not press on the wound. Tuck in the ends.*

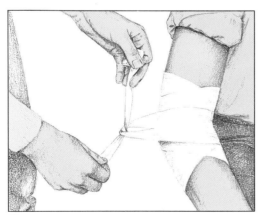

2 *Tie the two strips together with a single knot, pulling fairly tight at the bottom of the cut. This knot will stop the cut tearing further when you tie off the bandage. Make sure that the knot does not press on the wound.*

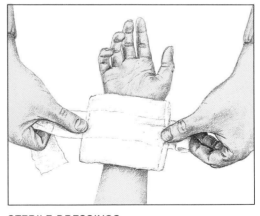

STERILE DRESSINGS
Sterile dressings or pads can be found in most drugstores. Sealed wrappers ensure their sterility. The dressing is applied to the wound and bound in place with a bandage.

piece of linen or cotton, about 3 ft. (1 m) square, in half diagonally.

Unfolded, triangular bandages can be used as slings (see page 121).

They can also be folded into a broad bandage suitable for strapping up a broken limb, or into a narrow bandage for holding a dressing in place over a wound.

A triangular bandage can also be made into a ring-pad for a wound which contains a foreign object, or to protect an open fracture when a broken bone is jutting from the wound.

Seamless tubular bandages are easier to apply than conventional bandages, because they do not need to be tied.

Tubular bandages resemble stockings without feet, and they are available from drugstores in various sizes to fit different parts of the body. They are all supplied with applicator tongs to slip them on over a dressing.

MAKING A RING-PAD

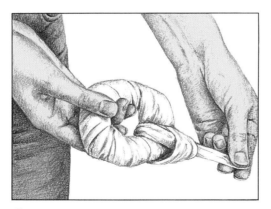

1 *Wind one end of a narrow bandage once or twice around your fingers, to make a loop. Bring the other end through the loop, under and back through again.*

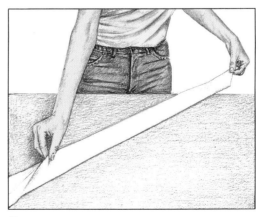

2 *Continue winding the free end around the loop until all the bandage is used up. You then have a pad to prevent pressure on a wound that has a foreign body, such as glass, in it.*

IMPROVISING WITH A TRIANGULAR BANDAGE

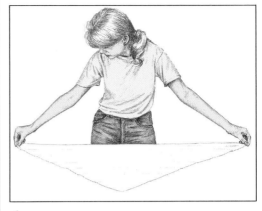

1 *To make a broad or narrow bandage in an emergency, spread the triangular bandage out on a flat, clean surface.*

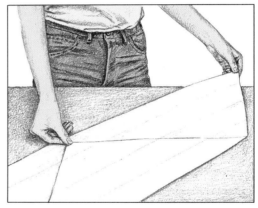

2 *Fold the apex of the triangle to the center of the base, and then fold it once more in the same direction. This makes a broad bandage.*

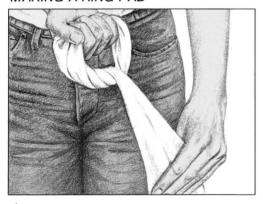

3 *To make a narrow bandage, fold a third time in the same direction. It can then be used like a traditional rolled bandage to bind wounds.*

PUTTING A TUBULAR BANDAGE ON A FINGER

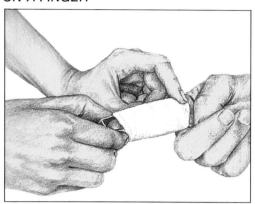

1 *Cut a piece of tubular bandage 2½ times as long as the finger. Put the applicator over the finger and slide the bandage over the tongs.*

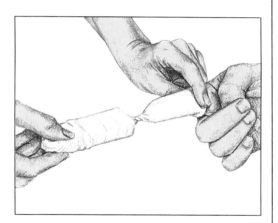

2 *Slip the applicator off the finger, together with one end of the bandage. Turn the tongs so that the bandage is slightly twisted.*

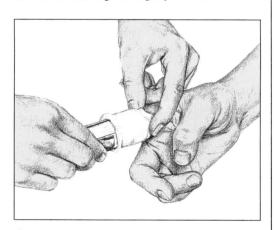

3 *Push the tongs gently back down the finger, sliding the bandage off them as you go and leaving the finger covered with two layers.*

Black eye

A blow to the eye socket and eyelid causes internal bleeding which colors the skin dark blue or black and produces a swelling.

Apply cold compresses immediately. Do not put raw steak on a black eye; it is ineffective and wasteful.

There is always a possibility of damage to the eye itself or to the head, so have the injury examined by a doctor.

What you should do
• Put a cold compress over the eye to limit the swelling and relieve the pain. To make the compress, put crushed ice or ice cubes into a plastic bag, add some salt to encourage the ice to melt, seal the bag and wrap it in a cloth. Alternatively, soak a small towel in cold or iced water and wring it out.
• Cool the eye for at least 30 minutes, replacing the compress if it becomes warm.
• Take the victim to a doctor as soon as possible to check that there is no serious damage to the eye or a fracture of the skull. A blow which is violent enough to blacken the eye may cause either.

First aid and medical emergencies

Bleeding

Although bleeding can be alarming and dramatic, most cases are not fatal, provided the injury is treated promptly.

Bleeding can usually be stopped by pressing down on the wound, which slows the flow of blood and allows clotting to take place. If there is a foreign object, such as a piece of glass, in the wound, apply the pressure alongside it. Maintain pressure until the bleeding stops. This may take as long as 45 minutes.

The clotting process can be assisted by raising the injured area, which also slows the flow of blood. If severe bleeding continues, it may be possible to stop it by pressing on the appropriate artery. But this is a last resort only (see page 62).

Detecting bleeding in the dark

Usually bleeding is obvious, but after an accident – particularly in the dark – a victim's position may conceal a serious wound. In this situation feel all over and under the body for patches of sticky dampness, and assume they are blood until you are sure that they are not.

Other warning signs of severe bleeding are:
- Pale skin which is moist and cold to touch.
- Profuse sweating.
- Fast but weak pulse (the normal adult pulse rate is 60-80 per minute).
- Victim complains of thirst.
- Victim's vision becomes blurred and he feels faint and giddy.
- Breathing becomes shallow, with yawning and sighing.
- Victim becomes restless and talkative.

A large foreign object in the wound

If a large object, such as a piece of glass, is embedded in a wound, do not try to remove it. You may make the injury worse. Moreover, the object may be plugging the wound, helping to restrict the bleeding.

Control the bleeding by pressing the sides of the wound together around the object. Then bind up the wound, using a ring-pad (see page 58) to keep pressure off the object.

Take the victim to a hospital emergency department. If you need assistance, call 911.

HOW TO STOP SEVERE BLEEDING

1 *Lay the victim down. Remove clothing from around the wound if you can without wasting time or causing distress. Press down hard on the wound with any absorbent material or your bare hands, unless something is embedded in it.*

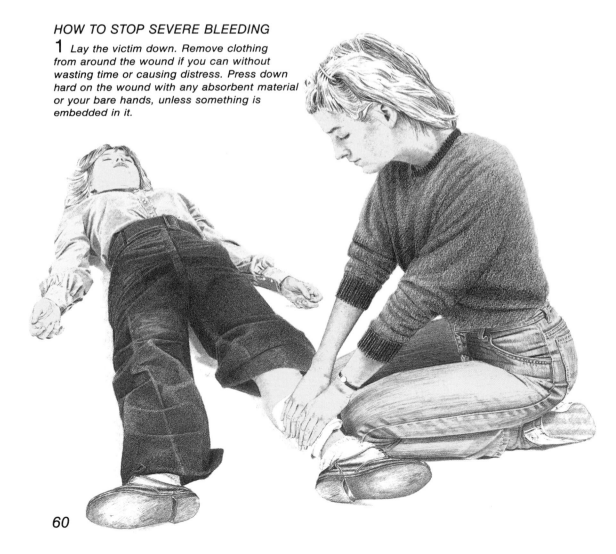

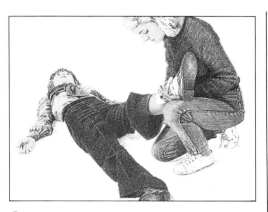

2 *If possible, raise the wounded area above the level of the heart to reduce the flow of blood. When the bleeding stops, put on an absorbent dressing, such as the inside of a clean, folded handkerchief.*

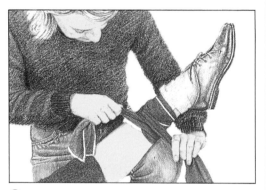

3 *If the blood seeps through the dressing, do not remove it. Put another dressing on top. Tie the dressing in place with a bandage or other material. Keep the victim as still as possible and do not give food or drink.*

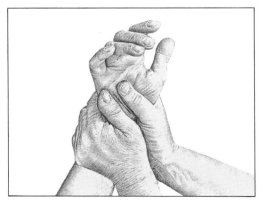

A LARGE WOUND
Squeeze the sides of a large wound together gently but firmly, and maintain the pressure for up to 10 minutes. Then treat as above and call an ambulance.

IF SOMETHING IS EMBEDDED

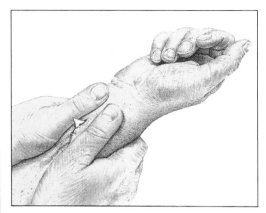

1 *To stop the bleeding, squeeze the edges of the wound together for up to 10 minutes. Do not try to remove the object.*

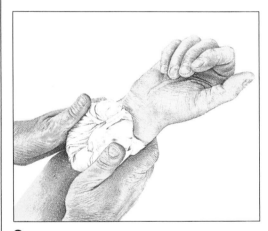

2 *Put a thick circular pad of clean material around the wound, preferably higher than the object, to prevent pressure on it.*

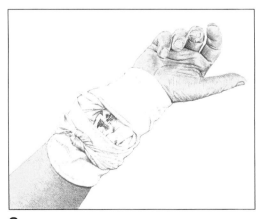

3 *Bandage the wound with diagonally applied strips of material that do not go over the object. Get the victim to hospital.*

61

Stopping blood flow at a pressure point

If severe bleeding from an arm or leg cannot be stopped by direct pressure on the wound, or if direct pressure cannot be applied successfully, it may be possible to stop the bleeding by pressing on a pressure point.

Pressure points are places where an artery can be pressed against an underlying bone to prevent the blood flowing past. Use a pressure point to reduce severe bleeding only as a last resort and then do so with extreme care. Never maintain maximum pressure for more than five minutes, for example. To do otherwise could cause irreparable damage to the tissues of the injured limb. Instead reduce the pressure after five minutes and continue alternating five minutes maximum pressure with five minutes reduced pressure for as long as necessary.

There are two main pressure points. One is on the inner side of the arm where the brachial artery can be pressed against the bone. The other is high inside the thigh, where the femoral artery can be pressed against the pelvis.

When a varicose vein bursts

If a varicose vein in the leg bursts or is injured, severe blood loss can occur rapidly. The bleeding must be stopped as quickly as possible and the victim taken to hospital.

• Lay the victim down and press on the wound with a cloth pad, such as the inside of a folded handkerchief. If no pad is available, press with your bare fingers.

• Raise the leg onto your thigh and maintain the pressure for up to 45 minutes to stop the bleeding.

• Put a dressing on the wound and tie it firmly in place with a bandage or piece of material.

• If bleeding continues, lay further dressings and bandages over the first.

• Tell the patient to rest, and prop up the leg with pillows or on a chair seat.

• Take the victim to the emergency department of your local hospital. Call 911, or an ambulance, if necessary.

When blood flows from nose, mouth or ear

If an injured person bleeds from the nose, mouth or ear, he may be suffering from a severe internal injury to the head or chest.

A fractured skull may cause blood to trickle from the nose or ear. An injury to the lungs, caused by a fractured rib, may cause the victim to cough up blood from the mouth.

Call for an ambulance as quickly as possible, and in the meantime place the patient in a half-sitting position with the head tilted toward the side from which the blood is coming.

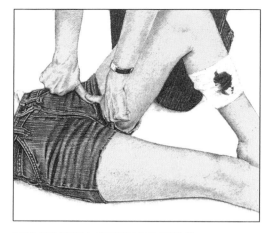

THE FEMORAL PRESSURE POINT
Lay the victim down and bend the injured leg at the knee. Press down firmly in the center of the fold of the groin, one thumb on top of the other, against the rim of the pelvis. Do not press forcefully for longer than five minutes.

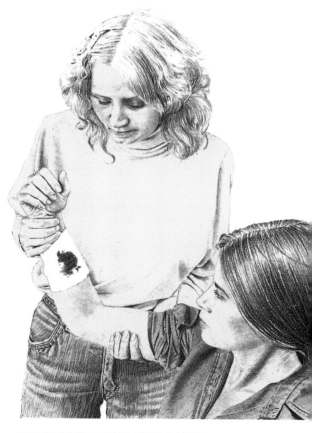

THE BRACHIAL PRESSURE POINT
Hold the victim's arm at right angles to the body. The brachial artery runs along the inner side of the upper arm. To control bleeding from the lower arm, put one hand under the upper arm and press your fingers against the bone.

BLOOD FROM NOSE, MOUTH OR EAR

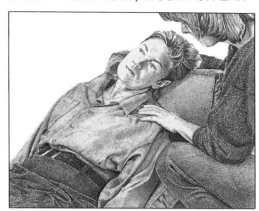

1 *Prop the victim in a half-sitting position, with the head tilted toward the side from which the blood is coming.*

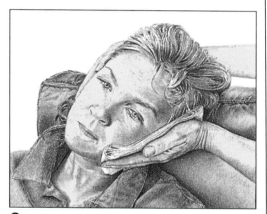

2 *Cover the bleeding point with a pad of clean material, but do not apply pressure. Call 911 and ask for an ambulance.*

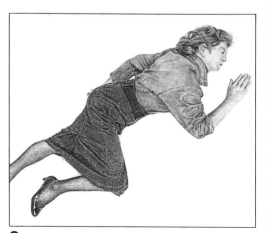

3 *If the victim becomes unconscious before the ambulance arrives, put her in the recovery position like this (see page 136).*

Blindness

Sudden blindness can occur in one or both eyes for a number of reasons, some much less serious than others.

Migraine
The most common cause is migraine, which can produce bright spots or zigzag lines in the vision, preventing the victim from seeing properly. The disturbances of the vision are seen with both eyes. The sight will return to normal in 30 minutes or less, and a severe headache is likely to follow.

After the first attack, see your doctor. Once the condition has been diagnosed it should not be necessary to see the doctor after subsequent attacks.

Snow blindness
People who spend long periods in the snow risk snow blindness if they do not protect their eyes with dark glasses. The ultraviolet rays from bright sunlight reflected from the snow inflame the cornea, causing pain and loss of vision.

Cover the victim's eyes with improvised pads, put in place tightly enough to keep the lids from moving, and get medical help as quickly as possible. With prompt treatment, normal vision should return in a day or two.

Circulation problems in the eye
High blood pressure and diabetes can bring about hemorrhages or clots in the blood vessels of the eye. These clots can cause sudden, painless loss of vision – either partial or total – in one eye.

Call an ophthalmologist immediately, or take the victim to the emergency department of the nearest hospital.

Detached retina
A sudden painless loss or change of vision, sometimes preceded by flashing lights, can be the main symptom of a detached retina, a potentially blinding ailment. Alternatively, the victim may have the sensation of a curtain coming across the field of vision.

Get medical help immediately. With prompt treatment, the eyesight can be successfully restored.

Acute glaucoma
Severe pain in and around the eye, with blurring of the vision and nausea, can indicate glaucoma, a serious eye ailment. It occurs most often in 50- and 60-year-old persons.

The main attack is often preceded by blurring of the vision and discomfort in the eye, which is better after sleep. Attacks often occur in the evening, and can be caused by excitement.

Call an ophthalmologist immediately or take the patient to the nearest emergency department. Treatment with drugs, laser and possibly surgery can lessen the damaging effects on the vision.

Blisters

Blisters caused by burns or friction to the skin usually heal within a week, whether they burst or not. A severe blister, affecting more than the outer layer of skin, will also heal completely but may leave a scar.

To burst or not to burst?
Do not burst a blister deliberately unless the taut skin is causing acute discomfort. Opening the skin increases the risk of infection.

If you decide to do so, observe scrupulous conditions of cleanliness.
• Wash the blistered area, and your hands, thoroughly.
• Pass a fine needle through a flame and let it cool for a moment. Do not wipe off any soot and do not touch the point.
• Hold the needle flat on the skin and press the point gently but firmly into the blister, just enough to burst it.
• Remove the needle and make a second puncture on the opposite side of the blister.
• Remove the needle and press gently on the blister with a clean piece of cotton wool.
• Wipe, and apply an adhesive dressing.

If a blister bursts by itself, expose it to the air as much as possible in hygienic conditions, but keep it covered with a bandage if there is a risk of dirt getting in.

See your doctor if a blister becomes infected, with a swollen, tender or inflamed area around it, or if blisters occur without any obvious cause. Multiple blisters are a symptom of several diseases, including shingles, chicken pox and impetigo.

How to avoid blisters
Blisters can be avoided by taking a few simple precautions.
• Take care when cooking or ironing. Cooks who do not wear oven mitts, for example, often receive burns on the arm when removing cooked food from the oven.
• Wear protective gloves for any heavy manual work to which you are not accustomed.
• Only buy shoes that fit well, and break them in with short periods of wear.
• On country hikes, or other outings where you will be on your feet a lot, wear comfortable shoes, with two pairs of socks to reduce friction on the feet. They can be a thin cotton pair next to the skin, with a thicker pair of woolen over-socks.

Boils

Most boils burst within a week of starting, but if the infection goes very deep it may take two weeks for the boil to "come to a head." The process can be speeded up by applying hot cloths or magnesium sulfate poultices to the boil.

While waiting for the boil to burst, try to rest the affected area, and move it as little as possible. This allows the body's defenses to work, and reduces the chance of the infection spreading below the skin.

Take acetaminophen or aspirin to relieve the pain. Do not apply creams or antiseptics to the skin; they will not penetrate and so will not help to cure the boil.

When the boil bursts, cover it with a clean, dry dressing to prevent infection entering the wound.

Why do they occur?
Boils tend to occur in hairy parts of the body and areas where friction takes place, such as the nostrils, armpits, back of the neck and between the legs and buttocks.

They are caused by infection from bacteria, particularly in people with low resistance due to excessive tiredness, poor nutrition, diabetes mellitus or a blood disorder.

The bacteria create pockets of infection in the skin, often around a hair follicle. The follicle and surrounding cells in the skin are killed by the bacteria and form pus, which increases (or "comes to a head") until it bursts through the skin and escapes.

A collection of boils, forming in several hair follicles, is called a carbuncle. The pocket of pus may be extensive, and can spread below the skin until two or more heads form and burst.

Boils tend to spread between members of a household, and sufferers should use their own towels and if possible sterilize underwear and handkerchiefs in boiling water or disinfectant while the boil is discharging.

It should be necessary to see a doctor only:
• If the boil is very painful.
• If the inflammation around the boil spreads without coming to a head.
• If the boil does not discharge pus, although a head has developed.
• If a person has many boils at the same time, or a sequence of infections.

The doctor may cut into the boil to release the pressure and ease the pain. Antibiotics may be prescribed to prevent the spread of infection. And tests may be made to discover any disease that is lowering resistance to infection.

To avoid boils in the future, eat a balanced diet and obtain plenty of rest to build up the body's resistance to infection. Control diabetes or any other disorders.

Bruises

Bruises are the visual sign of bleeding beneath the skin, usually as the result of a blow or a fall. Blood seeps into the tissues, causing swelling, soreness and discoloration. Swelling may be considerable whenever the bruise occurs on the head or shin or anyplace where the bone is just beneath the skin.

The bruise is usually red or pink to start with, turning bluish and then greenish-yellow in the seven to 14 days it may take to heal. These color changes are caused by the gradual degeneration of the components of the blood as the bruise starts to heal.

Before treating a bruise, check that there are no other injuries, particularly fractures.

Apply a cold compress to the bruised area to help to limit the swelling. The compress can be a small towel soaked in cold water and wrung out, or crushed ice cubes tied up in a plastic bag and wrapped in a cloth.

The cooling process slows down the blood flow. Apply the compress as soon as possible and keep it on for at least 30 minutes. Alternatively, instead of using a compress, hold the bruised area under cold, running water.

If a bruise has not faded away within two weeks, consult a doctor. See a doctor also:
• If the pain is severe, or if there is difficulty in moving the bruised part 24 hours later.
• If bruises occur without any apparent reason.
• If the lower leg is bruised in an elderly person or a person suffering from poor circulation.
• If the vision is disturbed as the result of a black eye (see page 59).

TREATING A BRUISED ARM

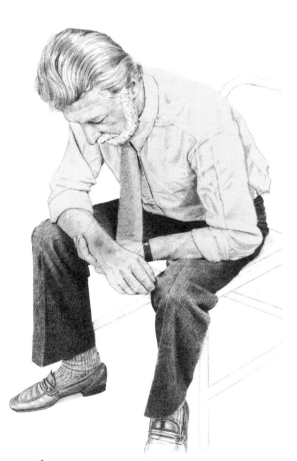

1 *Put the victim in a comfortable position and get him to support the injured part before and during treatment. This helps to reduce the bleeding within the tissues.*

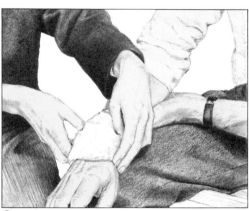

2 *Apply a cold compress at once to help minimize the swelling. If necessary, fix the compress in place with an elastic bandage, winding from below the injury to above it.*

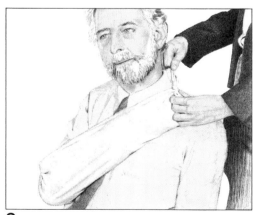

3 *Support a bruised arm with a sling (see page 121). If a leg is bruised, lay the victim down and prop up the leg on a pillow. For bruises on the trunk, lay him down with pillows beneath his head and shoulders.*

Burns and scalds

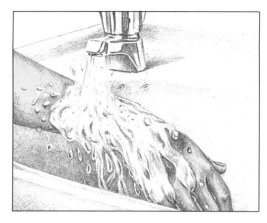

TREATING A MINOR BURN
A superficial burn smaller than a 25¢ piece can be treated by flooding it with cold water for at least 10 minutes, or immersing it in any cold harmless liquid, such as milk or beer.

The seriousness of a burn or scald depends on how deep it is and how large an area it covers. All but minor burns and scalds are potentially serious and should be seen by a doctor. The treatment for burns and scalds is identical.

Do not put butter, oil, ointment or lotion on a burn. It will have to be removed by hospital staff before they can give treatment, and may be a source of infection.

Do not apply any adhesive bandages, do not touch a burn and do not break any blisters. And do not remove anything that is sticking to a burn.

The first action in treating a victim is to remove him from the source of heat. If the source is electrical, pull out the plug or switch off the power, taking care not to injure yourself.

If the burn is caused by a dry chemical, such as caustic soda or quicklime, brush away as much as you can with a duster or soft brush, taking care to protect your own hands. Remove contaminated clothing and check that the victim is not lying on any of the chemical. For burns

REMOVING BURNED CLOTHING
When approaching a person with burning clothing, hold a blanket, rug or coat in front of you for protection. Wrap the material around him and lay him on the floor, burned side uppermost. When the fire is extinguished, remove any hot clothing that can be taken off easily, but leave fragments that have stuck to the skin.

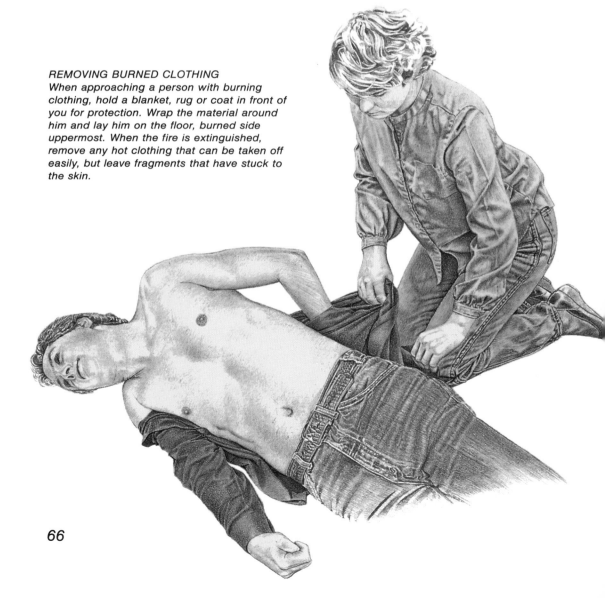

and scalds in the mouth, give the patient ice cubes or ice cream to suck.

Treating a minor burn

If the burn is extremely painful, it will probably be superficial. The outer layers of skin will be red, swollen and possibly blistered.

If a burn of this sort is smaller than a 25¢ piece, hold it under a slow-running cold water faucet or put it in cold water for at least ten minutes to cool the skin. If no water is available, use some other cold liquid, such as milk or beer.

Remove rings, watch or tight clothing before the area starts to swell, and finally cover it with a dressing of non-fluffy material.

Larger superficial burns

If a superficial burn is larger than a 25¢ piece, see a doctor or go to a hospital emergency department, because there is a danger of infection. Cool the burn in cold water and cover it with a clean dressing, but do not waste time before getting medical help.

Dealing with deep burns

If a burned area of skin appears gray and is peeling or charred, the burn may be deep. It may not be particularly painful, as the nerves will have been damaged.

Whatever the size of a deep burn, do not immerse it in water, and do not apply water or ice. Cover it with a clean, non-fluffy dressing and get medical help at once, because there is a strong risk of infection.

Widespread burns

Burns covering a large area of the body, such as an arm, a thigh or the chest, are medical emergencies which must be treated in hospital as quickly as possible with minimum interference to the damaged skin.

Remove rings, watch or tight clothing before the area starts to swell. Remove scalding clothing as soon as you can handle it. Then dial 911 and ask for an ambulance.

While waiting for the ambulance, cover the burn with clean, non-fluffy material, such as a freshly washed pillowcase. Fix it in place with a scarf or piece of clean cloth.

If the victim is unconscious but breathing, put him in the recovery position (see page 136), before calling for an ambulance.

When a person's clothes catch fire

A person with burning clothes should be laid flat to prevent the flames rising to the head, then rolled. You can also douse the fire with water or any nonflammable liquid such as milk or beer (but *not* alcoholic spirits such as whiskey or gin). If no liquid is available, wrap the victim in thick, non-synthetic material, such as a rug or coat, to smother the flames.

If your own clothes catch fire, lie down and roll on the ground.

DEEP OR WIDESPREAD BURNS

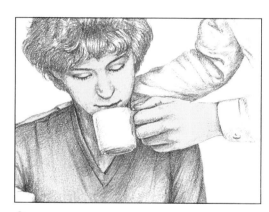

1 *Prevent infection by covering the burned area with a clean dressing, such as a clean handkerchief or pillowcase. Hold it in place with a soft towel or other material.*

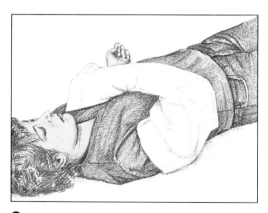

2 *Reassure the victim and give sips of water to replace lost fluid. Adults should sip half a cup of water over 10 minutes. Children should sip water continuously.*

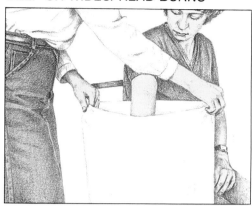

3 *If the burn is widespread, lay the victim down and treat for shock (see page 120). Call an ambulance as soon as possible. Do not try to cool deep or widespread burns with water.*

Chest injuries

Car accidents are the most common cause of chest injuries, particularly among drivers and passengers not wearing seat belts.

The other main causes are stab wounds and crushing by a heavy weight.

Serious chest injuries divide into two types, depending on whether the chest wall has been punctured.

"Sucking" chest wounds

If the chest wall has been penetrated by a sharp instrument, or by a fractured rib, the injury is known as a "sucking" wound. As the patient breathes, air is sucked into the chest through the wound, rather than down the airway, so that the lung does not inflate.

The lung on the uninjured side can also be affected, and the victim can be in danger of dying from asphyxiation because of an inability to get enough air into the lungs.

Symptoms of a "sucking" wound include:
- Pain in the chest.
- Difficulty in breathing.
- Blueness of the mouth and skin.
- Bubbles of blood-stained liquid emerging from the wound as the patient breathes out.
- The sound of air being sucked through the wound as the patient breathes in.

It is essential to seal the wound as quickly as possible so that the patient can breathe.

Begin by placing the palm of your hand over the injury to provide immediate relief. Then, if

HOW TO TREAT A "SUCKING" WOUND

1 *Rest the victim in a comfortable position. Make him sit up and lean him toward the injured side. Leaning the victim toward the injured side prevents blood draining across inside the chest and lessens the risk of the uninjured lung becoming affected. Lean him on cushions or against your thigh. Slacken belt or waistband.*

possible, apply a dressing and create an airtight seal by covering the dressing.

For the covering, use a piece of polyethylene, or plastic film of the type used to wrap up food, or kitchen foil, and seal the edges securely with adhesive tape.

Tell someone to dial 911 and ask for an ambulance.

Complicated fracture of the rib cage

A fractured rib may damage internal organs, such as the lungs, without penetrating through to the outside of the chest.

This will cause bleeding inside the chest. The victim will then cough up red, frothy blood.

Other symptoms include:

• Bruising and bleeding from the chest.
• Pain which may become worse if the victim coughs.
• Shallow breathing.
• A tight feeling in the chest. If several ribs are fractured, you may also be able to hear a crackling noise, which is caused by the bone ends rubbing together.

Ask someone to call for an ambulance as soon as possible, and if possible put the arm on the injured side in a triangular sling to support the fractured ribs.

Crushed chest

If the rib cage is fractured in several places – as can happen when the chest has been crushed

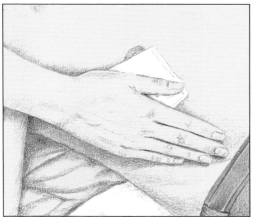

2 *Seal the puncture wound in the chest immediately with your hand — and a clean folded handkerchief if possible. Do not press hard if you suspect fractured ribs.*

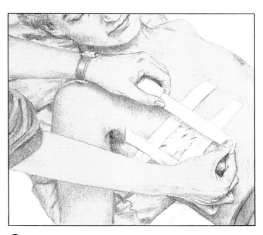

3 *To make a more permanent seal, cover the handkerchief with a sheet of polyethylene, plastic film or kitchen foil, securing it with adhesive tape to make it airtight.*

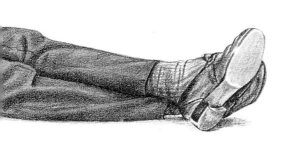

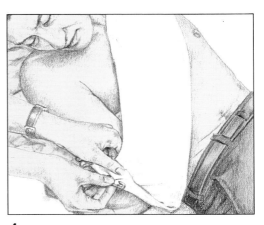

4 *While waiting for an ambulance, put the arm on the injured side across the chest to support the damaged area. Keep the arm in place with a triangular sling (see overleaf). Make the patient as comfortable as possible.*

by a heavy weight – a condition known to medical emergency teams as paradoxical breathing may occur. The fractured ribs will be sucked in when the patient breathes in, and pushed out as he breathes out. This is the reverse of the normal chest movement and can cause extreme difficulty in breathing.

A patient in this condition should be treated as for a complicated fracture of the rib cage.

TREATING A COMPLICATED FRACTURE OF THE RIB CAGE

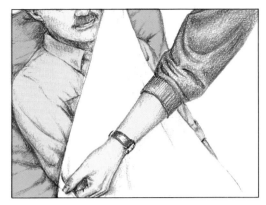

2 Put one end of the base of the sling over the shoulder on the uninjured side, with the point extended beyond the elbow. The sling should hang over the arm.

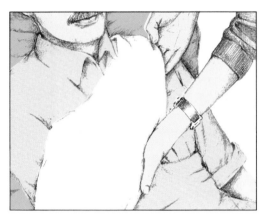

3 Tuck the base under the hand, forearm and elbow. Bring the lower end up and around the back. Tie the ends together just above the collarbone on the uninjured side.

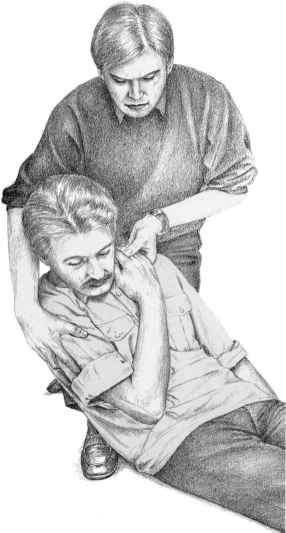

1 Rest the victim in a comfortable position. Make him sit up and lean him toward the injured side to help to drain blood and fluid away from the uninjured lung. Move the arm on the injured side diagonally across the chest, so that the hand rests on the opposite shoulder. The arm is now ready for a triangular sling.

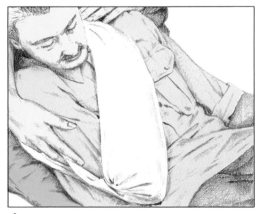

4 Fold the point of the sling at the elbow and fasten it with a pin or tape, or twist then tuck it in. Get the victim to support the sling with the other hand if possible.

First aid and
medical emergencies

Chest pain

Pain in the chest may be clearly related to breathing or quite unrelated to it.

In either case, the pain can be a danger signal of a serious condition – in the lungs or the heart – and should not be ignored.

Pain related to breathing

Painful breathing can be caused by chest injuries, which are usually obvious (see *Chest injuries*, page 68, and *Rib fractures*, page 120). It can also indicate a disorder of the lungs or their lining (the pleura), or of the bones, muscles or skin of the chest.

The pain forces the sufferer to take short and often rapid breaths. There is often a cough as well.

See a doctor as soon as possible if there is:
• Severe pain.
• Breathlessness.
• High temperature.
• Blood-stained spit.

Pain not related to breathing

Chest pain that is not associated with breathing may have a clear connection with exertion or with eating.

Pain brought on by exertion usually feels "crushing," and may radiate to the neck, shoulders or arms. It passes off with rest. It is usually a symptom of a heart disorder, and is known as cardiac or anginal pain.

If the pain is associated with eating, it may be caused by a problem in the digestive system such as indigestion or duodenal ulcer.

See a doctor immediately if:
• There is paleness of the skin and sweating.
• A heart condition is suspected – either because the patient has already suffered a heart attack or because the pain fits the description of cardiac or anginal pain given above (see also *Heart attack*, page 105).
• The pain is not improved after an hour's rest.

Treat indigestion by resting in a chair and taking an antacid or half a teaspoon of bicarbonate of soda in a glass of water.

Chicken pox

A highly irritating rash which starts on the body and spreads to the arms, legs, face and head heralds an attack of chicken pox.

The rash begins as raised pink spots which change to watery blisters. These then burst or shrivel up, and crust over to form scabs. The spots appear in crops over about four days, so that all stages of the rash may be on the body at the same time.

The patient has a raised temperature and may feel quite ill for three or four days.

What you should do

Most cases of chicken pox do not require medical attention, and can be treated at home.
• Keep the rash clean and dry by having a quick shower every day and patting the skin dry.
• Apply calamine lotion to the rash twice daily to ease the itching. Do not pick the spots, or they will leave little pockmarks.
• Drink plenty of liquid. It does not matter if the patient refuses food during the illness.
• Rest, and take painkillers in recommended doses to help reduce fever and discomfort. But avoid aspirin, which has been linked to the development of Reye's syndrome in children with chicken pox or influenza.
• There is no need to isolate an infected child from your other children, as it is better to have the infection in childhood than in adult life. But keep the patient away from children being treated for serious diseases such as leukemia, because chicken pox could be fatal to them.
• Try to avoid spreading the infection to babies under six months and to women in late pregnancy. If a woman has the disease within a few days before giving birth, the baby may have chicken pox and be quite ill. But chicken pox in earlier pregnancy does not affect the unborn child. Avoid spreading the infection to elderly people, too. They might develop shingles, a painful and sometimes long-lasting disease.

When to see the doctor

Chicken pox can be complicated by infected blisters and by pneumonia and encephalitis, which are rare but serious. See your doctor if:
• The patient has a high fever, is vomiting or is coughing excessively.
• There is some alteration in the patient's state of consciousness, or if he develops a severe headache or becomes confused.
• The eyes themselves (not simply the eyelids) are affected, or the spots become inflamed.

Chicken pox patients are infectious from about four days before the rash appears until all the blisters have formed scabs. The scabs disappear after about two weeks.

Chicken pox is mainly a disease of childhood, but it occasionally affects adults. It occurs in epidemics every two or three years. One attack ensures immunity to further attacks, but the virus may lie dormant in the body and cause shingles in later life.

Childbirth

Most babies are born without difficulty. So your most important task in coping with an emergency delivery is to stay calm and reassure the mother and anyone else present.

Normally supervision of childbirth is restricted to doctors in Canada, to doctors and nurse-midwives in the United States. But an unqualified person may have to take charge in an emergency.

Before doing so, however, every effort should be made to contact a doctor. Call 911 for help, if necessary.

There are three distinct stages in labor:

Stage 1 lasts for several hours – up to 14 hours in a first pregnancy, less in later births.

During this stage the muscles of the body of the uterus begin to contract, opening up the neck of the uterus (the cervix) to let the baby's head pass through. The contractions cause pain in the back and lower abdomen, and at first they occur about every 30 minutes. Blood may seep from the vagina at the start. Gradually the contractions become more frequent.

A watery fluid runs from the vagina. This is "the breaking of the waters" – the release of fluid which has surrounded the baby in the womb.

Stage 2, during which the baby is actually born, lasts between 15 minutes and an hour. The contractions become stronger and the mother feels an urge to bear down.

Stage 3 happens after the birth, and is vital to the health of the mother. The placenta, or afterbirth, to which the umbilical cord is attached, is expelled after further contractions.

What you should do to prepare

Between contractions, or before labor starts, try to make the following preparations (you may have to improvise):

• Line the bottom of a crib with a folded blanket, shawl or towel. Fold another blanket ready for when the baby is born. A baby's head is large in proportion to its body, so you do not need a pillow. If there is no crib, use a drawer or a cardboard box.

• Prepare a bed or a large clean surface such as a table for the mother to lie on. Spread a plastic sheet or newspaper over the surface and cover it with a clean sheet or towel.

• Using clean scissors, cut three pieces of string, each about 9 in. (23 cm) long.

• If possible, sterilize string and scissors by boiling them in water for about ten minutes. Wrap them in a clean cloth. Do not touch the sterilized scissor blades.

• Have a clean sheet ready to cover the mother's top during delivery, and a blanket to keep her warm afterward.

• Three or four more clean towels and several pieces of cloth or sheeting should be stacked ready, if available. You will also need a sanitary napkin for the mother to use after the birth, and a diaper for the baby.

Cleanliness is essential

• Wash your hands and scrub your nails under running water before assisting, and as often as necessary during the birth. Do not dry them on a towel. Shake them as dry as possible.

• Keep anyone with an open cut or infection away from the mother and baby.

• Make sure that bedding, towels, cloths and swabbing materials are as clean as possible. When they become soiled, discard them and get fresh ones if you can.

How you can help a mother during labor

• Give the mother occasional small drinks of milk or water, but nothing to eat. The body's digestive system shuts down during labor, so food will not be digested anyway.

DELIVERING THE BABY

1 *Tell the mother to lie on her back, or on her side if that is more comfortable, with her knees bent. Support her shoulders with pillows and cushions. When the baby's head first appears, put a clean towel or cloth under the mother's buttocks and a clean towel or sheet on the bed between her legs.*

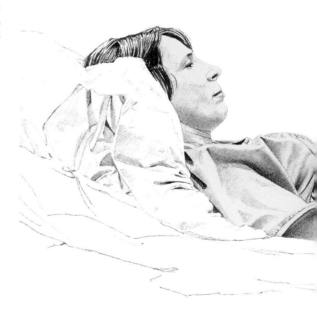

• As the contractions become more frequent, or if the waters break, tell her to lie on the bed (or other prepared surface) in the position most comfortable for her.

• If the pains are bad, it may help if she breathes deeply, in and out, with each contraction, and does not hold her breath.

• If she complains of tingling fingers or a trembling sensation when she does this, she is taking in too much oxygen. Cup your hands loosely over her mouth and nose during the contraction so that she rebreathes some of her own air. The tingling sensation should stop.

• During this first stage, encourage her to relax as far as possible between and during the contractions, and not to bear down.

As the second stage of labor begins, the mother will feel an unmistakable urge to bear down. By this time the contractions may be coming every two or three minutes, and the birth is imminent – though it may still take up to an hour to complete.

• Encourage her to lie on her back or side – whichever is more comfortable – and, with each contraction, tell her to hold her breath and bear down hard.

• Tell her to grip her thighs behind her knees, and pull her legs at the same time as she is bearing down.

Delivering the baby
Your first sight of the baby will usually be the top of its head, and it will usually become visible at the height of a contraction.

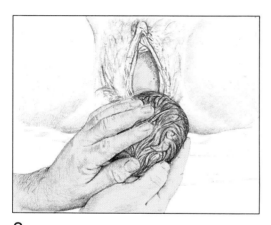

2 *When the baby's head is fully out, support it with clean, cupped hands. If a caul, or membrane, covers the baby's face, remove it gently but quickly.*

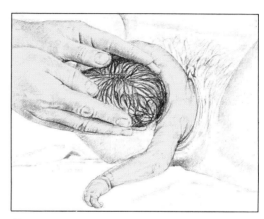

3 *As the shoulders emerge, support them gently but do not pull. One shoulder appears first. The second will follow easily if you gently raise the baby's head.*

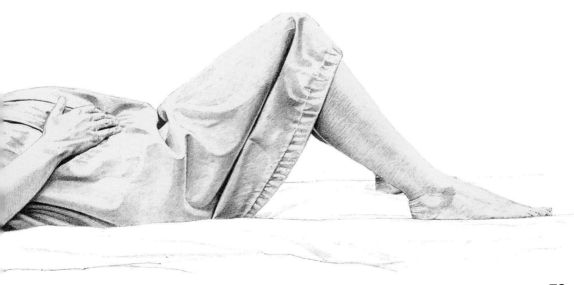

Between contractions the head may slip back out of sight at first. This is normal.

Do not touch the baby's head as it emerges. Tell the mother to stop bearing down, and to pant in quick breaths to prevent the baby being thrust out too forcefully.

Once the shoulders are out, the rest of the baby will be born without difficulty.

Tying the umbilical cord

When the baby is breathing normally, use two pieces of string to tie off the umbilical cord and cut the cord between the two ties with clean scissors.

After the birth

Some 5 to 15 minutes after the birth, the uterus will contract again to expel the placenta.

• When these contractions start, place a bowl between the mother's legs. It will take between 5 and 20 minutes for the placenta to be pushed out.

• Do not pull the umbilical cord to speed delivery of the placenta – it will deliver itself.

• When the placenta is fully out, put it aside in the bowl, with the cord, so that it can be examined later by a doctor.

• Wash the mother, fix a sanitary pad or an improvised pad in place and give her fresh clothes if possible.

• Tidy up the room. If the mother wants something to eat or drink, she can now have it.

• Put the baby to the mother's breast if she wants to feed it.

If the mother is asleep, lay the baby in a crib on its side (to drain any remaining mucus from the lungs) and with the head low (to ensure a good flow of blood to the brain).

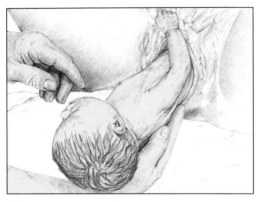

4 *The rest of the baby will be born without difficulty. Support the body with one hand. When it is fully born, wipe away any mucus or blood from the mouth with a clean cloth.*

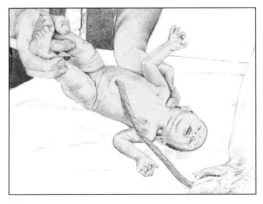

5 *If the baby does not breathe immediately, hold it with the head lower than the body to drain any mucus. Do not slap the baby. If necessary, blow hard on its chest.*

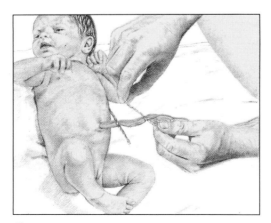

6 *Once the baby is breathing normally, which usually happens within a few seconds of birth, tie the cord with two pieces of clean string as tight as you can about 6 in. (15 cm) and 8 in. (20 cm) from the baby's navel.*

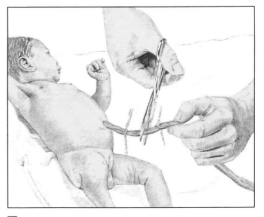

7 *Cut the cord with clean scissors between the two ties. Make a further secure tie about 4 in. (10 cm) from the baby's navel. There is no need to cut the cord closer to the baby's navel. It will fall off on its own in a few days.*

Unusual deliveries

Most babies emerge head first and face down. Occasionally the baby emerges face up. Deliveries in this position tend to be slower, but present no special problems.

• In a small number of cases, the baby may appear with the umbilical cord around its neck. Hook a finger round the cord and loop it over the baby's head.

In a very small number of cases, the baby may appear bottom first (breech birth). Support but do not pull the baby as it emerges. When the shoulders are out, support them with your hands and ease the body up so that the mouth is clear to breathe.

If the baby does not breathe

A baby usually begins to breathe within a few seconds of birth.

• If it does not, hold it with the head down and blow hard on its chest. If it still does not breathe, open its mouth and clear out any mucus with your little finger. Clear the nose with a cloth, and lay the baby on one side with the head slightly lower than the body.

• Flick the bottom of the baby's feet sharply with your index finger to stimulate it into breathing. The child should breathe after a few taps. Do not smack the baby's bottom.

If the baby fails to respond, give artificial respiration (see page 50), using gentle puffs.

If the placenta fails to appear

Should the placenta not be expelled, or if it looks as though only part of the placenta has been expelled, get medical help as soon as possible. It may mean that the mother has serious internal bleeding.

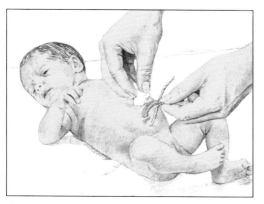

8 *Put a clean dressing over the end of the cord attached to the baby. Wrap the baby warmly. It will lose heat rapidly if left uncovered – particularly from the top of the head.*

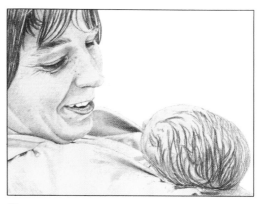

9 *Give the baby to the mother and wrap her warmly in blankets. Now wait for the placenta to appear. Do not pull on the cord to speed delivery; it will deliver itself.*

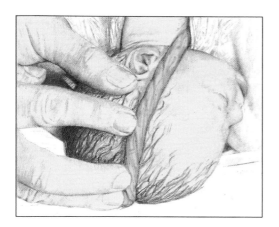

CORD AROUND THE NECK
If the baby appears with the cord around the neck, just hook a finger around the cord and loop it over the baby's head. Do not pull the baby or the cord.

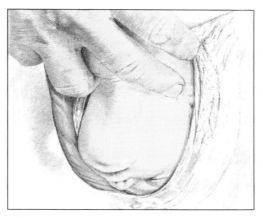

BREECH BIRTH
If the baby's bottom appears first, do not worry. Support it as it emerges, but do not pull. When the shoulders are out, ease the body up so that the mouth is clear to breathe.

75

Childhood illnesses

If you are worried that your child may be dangerously ill, ask yourself the following five questions. If the answer to any of them is "yes," contact your doctor without delay.

1 Is the child not fully conscious or unnaturally drowsy?
2 Has the child's color become *and stayed* very pale?
3 Is there blueness around the face or lips?
4 Does the child have serious difficulty in breathing?
5 Is there a rash that looks like bleeding under the skin,
 and which does not go pale when you press firmly?

If the answer to all five questions is "no," but the child still seems off-color, use the charts on the following six pages to discover the best course of action. Begin by choosing the most appropriate major symptom, which is listed in capital letters at the head of each chart. Then start at the red box and follow the arrows, answering each question either "yes" or "no," to find the likely cause of the child's symptoms. Where painkillers are in order, use acetaminophen. Avoid aspirin, which has been associated with the development of Reye's syndrome in children who have chicken pox, the flu or other viral infections.

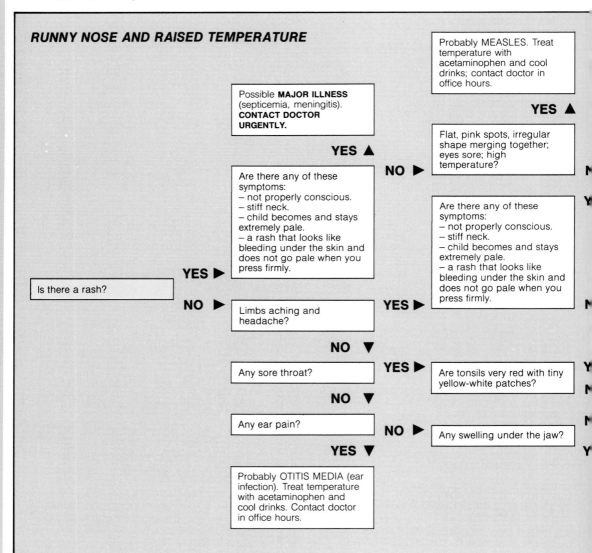

RUNNY NOSE AND RAISED TEMPERATURE

Probably MEASLES. Treat temperature with acetaminophen and cool drinks; contact doctor in office hours.

YES ▲

Possible **MAJOR ILLNESS** (septicemia, meningitis). **CONTACT DOCTOR URGENTLY.**

YES ▲

NO ▶

Flat, pink spots, irregular shape merging together; eyes sore; high temperature?

Are there any of these symptoms:
– not properly conscious.
– stiff neck.
– child becomes and stays extremely pale.
– a rash that looks like bleeding under the skin and does not go pale when you press firmly.

YES ▶

Are there any of these symptoms:
– not properly conscious.
– stiff neck.
– child becomes and stays extremely pale.
– a rash that looks like bleeding under the skin and does not go pale when you press firmly.

Is there a rash?

NO ▶   Limbs aching and headache?   YES ▶

NO ▼

Any sore throat?   YES ▶   Are tonsils very red with tiny yellow-white patches?

NO ▼

Any ear pain?   NO ▶   Any swelling under the jaw?

YES ▼

Probably OTITIS MEDIA (ear infection). Treat temperature with acetaminophen and cool drinks. Contact doctor in office hours.

DIARRHEA

Are there any of the following symptoms: listlessness, sunken eyes, very dry mouth, not properly conscious?

YES ▶ Possible **MAJOR ILLNESS** (gastroenteritis with dehydration, meningitis, septicemia). **CONTACT DOCTOR URGENTLY.**

NO ▶ Is there sore throat, ear pain or aching limbs and headache?

NO ▶ Probably GASTROENTERITIS without dehydration. Give plenty to drink — fruit juice, squash, clear soup, water, but not milk. Contact doctor if no improvement in 6–8 hours, or immediately if signs of dehydration appear (see first question).

YES ▶ Could be TONSILLITIS, EAR INFECTION or FLU. Treat temperature with acetaminophen and cool drinks. Contact doctor in office hours.

Probably RUBELLA (GERMAN MEASLES). Treat as for measles and keep patient away from women in early pregnancy.

YES ▲

Tiny pink spots starting on face; tiny lumps behind ears; not very ill?

NO ▶ Raised blisters appearing in crops. High temperature?

NO ▶ Rash on face *only*?

YES ▼

YES ▼ Probably CHICKEN POX. Treat as for measles. Use calamine on skin.

Probably IMPETIGO. Make appointment with doctor for same or next day. Avoid contagion by reserving a facecloth, towel, etc., for affected child.

Probable **MAJOR ILLNESS** (meningitis, septicemia). **CONTACT DOCTOR URGENTLY.**

Possibly FLU. Give acetaminophen and cool drinks. Call doctor in office hours.

Probably TONSILLITIS. Treat temperature with acetaminophen and cool drinks, and call doctor in office hours.

Probably COMMON COLD. Treat temperature with acetaminophen and cool drinks.

Probably MUMPS. Contact doctor in office hours; treat temperature with acetaminophen and cool drinks.

JERKY MOVEMENTS OF LIMBS

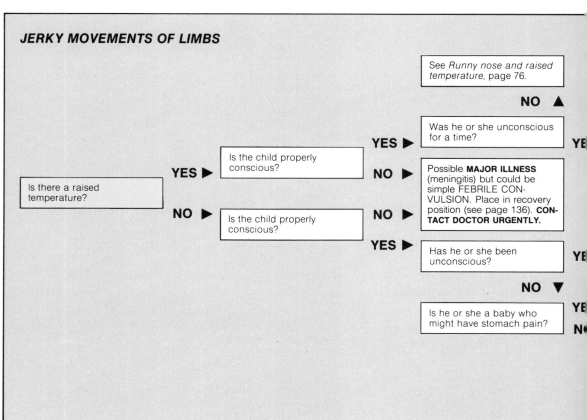

See *Runny nose and raised temperature*, page 76.

NO ▲

Is there a raised temperature?

YES ▶ Is the child properly conscious?

YES ▶ Was he or she unconscious for a time?

YE

NO ▶ Possible **MAJOR ILLNESS** (meningitis) but could be simple FEBRILE CONVULSION. Place in recovery position (see page 136). **CONTACT DOCTOR URGENTLY.**

NO ▶ Is the child properly conscious?

NO ▶

YES ▶ Has he or she been unconscious?

YE

NO ▼

Is he or she a baby who might have stomach pain?

YE

N

ABNORMAL BREATHING

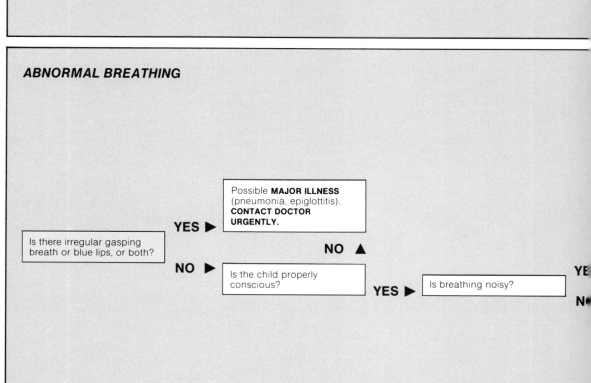

Is there irregular gasping breath or blue lips, or both?

YES ▶ Possible **MAJOR ILLNESS** (pneumonia, epiglottitis). **CONTACT DOCTOR URGENTLY.**

NO ▲

NO ▶ Is the child properly conscious?

YES ▶ Is breathing noisy?

YE

N

Probably FEBRILE CONVULSION. Remove clothes; sponge body down with lukewarm water; give acetaminophen. If this is the child's first attack, **CONTACT DOCTOR URGENTLY.** But if the child has had similar attacks before, contact doctor in office hours.

Possibly CONVULSIONS. If this is the child's first attack, **CONTACT DOCTOR URGENTLY.** But if the child has had attacks before, and the symptoms are unchanged, contact doctor in office hours.

Possible **MAJOR ILLNESS** (dehydration). **CONTACT DOCTOR URGENTLY.**

Probably GASTROENTERITIS. Is there listlessness, sunken eyes, very dry mouth?

YES ▶

NO ▶

Give plenty to drink (not milk). Contact doctor if no improvement in 6–8 hours.

Is there diarrhea or vomiting?

YES ▶

NO ▶

Probably COLIC. Give usual medicine; try rocking or cuddling. If very upset discuss with doctor when you next visit his office.

Probably not serious; wait and see.

Probably ASTHMA. Use your regular asthma medicine and contact doctor without delay unless the wheezing is mild only.

YES ▲

Probably BRONCHITIS. Contact doctor during day unless you are very worried; then you should not delay.

NO ▶

Musical note to breathing with rapid breathing and/or cough? Has the child had this before?

Could be **MAJOR ILLNESS** (epiglottitis). **CONTACT DOCTOR URGENTLY.**

NO ▲

Does the child look very ill?

YES ▶

NO ▶

Hoarse sound with ringing or "cow-like" cough?

YES ▶

Probably CROUP. Nurse in steamy room and contact doctor if no better in 2 hours.

Probably **MAJOR ILLNESS** (pneumonia). **CONTACT DOCTOR URGENTLY.**

Very rapid breathing with high temperature and/or chest pain?

YES ▶

NO ▶

Severe paroxysms of coughing, which may cause vomiting or going blue in the face, indicate WHOOPING COUGH. See doctor in office hours.

STOMACH PAIN

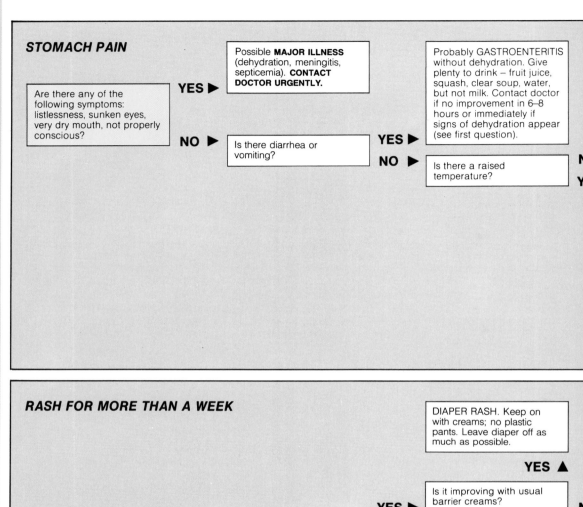

Are there any of the following symptoms: listlessness, sunken eyes, very dry mouth, not properly conscious?

YES ▶ Possible **MAJOR ILLNESS** (dehydration, meningitis, septicemia). **CONTACT DOCTOR URGENTLY.**

NO ▶ Is there diarrhea or vomiting?

YES ▶ Probably GASTROENTERITIS without dehydration. Give plenty to drink – fruit juice, squash, clear soup, water, but not milk. Contact doctor if no improvement in 6–8 hours or immediately if signs of dehydration appear (see first question).

NO ▶ Is there a raised temperature?

N
Y

RASH FOR MORE THAN A WEEK

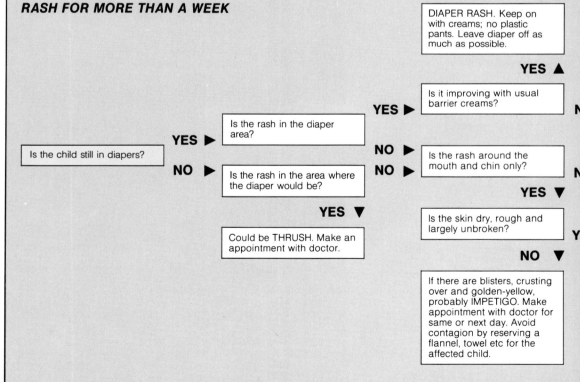

Is the child still in diapers?

YES ▶ Is the rash in the diaper area?

NO ▶ Is the rash in the area where the diaper would be?

YES ▶ Is it improving with usual barrier creams?

YES ▲ DIAPER RASH. Keep on with creams; no plastic pants. Leave diaper off as much as possible.

N

NO ▶ **NO ▶** Is the rash around the mouth and chin only?

N

YES ▼ Could be THRUSH. Make an appointment with doctor.

YES ▼ Is the skin dry, rough and largely unbroken?

Y

NO ▼ If there are blisters, crusting over and golden-yellow, probably IMPETIGO. Make appointment with doctor for same or next day. Avoid contagion by reserving a flannel, towel etc for the affected child.

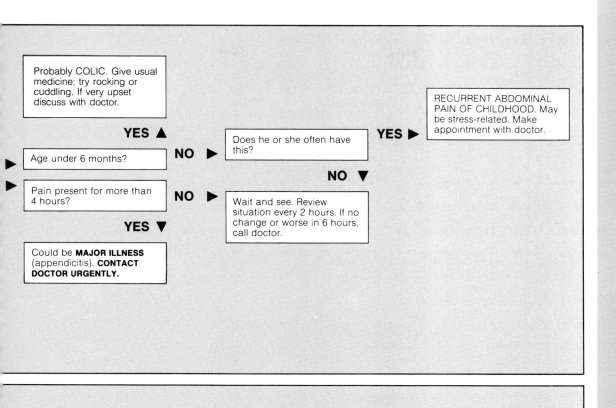

Probably COLIC. Give usual medicine; try rocking or cuddling. If very upset discuss with doctor.

YES ▲

Age under 6 months?

NO ▶

Does he or she often have this?

YES ▶

RECURRENT ABDOMINAL PAIN OF CHILDHOOD. May be stress-related. Make appointment with doctor.

NO ▼

Pain present for more than 4 hours?

NO ▶

Wait and see. Review situation every 2 hours. If no change or worse in 6 hours, call doctor.

YES ▼

Could be **MAJOR ILLNESS** (appendicitis). **CONTACT DOCTOR URGENTLY.**

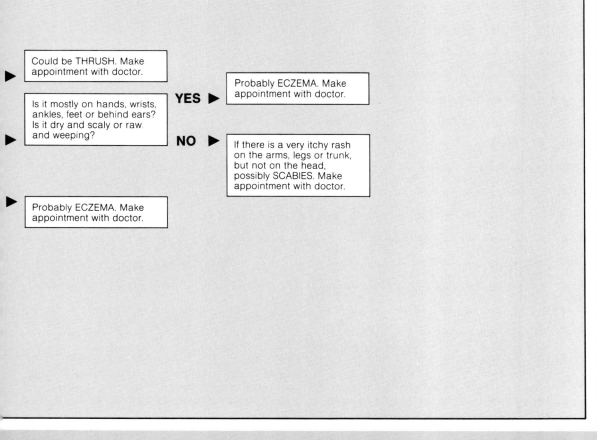

Could be THRUSH. Make appointment with doctor.

Is it mostly on hands, wrists, ankles, feet or behind ears? Is it dry and scaly or raw and weeping?

YES ▶

Probably ECZEMA. Make appointment with doctor.

NO ▶

If there is a very itchy rash on the arms, legs or trunk, but not on the head, possibly SCABIES. Make appointment with doctor.

Probably ECZEMA. Make appointment with doctor.

Choking

A piece of food or some other object stuck in the airway will cause choking. In severe cases the victim cannot breathe at all, and if left untreated will die within minutes. It is vital, therefore, to act promptly.

Suspect choking if a person who is unconscious and not breathing is found anywhere near an eating area. However, choking can happen away from eating areas when the victim has been eating candy, chewing gum or peanuts. Peanuts are a common cause of choking in young children, and should not be given to them. Children can also choke on toys that they put in their mouths, and adults can choke on dislodged dentures.

When choking occurs, the victim may have a fit of coughing, his face turns blue and the veins on the head and neck are swollen. He will instinctively make violent efforts to breathe, but the harder he tries, the more firmly lodged the obstruction will become. Instant action is vital.

Treating a conscious victim
• Encourage the victim to cough. It may be enough to dislodge the obstruction.
• If this fails, and the victim can neither breathe nor cough, quickly ask him if he is choking. If he is unable to speak or nods his head ''yes,'' apply the Heimlich maneuver. To do so, stand behind the victim whether he is standing or sitting, and put both arms around his waist.
• Make a fist with one hand and place the thumb side against the victim's abdomen, just above the navel but below the breastbone.

ABDOMINAL THRUST ON A CONSCIOUS ADULT

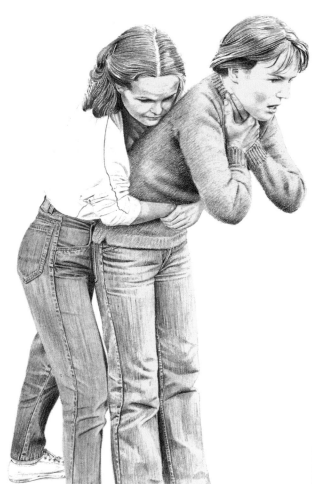

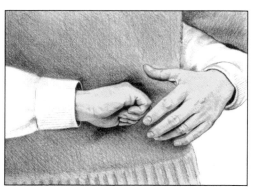

MAKING A FIST
Clench your fist in such a way that the tip of your thumb is contained by your fingers and the first knuckle of your thumb is pressing into the victim's abdomen.

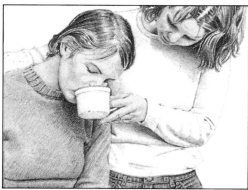

1 Put your arms around the victim, make a fist (see illustration, top right) and, with your other hand, hold the fist against her stomach, just above the navel but below the breastbone. Give quick inward-and-upward thrusts.

2 When the throat is clear, reassure the victim. Rest her in a comfortable position and give her water to sip if she asks for it. She should see her physician to make sure she has suffered no injuries from the abdominal thrusts.

First aid and
medical emergencies

• Grasp your fist with the other hand and press it forcefully into the abdomen with a quick inward-and-upward thrust. You are trying to pull the upper abdomen against the bottom of the lungs to drive out the remaining air and force out the obstruction.

• Repeat as often as necessary.

• Even if the thrusts are successful, the victim may be winded by the force and unable to breathe for a few moments.

• Check in his mouth to see if the obstruction has come up. If so, remove it.

• When he begins to breathe again, get him to sit quietly and, if he wants, let him sip water.

• Even though the Heimlich maneuver may be necessary to restore a victim's breathing, abdominal thrusts can damage the liver and other internal organs. For this reason, anyone who has been revived by this technique should see his physician.

Children and infants

• Watch closely but do not interfere as long as the youngster can breathe, speak or make sounds, and is coughing. These are all signs that he is getting some air in his windpipe and so may be able to expel whatever is causing the partial blockage. Be ready to act quickly the minute he stops breathing or making sounds.

• Rescue a child, 12 months and older, the same way you would an adult: the steps are outlined above. Apply the Heimlich maneuver gently if the child is small. In such cases, you may also administer the thrusts with the child

REVIVING A CHOKING CHILD

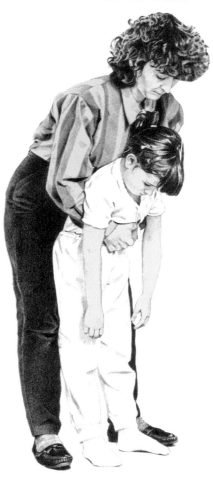

If you are sure that a child 12 months or older is choking, apply the Heimlich maneuver as you would for an adult. With arms wrapped around the victim, give quick abdominal thrusts. Bend your arms at the elbows to avoid squeezing too much on the youngster's ribs.

IF AN INFANT IS CHOKING

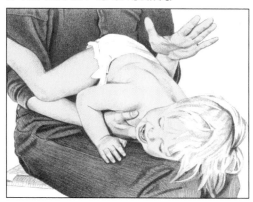

1 Lay the infant face down on your forearm, which you support on your thigh. With the heel of your other hand, give four rapid but light blows between the shoulder blades.

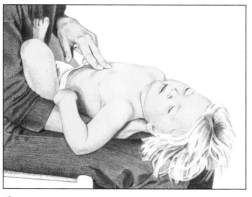

2 If back blows fail to dislodge the blockage, turn the infant on his back. Put two fingers on the breastbone, one finger's width below the level of the nipples, and depress the chest 1 to 1½ in. (2.5 to 4 cm). Press quickly four times.

lying down. In adults and older children this position is used only if the victim is unconscious.

• If the victim is one year old or less, however, place him face down on your forearm, which you rest on your thigh.

• While thus supporting the infant's head and body with one hand, slap him rapidly but lightly on the back between the shoulder blades with the heel of the other hand. Do this up to four times.

• If the blows fail to expel the object, turn the infant over on his back and, using only the index and middle finger of one hand, compress the chest rapidly four times. Use a point in the center of the chest, just below the nipples.

• Repeat this sequence of back blows and chest thrusts until the obstruction is dislodged.

• Be extremely careful when removing anything from a baby's mouth. Put your finger into his mouth only if you can actually see the object. Take care not to push it farther down the throat.

An unconscious victim

• Have someone call 911 or an ambulance as soon as a victim becomes unconscious.

• Place the victim on her back immediately and open her mouth.

• With your thumb on her tongue and your fingers under her chin, lift the victim's lower jaw with one hand while you perform a sweeping

ABDOMINAL THRUST ON AN UNCONSCIOUS ADULT

1 *Turn the victim face up, and perform a finger sweep of her mouth to remove any obstructions. Kneel astride her hips, and put the heel of one hand slightly above the navel and well below the bottom of the breastbone. Cover one hand with the other and, with your arms straight, give a quick upward thrust. Repeat up to 10 times.*

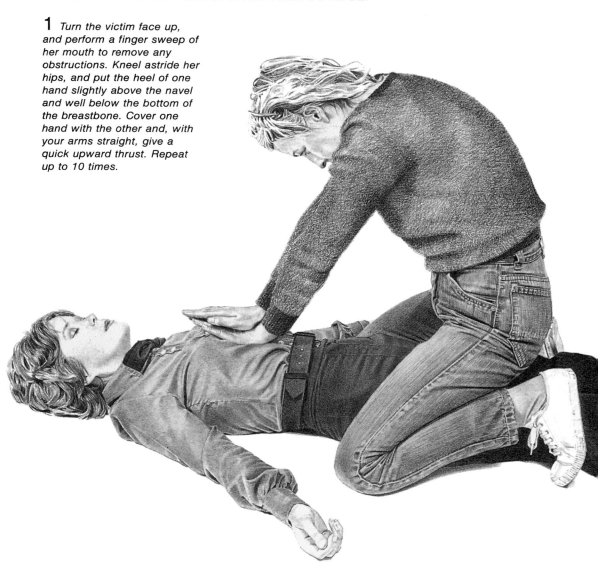

movement with the index finger of your other hand along her cheeks and deep into the throat. Try to hook and remove the obstruction. Use extreme care lest you push a foreign object deeper into the throat.

• If breathing is not restored, position the head for mouth-to-mouth respiration (see page 50).

• With the nose pinched shut, blow two full breaths into the victim's mouth, taking a breath of air yourself between ventilations.

• Watch for the rise and fall of the chest. Even a little air getting past the obstruction may be enough to keep the victim alive. If you succeed in inflating the lungs, continue mouth-to-mouth respiration until normal breathing resumes.

• If the lungs do not inflate with the first two breaths, prepare to continue the Heimlich maneuver. Kneel astride the victim and position the heel of one hand, fingers raised, just above the victim's navel, well below the breastbone. With arms straight and one hand on top of the other, fingers intertwined, give a quick inward-and-upward thrust. Repeat up to ten times.

• Check if the obstruction has been dislodged. If it has, hook it out with a finger.

• If not, try mouth-to-mouth respiration again. If the lungs do not expand after the first two breaths, repeat the sequence of thrusts, finger sweep, and mouth-to-mouth respiration. Continue as long as necessary.

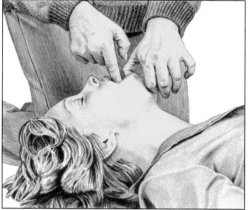

2 *With your finger, check the victim's mouth again and clear away any object that has been expelled by the abdominal thrusts. Once her breathing has returned to normal, put the victim into the recovery position (see page 136).*

TWO METHODS OF SELF-HELP

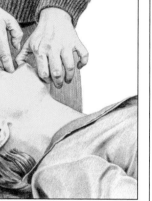

1 *Someone choking can perform abdominal thrusts on herself. Clench a fist and place it, thumb side against the stomach, slightly above the navel. With the other hand, jerk the fist firmly inward and upward.*

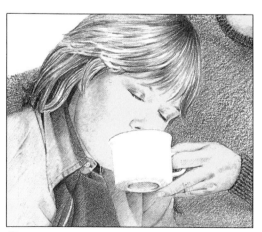

3 *Should it happen that the victim becomes fully conscious before the ambulance arrives, let her sit up, supporting her if necessary. If she wants something to drink, she could sip some water.*

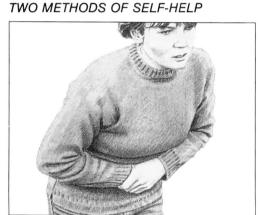

2 *Alternatively, lean over the back of a chair, supporting yourself by holding on to the sides with your hands. With the top sticking into you just above the navel, pull yourself downward and forward onto the back of the chair.*

Concussion

A blow to the head or a heavy fall onto the feet can shake and disturb the brain, causing concussion. There is usually a brief period of unconsciousness, but it may be so short that it goes unnoticed.

If the victim is unconscious for any length of time, his breathing may be shallow, his face pale and his skin cold and moist.

After the spell of unconsciousness – however brief – the victim may suffer from nausea and vomiting and may remember nothing about the incident.

Anyone suffering these symptoms should see a doctor for examination in case a more serious condition called compression should develop.

While a person is unconscious, treat as described on page 136.

If a person feels very weak after a blow to the head, treat for shock (see page 120).

Recognizing and treating compression

Any pressure on the brain – either from blood or fluid, or from a fracture of the skull – can cause the more serious condition of compression, which may develop up to 48 hours after the victim appears to have recovered from concussion.
• The victim's alertness and level of consciousness fall.
• There may be weakness or paralysis of one side of the body.
• Breathing may become noisy.
• The face may be flushed, and the victim's temperature high.
• The pulse may be slow.
• The pupils of the eyes (the dark parts) may be unequal in size.

Usually most of these symptoms occur, but the absence of any of them does not mean that compression is not present.

Telephone 911 and ask for an ambulance. If the victim is unconscious, treat as described on page 136.

Cramp

The sudden, involuntary spasm of muscles known as cramp causes acute pain, but it is usually dangerous only if a swimmer is affected (see *If you get into difficulties while swimming*, page 222). Cramp may be caused by chilling during or after exercise such as swimming, by poor muscular coordination during exercise, or by loss of salt through severe sweating, vomiting or diarrhea. It can also occur during sleep for no apparent reason.

The spasm is generally relieved by stretching the affected muscles. This can be done by the sufferer, but it is often easier if another person can help gently to force the limb straight.

Cramp in the hand
• Straighten your fingers, using gentle force if necessary.
• Spread your fingers and press down on the outstretched tips.
• Massage the affected muscles as you stretch them.

Cramp in the calf
• Straighten your leg and stand up.
• Press down on your heel and toes alternately. Lean forward slightly to stretch the calf muscles.
• Massage the muscles as you stretch them.

Cramp in the foot
• Stand on the ball of the foot so that your toes are forced up. Alternatively, sit down and pull

HELPING A CRAMP VICTIM
To relieve cramp in the calf, the foot or the thigh, lay the victim down, straighten the knee and toes, and press the foot firmly up toward the shin. Massage the affected muscles.

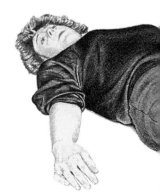

your toes up toward the shin with your hand.
• Massage the muscles as you stretch them.

Cramp in the thigh
• Sit on the floor and straighten the leg. Then bear down at the knee to stretch the thigh muscles. If there is someone to help, get him to raise your leg by the heel and press down on the knee with the other hand.
• Massage the muscles.

If cramp persists
Cramp caused by loss of salt from the body – through sweating, vomiting or diarrhea – can persist for some time. It is often felt as a gripping pain in the stomach.

To treat it, drink plenty of slightly salted water. Use about half a teaspoon of salt to two cups of water.

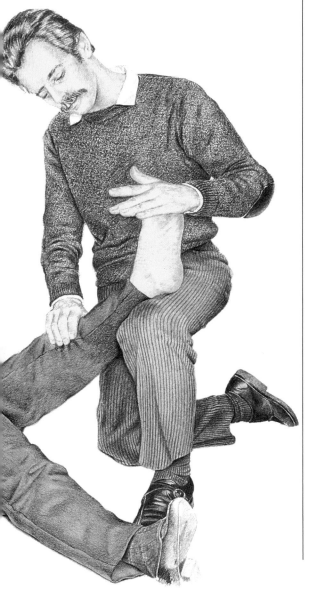

Crush injuries

Someone who has been trapped for more than a few minutes under a heavy weight, such as fallen masonry or a car, may suffer severe internal damage, even if there is little external sign of injury. Without treatment, the damage can lead to shock, kidney failure and death.

The warning signs
• Redness, swelling, bruising or blistering of the trapped part.
• Numbness or tingling.
• Continued swelling and hardening of the injured tissue.
• Shock – symptoms can include pallid clammy skin, dizziness, fainting, blurred vision, nausea, vomiting, thirst, anxiety and restlessness.

What you should do
• Treat severe injuries as far as possible while the victim is still trapped.
• Once he has been released, keep the victim on his back with his legs raised if possible.
• Do not let him move.
• If the victim is unconscious, place him in the recovery position (see page 136).
• Get medical attention as quickly as possible. Make sure that the doctor or ambulance attendant is told that there may be crush injuries. Tell him how long the crushing lasted.

Minor crushing – what to do
• If fingers, hand or foot are crushed for a short time only, hold the injured part under cold running water.
• Show the injured part to a doctor in case it is fractured.

First aid and medical emergencies

87

Crying baby

Normal babies generally cry only when they are hungry, angry, lonely, uncomfortable or in pain, and the crying will stop when you put right whatever is upsetting them.

It takes time for a new parent to learn what the different sorts of crying mean. The only way to find out is by discovering what stops it. There are some babies, however, who cry for no obvious reason.

What you should do
- Consult the chart and see if you can find a remedy.
- If you are feeling jumpy and nervous yourself, remember that this can affect the baby.
- Find some way to keep calm.
- Be sure to get enough rest. Perhaps you can persuade your partner to help out more than usual. Alternatively, get help from relatives,

ELEVEN REASONS WHY A BABY CRIES

Reason	Evidence
Hunger	Some hours since feed, or last feed not large enough.
Thirst	Hot weather. Baby feverish or sweating.
Passing urine	A sudden shriek.
Discomfort	Diaper rash, eczema, wet diaper, cold fingers and toes.
Colic	Restless, draws up legs, sudden cry, then relaxes. Passes a lot of wind.
Loneliness and boredom	Cries when he is alone, stops when you come in.
Habit	Usually cries at night. Stops when you come in.
Teething	May cause crying but less often than most people think.
Tiredness	Has missed a nap. A particular sort of moaning cry.
Personality	No other cause found.
Illness	Off feeds. Feverish. Signs of cold. Pulls at ear. Vomiting, diarrhea. Pain is suggested if crying is severe, fails to stop when baby is picked up and comforted, or is accompanied by pale skin or drawing up of legs.

Cuts

Minor cuts do not need medical help unless infection has set in or the wound was caused by a dirty or rusty object.

The amount of blood lost and the extent of the injury usually show whether the wound is serious, but puncture or stab wounds are deceptive because the surface damage may be small. Get medical help for a puncture wound after giving first aid (see *Stab wounds*, page 133).

When treating a minor cut, first stop the bleeding by pressing on the wound with a piece of clean cloth. Then clean the skin around it with gauze or cotton swabs and lukewarm water with soap or a mild antiseptic. Wipe outward and away from the cut and make sure the water you are using does not run into it. Use each swab once and then change to a fresh one.

If the bleeding is severe, see page 60.

HOW TO TREAT A CUT

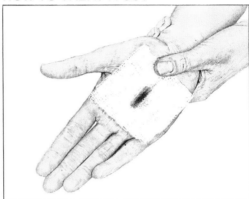

1 *Press a clean piece of cloth on the cut, or around the edges if a foreign body is present. When bleeding stops, take the pad away and remove any foreign bodies that come out easily.*

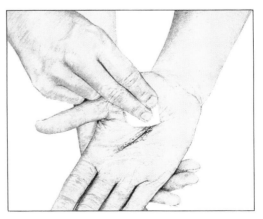

2 *Gently wipe the wound outward with a swab soaked in warm, soapy water. Renew the swabs frequently. Dry around the wound with a new swab. Apply an adhesive bandage.*

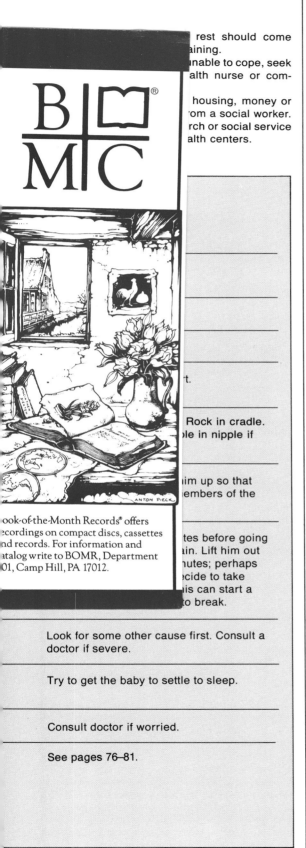

Diabetic coma

A diabetic who appears to be drunk may be suffering from low blood sugar, a condition known as hypoglycemia. It is brought on by taking too much insulin or eating too little food. It can also occur after exercise has burned up the sugar in the blood.

Low blood sugar affects the brain and leads to coma. Death could possibly follow in as little as 20 minutes.

The condition can be distinguished from drunkenness by the person's breath, which will have no smell of alcohol.

Low blood sugar can lead to rapid deterioration in the diabetic, with the following symptoms:
• Pale appearance, with sweating, rapid pulse, shallow breathing and possibly trembling.
• Confused state, sometimes resembling drunkenness.
• Faintness, leading to unconsciousness in 15 to 20 minutes.

What you can do

If a diabetic collapse comes on quickly, you can assume that the patient needs sugar. If he is conscious, give him three or four teaspoons of sugar, some cake or cookies, honey, jam, chocolate, or a sweet soft drink.
• If the patient is unconscious, put him in the recovery position (see page 136), then call 911 and ask for an ambulance.

The opposite condition of too much sugar in the blood (hyperglycemia) can also eventually lead to coma, but it comes on much more slowly, and the diabetic will usually become aware of it and treat himself by taking insulin. If he does not take insulin, the symptoms will be:
• Flushed appearance with dry skin.
• Deep, sighing breathing, with the breath having the fruity smell of acetone.
• Eventually unconsciousness.

If the person becomes unconscious, put him in the recovery position (see page 136) and get immediate medical attention. If he is conscious, tell him to take some insulin at once.

What the patient can do

A person who is subject to hypoglycemic attacks should carry a card or wear a bracelet giving his condition and emergency instructions. This can avoid the danger of being mistaken for being drunk when, in fact, all he really needs is some sugar.

A diabetic on insulin should avoid driving or using dangerous machinery unless he has had some food in the previous two hours. Consequently, regular mealtimes are important.

Dislocated joints

A bone that is wrenched out of place at a joint is said to be dislocated. The injury is usually accompanied by torn ligaments (a sprain) and sometimes by a fracture.

The symptoms may include severe pain, swelling and bruising, deformity of the joint and difficulty in moving the joint. Never try to push a dislocated bone back into place, but treat it as though it were broken.

In a case of dislocation, always assume there might be a fracture as well – the symptoms are similar (see page 98).

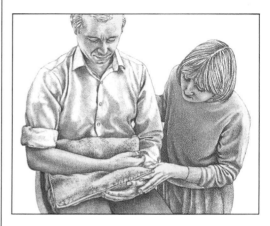

TREATING A DISLOCATION
Put the victim into the most comfortable position possible, and support the dislocated joint with pillows or a rolled blanket. Call 911 and ask for an ambulance. If the dislocation is in the arm, you may be able to support it with an arm sling (see page 121).

Drowning

Death by drowning happens because, as the victim struggles for breath, water enters the airway. The water causes a spasm of the epiglottis, a cartilage flap at the back of the tongue, and this spasm blocks the air supply. Quick action can still save a victim's life.

In North America each year, there are nearly 7,000 deaths from drowning. In most cases, the victim did not know how to swim and did not intend to go into the water. Some unexpected occurrence – a boat capsizing, a fall from a dock – is responsible for his plight. Indeed most drownings occur within 15 ft. (5 m) of a boat, a dock or the shore. Eighty-five percent of the victims are male.

Assume that anyone you see in the water fully clothed is a potential victim, and be ready to help. A swimmer who develops cramp or becomes exhausted is less easy to recognize. If he is having breathing problems, he may be unable to draw attention by shouting.

Warning signs
• As he gets more tired, the victim's body tends to sink until it is vertical and only his head shows above the water.
• The victim's strokes become erratic and his movement through the water appears jerky or simply stops.
• The victim's face – particularly the lips and ears – may turn a bluish-purple color.

Rescuing a drowning person
For methods of getting a drowning person out of the water in a variety of different situations, see pages 221 and 228.

REVIVING A DROWNING PERSON

1 *If the drowning person has stopped breathing, start mouth-to-mouth resuscitation as quickly as possible (see page 50). Begin while still in the water if necessary – as soon as you can stand up or sooner if you are a strong swimmer. Remove any debris from the mouth with your index finger, tilt the head back and begin breathing into the mouth. Either press your cheek against the victim's nose to stop air escaping, or pinch the nose between finger and thumb. Move toward land between breaths. Once out of the water, continue artificial respiration, or begin if it is not already under way.*

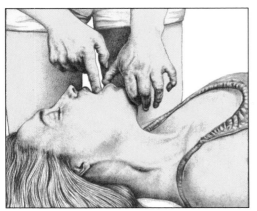

2 *Victims of drowning sometimes swallow water, which is brought up with food during artificial respiration. Turn the head to one side and regularly clear the mouth of any debris.*

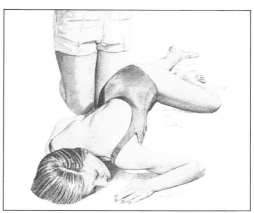

3 *Once breathing has re-started, turn the victim into the recovery position (see page 136). Cover her and treat any injuries. Get medical help as soon as possible.*

Drug overdose

Anyone who has taken a drug overdose will likely need immediate medical attention. This applies to an overdose of a prescribed medicine as much as an addictive drug such as heroin.

A drug overdose is likely to cause a stronger than normal reaction in a person who suffers from asthma, kidney disease or hypersensitivity to certain medicines.

Your poison control center will tell you what to do while waiting for medical help to arrive. Before calling the center, gather any information you can about the drug by talking to the victim, collecting pill bottles or taking samples of vomit.

Generally, do not try to induce vomiting. Inducing vomiting is worth doing only if you know that the overdose has been caused by barbiturates or tranquilizers. For details of how to treat overdoses of either of these drugs, see *Barbiturates*, page 336.

Do not try to keep the victim awake by giving him black coffee or walking him about. Physical activity will only speed up the absorption of the drug into the body.

How to recognize an overdose
Symptoms depend on the size of the overdose and the type of drug, but they can include any of the following:
• Vomiting.
• Difficulty in breathing.
• Unconsciousness.
• Sweating.
• Hallucinations.
• Dilation or contraction of the pupils of the eyes (the dark parts).

What you should do
• Ask the victim what has happened. Obtain any information about the drug as soon as possible, because the victim may become unconscious at any time.
• If the victim is unconscious, put him in the recovery position (see page 136).
• Call 911 and ask for an ambulance.
• Collect a sample of vomit and any bottle, pill container, hypodermic syringe or glue container that is near the victim. Send them to hospital with him as evidence to assist treatment.

Alcohol poisoning
If a person collapses unconscious after drinking a large amount of alcohol, put him in the recovery position so that he does not choke on his vomit (see page 136).

Then telephone 911 and ask for an ambulance (see also *Spotting and coping with alcoholism*, page 328).

Ear injuries

Damage to the middle or inner ear can be caused by injuries to the head, loud noise, explosions, or probing in the ear – to remove a foreign body, for example.

The most serious injury to the ear itself is a perforated eardrum, but bleeding from the ear or discharge of watery, straw-colored fluid can be a sign of a fractured skull (see page 102).

Symptoms of ear injury
• Severe earache.
• Dizziness and loss of balance.
• Deafness in one ear following an injury.
• Headache.
• Possible unconsciousness.
• Discharge of blood or watery fluid.

What you can do
• If the victim is conscious, stop him from hitting the side of his head to try to restore hearing; this will only make the damage worse.
• Sit the victim up with his head tilted over on the injured side so that blood or fluid can drain out.
• Cover the injured ear with a piece of clean cotton or gauze as protection. Bandage it lightly in place. Get medical attention.
• Do not attempt to plug the ear. This can cause a buildup of pressure in the middle ear.
• If the victim is unconscious but breathing, place him in the recovery position with the injured ear downward and a clean pad underneath (see page 136). Get medical attention.
• If the victim's breathing stops, begin artificial respiration (see page 50).

Foreign body in the ear
Children often push objects into their ears. This usually causes no more than temporary deafness, but if the object is pushed hard and deep into the ear, the eardrum may be perforated. The symptoms are variable.
• There may be no symptoms at all, just the knowledge that something is in the ear.
• Discharge from the ear.
• Pain or buzzing in the ear.
• Deafness on the affected side.
Do not attempt to remove a foreign body. If there are no symptoms, get medical attention in 24 hours. Go sooner if there are symptoms.

Insects in the ear
If an insect crawls or flies into a child's ear, its buzzing can sound frighteningly loud.
• Calm and comfort the child.
• Stop him from putting a finger in the ear. If the insect has a sting, this may provoke an attack.
• Hold his head still with the ear angled toward the ground. The insect may crawl out.
• If, after a minute or two, it has not come out, gently flood the ear with tepid water.
• If all attempts fail, or if it stings while inside, get medical help.

Electric shock

Electricity can kill or produce a wide range of injuries, including severe burns and asphyxiation. The extent of the injuries it will cause depends on three main factors: the strength of the charge; how long the victim was exposed to it; and how well he was insulated – by wearing rubber-soled shoes, say, or standing on a dry wooden floor.

• Never touch the victim of an electrical accident until you are certain you are not risking a shock yourself. If the victim is still touching the source of the electricity – such as an electric drill that has "shorted-out" – cut off the power first. Unplug the appliance or turn off the power at the main fuse box.

• If you cannot turn off the electricity, and the victim is still in contact with it, move him away using a piece of wood, such as a broom handle, or fabric, such as a towel. Neither wood nor fabric conducts electricity. Use a broom handle to lever the victim from the spot or loop a dry towel around an arm or leg and pull him.

• Because water is an excellent conductor of electricity, use only dry wood or cloth.

High-voltage electricity

Electricity from high-voltage sources, such as power lines and some industrial equipment, can give a fatal shock up to 20 ft. (6 m) away. Where railway, subway or streetcar systems are concerned, 10 ft. (3 m) away is considered a safe distance.

When confronted with any emergency involving high-voltage electricity, call 911 and ask for help. Stay clear until you can get an expert to cut off the power.

When lightning strikes

Another form of high-voltage electricity is lightning, which can do anything from merely stunning the victim to killing him (see *If you are caught in a lightning storm*, page 278).

HOW TO RESCUE A VICTIM OF ELECTRIC SHOCK

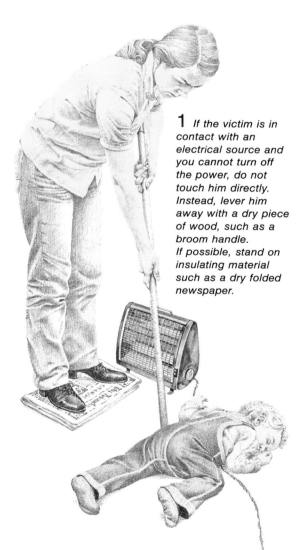

1 *If the victim is in contact with an electrical source and you cannot turn off the power, do not touch him directly. Instead, lever him away with a dry piece of wood, such as a broom handle.*
If possible, stand on insulating material such as a dry folded newspaper.

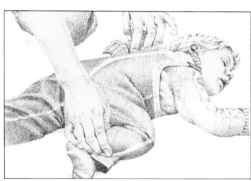

2 *If the victim is unconscious and not breathing, give artificial respiration. If he is breathing, put him in the recovery position (see page 136). In either case, call 911 for help.*

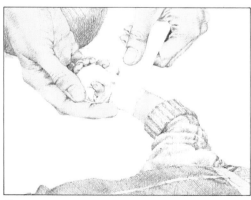

3 *Treat burns by cooling them with cold water. Then cover them with a dressing, such as the inside of a folded handkerchief, and secure it with a piece of clean cloth (see page 66).*

Epileptic seizure

A major epileptic seizure, also called *grand mal*, involves unconsciousness, convulsions and noisy breathing. Sufferers from epilepsy often wear a bracelet which identifies their illness, and a card with emergency telephone numbers.

A series of seizures, without the victim regaining consciousness in between, is called *status epilepticus*, and is a serious condition which requires hospital treatment.

A minor epileptic seizure, also called *petit mal*, usually involves only momentary inattention or confusion without loss of consciousness. Make sure that the sufferer is not in danger (from traffic, for example) and stay with him until he is once more quite alert.

The warning signs
• A sufferer from major epilepsy sometimes experiences a few seconds' warning of an attack. The warning may involve seeing flashing lights, or a sensation of noise, taste or smell.
• Loss of consciousness occurs.
• The limbs and neck stiffen for a few seconds; then the whole body is overcome by rhythmic and often violent twitching.
• The victim may bite his tongue, froth at the mouth or urinate involuntarily.
• Finally the muscles will relax and the victim may remain unconscious for some minutes.
• When consciousness returns, the victim may be drowsy and confused for as much as an hour.

What you can do
• Do not try to restrain a victim of a major epileptic attack. Try only to stop him from hurting himself.
• If he is about to fall, catch him and lay him gently on the ground, or cushion his fall.
• Clear a space around him. Remove furniture and other objects that he may bump into.
• If possible, loosen clothing around the neck and place something soft under the head.
• Do not put anything in the mouth or try to force it open.
• When convulsions end, place the victim in the recovery position (see page 136), and wait for him to regain consciousness. Do not leave him alone until he is fully recovered.
• Do not give him anything to drink until you are sure that he is quite alert.
• Call an ambulance if someone has seizures for the first time; if he has a series of seizures without regaining consciousness in between; if he injures himself; or if he takes longer than 15 minutes to regain consciousness.

Eye injuries

The most common injury to the eye is a small object, such as an eyelash or a piece of grit, lodged in it. Other injuries can be caused by corrosive chemicals or sharp objects, such as flying fragments of glass or metal.

Injury can also occur if contact lenses get displaced or stuck to the eyeball. If you have any difficulty with a contact lens, get medical help rather than risk hurting the eye.

Foreign body in the eye
If a person has something in his eye, tell him not to rub it. Turn the victim's face up to the light. With your thumb and forefinger, push the eyelids away from the eyeball. Ask the victim to look left, right, up and down while you look for the object.

REMOVING GRIT FROM THE EYE

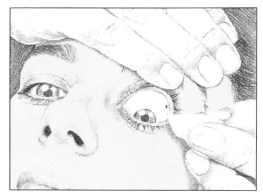

1 *Tilt the head back, and gently raise the eyelid with your finger (or draw down the bottom eyelid). Lift off the piece of grit or eyelash with the corner of a clean handkerchief.*

TREATING CHEMICAL BURNS

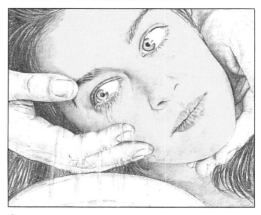

1 *Tilt the victim's head, injured eye downward. Flood the open eye with gently running water from a faucet or jug for at least 20 minutes. Or splash water onto it from a basin.*

Do not attempt to remove anything if it is on the pupil or iris (the black or colored parts of the eye), or if it is sticking firmly to the eye. Leave the object and cover the eye with a clean, non-fluffy pad, such as the inside of a clean, folded handkerchief. Bandage it loosely in place and get medical help.

If you can see the object, try to wash it out. Tilt the victim's head to the injured side, and gently run cold or lukewarm water over the eye from a faucet or jug. Alternatively, get the victim to blink his eyes underwater.

If no water is available, or flushing is not effective, try to lift the object off the eye with a moistened piece of clean gauze or the corner of a clean handkerchief.

If you are still unsuccessful, see a doctor.

Chemical burns to the eye

• If chemicals — either liquid or solid — get into the eye, flood the eye with water immediately and continuously for 20 minutes.

You may need to force the eyelids open if they are shut tight in a spasm of pain.

Object impaled in the eye

Do not attempt to remove any object which is embedded in the eye, because you might cause irreparable damage. First, protect the eye, taking great care not to touch it or apply any pressure, by covering it with a paper or plastic cup. Then put a bandage over both eyes so that the victim is not tempted to move them.

Call 911 and ask for an ambulance. Reassure the person while you wait for it.

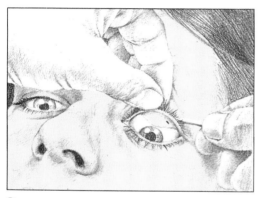

2 *If the grit is on the underside of the eyelid, press down the lid with a matchstick and pull up the lid against the matchstick with your finger and thumb.*

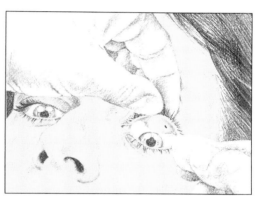

3 *Remove the grit with the corner of a clean handkerchief. Replace the lid by pulling down gently on the lashes. The same treatment can be used for the bottom lid.*

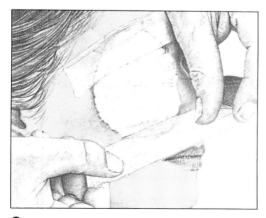

2 *When you have thoroughly flushed the chemical from the eye, dry the face and put a clean dressing lightly over the eye. Get the victim to hospital as soon as possible.*

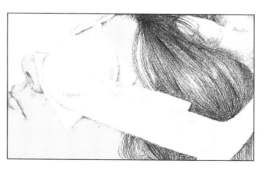

*DEALING WITH AN IMPALED OBJECT
Do not try to remove any embedded or impaled object from the eye. Instead, cut a hole in a piece of clean cloth and put it over the eye. Place a paper or plastic cup or a ring-pad (see page 58) over the cloth and hold it in place with a bandage. Cover the uninjured eye with the bandage as well. Call an ambulance.*

Fainting

If the blood supply to the brain is suddenly and temporarily reduced, a person may faint. Fainting is usually the result of the victim being in a hot, stuffy atmosphere.

But an emotional stimulus, such as an unpleasant sight, a fright or bad news, can also cause fainting. So can a drop in blood sugar due to missed meals or dieting, or standing still for long periods of time.

Sometimes there may be a more serious cause such as illness or injury, in which case a doctor should be consulted.

Someone who is standing still for a long time can reduce the risk of fainting by rocking gently from the heels to the balls of the feet.

The warning signs
• A person who is about to faint becomes pale or greenish-white. He may yawn frequently, showing that he is lacking oxygen.
• The skin is cold and clammy. Beads of sweat appear on the face, neck and hands.

What you can do
If someone says he is about to faint, tell him to sit down. Loosen tight clothing at the neck and waist, and put his head down to his knees.

If someone actually faints, first make sure he is breathing. Then raise his feet above the level of the head to increase the blood circulation to the brain.

Recovery from a faint is usually rapid and complete, but check for any injury that may have been received during a fall. If the fall resulted in a blow to the head that was hard enough to

cause a cut or wound, the victim should see a doctor, because there is risk of a fractured skull or concussion (see page 86).

Do not give the victim anything to eat or drink until full consciousness returns, and then only sips of cold water. Do not give the victim any alcohol, such as brandy. It lowers the rate of the body's vital activities, and may make the condition worse.

If you are in any doubt about the victim's condition, get medical advice.

TREATING SOMEONE WHO FAINTS
Lay an unconscious victim on her back with her legs raised above the level of her head. Hold the legs up, or prop them on a chair or anything suitable. Loosen clothing at the neck, chest and waist, and ensure that the victim gets plenty of fresh air. If she is indoors, open the windows; outside, protect her from the sun. She should recover after a few minutes, but tell her to stay seated for a few minutes more.

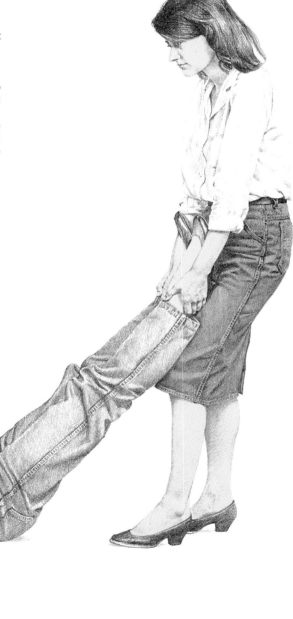

Flu

Epidemics of influenza (commonly called flu) occur during most winters. The illness is a virus infection, which spreads rapidly through an area for two or three weeks and then quickly subsides.

Flu leads to high temperature and aching muscles, and can be an emergency if it strikes a person with heart disease, chronic lung disease or diabetes, or someone over 65. The doctor should be consulted about a patient in any of these categories.

The warning signs
- Headache.
- Aching muscles and back.
- High temperature with the sensation of feeling cold.
- Sweating.
- General weakness.
- Coughing, and pain behind the breastbone which is made worse by coughing.
- Runny nose and sneezing.

What you can do
- Put the patient to bed.
- Give extra fluids to replace losses caused by fever.
- Give aspirin to an adult, acetaminophen to children and teenagers. In both instances, follow the recommended dosage.
- To help ease coughing and chest pain, give hot lemon-and-honey drinks or a cough medicine.
- Do not allow the patient to return to work or school until the main symptoms are over – usually in about three days. Otherwise, it will increase the risk of pneumonia, and will spread the flu to others.

How long will it last?
The worst of the illness will be over in two or three days, but aching muscles, headache and fever may persist for a week.

General weakness may continue for a few weeks more, possibly accompanied by a period of depression.

Preventing an attack of flu
Each year a vaccine is produced against the viruses that are expected to cause flu in the following winter. Anyone over 65, and sufferers from heart disease, lung disease or diabetes, should be immunized in September or October. But if an epidemic is caused by a new strain of virus, immunization may not be effective.

Food poisoning

Severe vomiting and diarrhea, usually with pain in the abdomen, are the main symptoms of food poisoning, a form of gastroenteritis.

Two main types of bacteria cause the ailment. Staphylococcal bacteria multiply in reheated or half-cooked food and produce severe vomiting. This occurs two to eight hours after the food is eaten, and rarely lasts 24 hours.

Salmonella bacteria usually come from food handlers (the bacteria are present on the hands of half the population), flies or unhygienic cooking utensils. The bacteria multiply in the victim's bowel, and the symptoms begin with severe diarrhea after 12 to 36 hours.

What you should do
- Give the patient sips of water. Do not give food or milk drinks. The stomach is trying to get rid of an irritant; do not irritate it any more. Let it rest.
- An antidiarrheal medicine may be given to an adult.
- After the stomach has begun to settle for a few hours, give the patient toast, crackers, jelly or clear soup. Avoid tea or coffee, or acid drinks such as lemon or orange; they may cause irritation, and vomiting could recur.
- Most attacks of food poisoning settle after two or three days, and the patient can be put back on a fuller, nonirritating diet.
- Call the doctor if there is abdominal pain, blood in the feces, other unexpected symptoms, or if the symptoms are severe and last longer than three days.

Botulism
Hospitalization is essential for botulism, a serious but rare food poisoning produced by the bacterium *Clostridium botulinum*. The organism grows slowly in low-acid foods, such as improperly processed home preserves and canned foods that have spoiled.

Symptoms include abdominal pain, vomiting, blurred vision, muscle weakness and eventual paralysis. Treatment is by antitoxin injections.

How to avoid food poisoning
- Avoid any creamy foods, processed meat or fish which have been left for any length of time at room temperature. Just how long they can be safely left depends on the air temperature, but a good rule of thumb is to keep all such foods in the refrigerator except when required for food preparation or serving.
- Avoid food which you suspect has been unhygienically prepared. This is especially important in hot climates.
- When heating up cold meat, make sure that it is thoroughly re-cooked.
- Discard any containers of food whose contents show signs of spoiling.

First aid and medical emergencies

97

Fractures

A fracture is a cracked or broken bone. It can be caused by direct force, as when a car hits a person on the thigh, or by indirect force, as when a person falls on an outstretched hand and breaks the collarbone at the top of the arm.

There are three main types of fracture. A closed fracture leaves the skin unbroken, although it may be heavily bruised. An open, or compound, fracture either has a bone protruding through the skin or a deep gash leading down to the bone. In either case germs may enter the wound, causing serious infection. A greenstick fracture, most common in children, involves a bone splitting as it bends.

The warning signs

Often, the victim will have heard or felt the bone break. There may be the feeling of broken bone ends grating together, which can sometimes be heard.

The victim may not be able to use the injured part of the body, and will feel pain when he attempts to do so.

The area around the break may be tender to the touch, swollen or bruised.

A limb may be in an unnatural position or deformed when compared to the uninjured side.

What you should do

All doubtful cases of injured bones should be considered as fractures. The principles of treatment are the same in all cases.

TREATING AN OPEN FRACTURE OF THE LEG

1 *If the ambulance is going to take more than half an hour, or if you have to carry the victim, you must protect the wound and immobilize the leg. First gently remove clothing from the area of the fracture.*

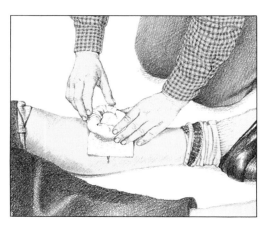

2 *Cover the wound with a piece of clean non-fluffy cloth (not cotton wool). Then put a ring-pad (see page 58) or two crescent-shaped pads of material around the protruding bone.*

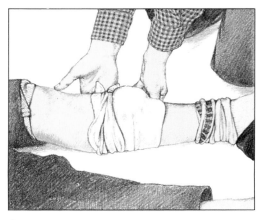

3 *Put a bandage around the leg, over the ring-pad. Try to get a helper to support the leg carefully as you do so. The pad will reduce pressure on the wound.*

- Do not move the victim unless it is absolutely necessary.
- Call 911 and ask for an ambulance.
- Deal with any severe bleeding (see page 60), unconsciousness (see page 136) or difficulty in breathing (see page 50) before doing anything to the fracture.
- Put the victim in the most comfortable position possible, and provide support for the injured limb with a rolled-up blanket or coat, or with cushions.
- Do not move the fractured part unnecessarily.
- To limit the dangers of shock, see page 120.
- If it is essential to move the victim – and time allows – immobilize the injured limb by bandaging it to an uninjured part of the body.

Supporting a fractured leg
Tie a fractured leg to the other leg (see page 128), using scarves, neckties or any other piece of material, preferably something that is at least as wide as a tie. This will support the leg until an ambulance arrives. If you need to improvise a stretcher, see page 115.

If a knee is broken, it will be extremely painful and may be bent in an unnatural way. Do not try to force it straight. Lay the victim down with the leg in the most comfortable position.

Then put a cushion or folded jacket under the knee, and other soft supports such as rolled-up coats or rugs around the leg for further support. Call an ambulance.

Treating a broken arm
Support a broken arm in an arm sling (see page 121). Secure the arm to the chest by tying a broad bandage around the body, passing over the arm. Then take the victim to hospital.

Never use force to bend a broken arm. If it will not bend, strap it to the body (see page 127) and wait for an ambulance.

Frostbite

In freezing weather, exposed parts of the body, such as the nose, ears, cheeks and chin, may develop frostbite as the skin cools and the blood vessels become constricted, cutting off the blood supply. The hands and feet can also become frostbitten, even when they are enclosed in gloves and boots. In severe cases, gangrene may develop unless the affected part is warmed up and the circulation restored.

The warning signs
- The affected part of the body feels cold and stiff, with a prickling pain.
- The skin becomes hard, and turns blue or white. The area becomes numb, and the feeling of cold and pain disappears.

What you should do
- If possible, get the victim into shelter.
- Remove clothing from the frostbitten area; take off rings and watch from an affected hand.
- Warm the area with skin-to-skin contact. The victim can put a frostbitten foot into your armpit, for instance. Cover ears, nose or cheeks with warm hands. You can also immerse the frozen part in tepid water.
- Do not warm the area with dry or radiant heat. Slow thawing is essential.
- Do not rub or massage the frostbitten area.
- When warmth returns, wrap a frostbitten foot or hand in a towel or other cloth, and then cover that with a blanket or sleeping bag.
- To relieve the inevitable swelling and pain, raise the affected area above the level of the victim's chest.
- As the area thaws, it may become blue and develop blood-filled blisters. Do not break the blisters or apply any medication.
- Call 911 and ask for an ambulance, or get the victim to the emergency department of the nearest hospital.

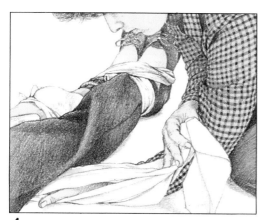

4 *Immobilize the leg by tying the two legs together with bandages, putting padding between the ankles and knees. Tie below, then above the fracture – but not on it.*

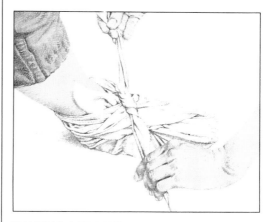

THAWING A FROSTBITTEN FOOT
When feeling begins to return, wrap the foot in a triangular bandage, towel or sweater, then cover it again with a sleeping bag or jacket.

Gas poisoning

Natural gas is not toxic. But many other things are, including ammonia, used in refrigeration plants and as an agricultural fertilizer; the fumes from burning polyurethane foam, sometimes found in mattresses and upholstered furniture; and carbon monoxide from car exhaust. The signs of poisoning:
• The victim may suffer from unsound judgment and may be difficult and uncooperative.
• The victim may be confused, stupefied or unconscious.

What you should do

With ammonia, which has a particularly strong smell, poisoning mostly occurs when people are trapped in an enclosed area. Ventilation will be a slow process. Meantime, do not enter the affected area without a face mask.

The fire department should handle burning polyurethane foam. Be aware that fumes from this substance can kill in minutes. If you suspect that a car or garage is filled with carbon monoxide, open the doors and ventilate the area thoroughly. Then get the victim into the open air.

If possible, before attempting a rescue, tell someone else to call expert help.

RESCUING AN UNCONSCIOUS VICTIM

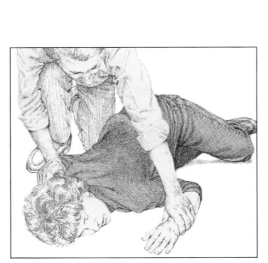

1 *Once a carbon monoxide-filled area has been ventilated, take a few deep breaths of clean air, then drag the victim into the open air. Pass your arms under her armpits and link them across the chest. Use the same technique but wear a face mask in an ammonia-filled area.*

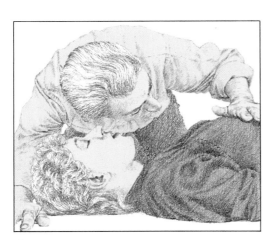

2 *Tilt the victim's head back to open the airway. Listen for breathing, feel any exhaled air, and watch the chest. If she is not breathing, give artificial respiration (see page 50).*

3 *Once she is breathing normally again, turn her into the recovery position (see page 136). Call an ambulance. Continue to check her breathing until help arrives.*

German measles

The main danger of German measles, known medically as rubella, is that it may affect an unborn child if contracted by a woman in early pregnancy. About 25 percent of babies whose mothers get German measles in the first 16 weeks of pregnancy are born deaf or blind – sometimes with heart disease as well – or are stillborn. The risk is as high as 60 percent in very early pregnancy.

The disease, which is otherwise not serious, is spread by contact with someone who has already been infected.

The warning signs
• The patient may feel unwell for a few days without any obvious symptoms.
• A rash of tiny pink, slightly raised spots then appears behind the ears or on the face, spreading downward to the rest of the body.
• The glands become swollen, particularly behind the ears. The joints may swell and become painful, sometimes severely so, especially in young women.

Duration of the disease
The patient is infectious to others from five days before and until four days after the rash appears. The rash lasts from one to five days, but the joint pains may last for up to 14 days.

What you should do
A patient with German measles should be kept away from pregnant women, and should stay indoors for four days from the onset of the rash. If necessary, acetaminophen can be given to ease the discomfort.

You should consult your doctor if the joint pains become severe or if the patient develops a high temperature, a severe and persistent headache or becomes drowsy.

A woman who is in contact with German measles in early pregnancy, and does not know if she is immune, should also see her doctor. Blood tests will confirm whether she has been infected. If so, the doctor may ask the patient if she wishes to terminate her pregnancy, rather than risk having a child with deformities.

Developing immunity
German measles is very serious in pregnant women, so children should be immunized against it and thus help eradicate the disease. The vaccine is usually given at 15 months but girls who did not receive it, and who have not had the disease, should be immunized at about 12 years.

Women of childbearing age who have not already had German measles, and who may wish to become pregnant, should be immunized. Pregnancy should be avoided for at least two months after the injection, as immunization might affect the unborn child during this period. Older women who do not know if they have had the disease can have a blood test.

Grazes

Minor grazes of the sort usually suffered by children rarely need medical attention. But if dirt or grit is embedded in the wound, there is a risk of infection, and the victim should see a doctor.

What you should do
• Wash your hands before treating the wound.
• Clean the area around the graze with a clean gauze or cotton swab which has been dipped in lukewarm soapy water.
• Wipe outward, away from the wound.
• Carefully remove any loose dirt or gravel, either by washing or with tweezers.
• Dry the area with a clean swab.
• Cover a small graze with an adhesive bandage and a large graze with a sterile dressing. If you do not have a sterile dressing, dress the wound with a clean, folded handkerchief turned inside out so that the untouched side is on the wound. Fix it in place with a bandage or tape.
• Do not cough on the injury or on the dressing. You could introduce infection.
• Do not dress the wound with cotton wool, because the fibers will stick to it.
• See a doctor straightaway if the wound is very dirty or if it was caused by a rusty object. The victim may need a tetanus injection or a course of antibiotics.
• If pus starts to ooze from the wound later, or the wound becomes sore and inflamed, see a doctor about it.

First aid and medical emergencies

Gunshot wounds

Handguns, shotguns and rifles are often the cause of accidental wounds. In fact every day a child somewhere in the United States dies from an accidental handgun blast. But even air guns are potentially dangerous.

In all types of gunshot accidents the bullet or shotgun pellet may leave two wounds – one at the point of entry into the body and another, larger one, at the point of exit.

When treating a gunshot wound, check both the point of entry and the other side of the victim's body for an exit wound. The victim may be aware only of the entry wound. If there is no exit wound, the pellet has either deflected off the body, leaving a wound similar in appearance to an entry wound, or it is lodged inside.

A bullet will cause a great deal of tissue damage, and it may hit and splinter a bone. All gunshot wounds require expert medical attention immediately.

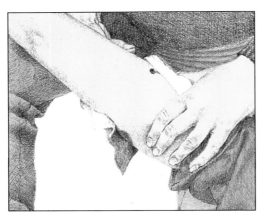

FIRST AID FOR A BULLET WOUND
Cover the wound with a clean pad or your bare hands to stop the bleeding. If there are entry and exit wounds, cover both. Once the bleeding has slowed, dress and bandage the wound (see page 56) and get medical help.

Head and face injuries

Any head injury which is severe enough to cause bleeding or a bruise could also fracture the skull or cause concussion (see page 86). So anyone who has suffered a head injury should be taken to a doctor or to the emergency department of a hospital for examination – even if, superficially, the injury does not appear to be serious.

Head injuries are common in road accidents, but they are also caused by falls – off a ladder or down a flight of stairs, for example. Old people are particularly prone to falls.

Sports such as cycling, hockey and baseball are also a source of head injuries. Cyclists often

HOW TO BANDAGE A SCALP INJURY

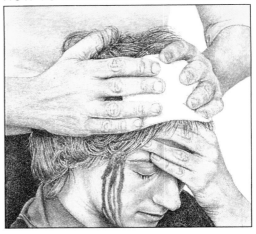

1 *Gently feel the skull around the wound. If part of it seems to move, suspect a fracture and do not press on it. Otherwise, press a clean pad on the wound to stop the bleeding.*

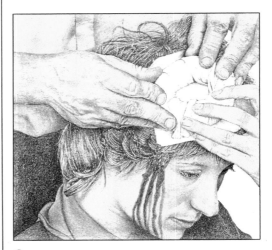

2 *Put a fresh cloth pad over the first. If you suspect a fracture, or if something is embedded, put the dressing on lightly, with a ring-pad to lessen pressure (see page 58).*

sustain head wounds in accidents, and team sport players can be hit on the head by balls, pucks and hockey sticks. Golfers, too, can be at risk.

Brain damage can occur without any obvious sign, except perhaps for brief unconsciousness. In elderly people, particularly, any slight knock to the head may cause internal bleeding.

The warning signs
If you suspect that someone may have suffered a blow to the head, look for any or all of the following symptoms:
• The eye pupils (the black parts) may be unequal in size, and the victim may have double vision and noisy breathing.
• Cuts, bruises and swellings on the scalp, face or jaw.
• Headache.
• Confusion or drowsiness, which may be followed by unconsciousness.
• Loss of memory of events before or at the time of the accident.
• Weak pulse and shallow breathing.

Bleeding scalp and face injuries
An injury to the scalp may bleed profusely because the scalp has a rich supply of blood.

First aid and medical emergencies

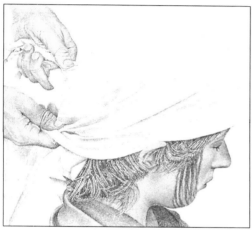

3 *Secure the dressing with a triangular bandage. Put the long edge across the forehead and the point at the neck. Bring the two ends around to the neck and cross them.*

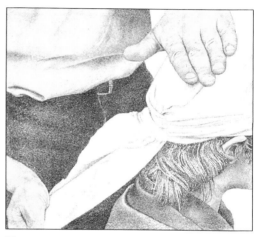

5 *Gently place one hand on the bandage to stop it slipping. With the other, draw the point downward, parallel with the back of the neck, so that the bandage is snugly over the scalp.*

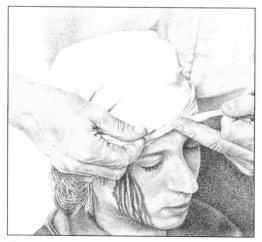

4 *Bring the two ends around to the forehead and tie them together, securing the bandage. Keep the victim's head as steady as possible while you put the bandage on.*

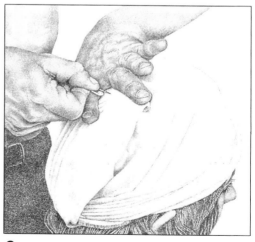

6 *Bring the point of the bandage up to the crown and fix it lightly in place with a safety pin or adhesive tape. Alternatively, tuck the point into the edge of the bandage at the front.*

Because the skin is stretched tight over the head, the wound may also gape open and look much more serious than it really is.

However, there is always the danger of a fracture to the skull, and the victim should be examined by his doctor or at the emergency department of a hospital. In the meantime, control the bleeding by holding your hand or a cloth pad, such as the inside of a clean, folded handkerchief, on the wound.

A wound on the face will also bleed profusely, and may look much worse than it really is. But if it is deep, take the victim to hospital because the wound may need to be stitched. If the wound followed a blow to the head, also get medical treatment at once.

A broken jaw

A person who has suffered a broken jaw will often have a wound inside the mouth. The victim may have difficulty in speaking and there may be an excessive flow of saliva, often tinged with blood, and broken teeth. Usually only one side of the jaw will be broken.

Put a bandage under the victim's chin and tie it in place on top of the head to support the jaw while you get the victim to hospital. Do not tie the bandage too tightly.

TREATING A BLEEDING FACE

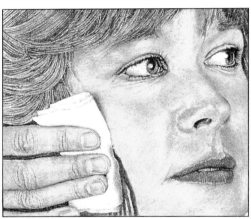

1 *A cut face may produce such severe bleeding that the wound may look worse than it really is. Press the inside of a clean, folded handkerchief, or a pad of tissues, against the wound. Do not use cotton wool.*

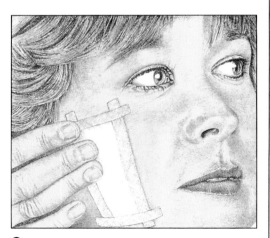

2 *When the bleeding slows (which may take 15 minutes), put a fresh handkerchief or pad on the wound – on top of the old one – and fix it in place with adhesive tape. If blood seeps through, put another pad on top.*

SUPPORTING A BROKEN JAW

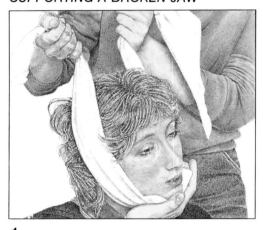

1 *If the jaw is broken or dislocated, make sure first that the mouth is clear of blood and broken teeth to avoid the risk of choking. Then put a pad of cloth under the point of the chin, and get the victim to hold it in place.*

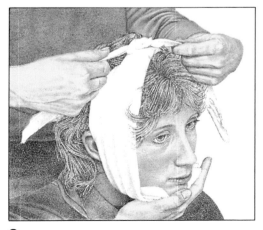

2 *Put a bandage or scarf over the pad, bring the ends to the top of the head, and tie them together in a reef knot. The bandage should be tight enough to support the jaw, but not so tight that the teeth are clenched.*

Heart attack

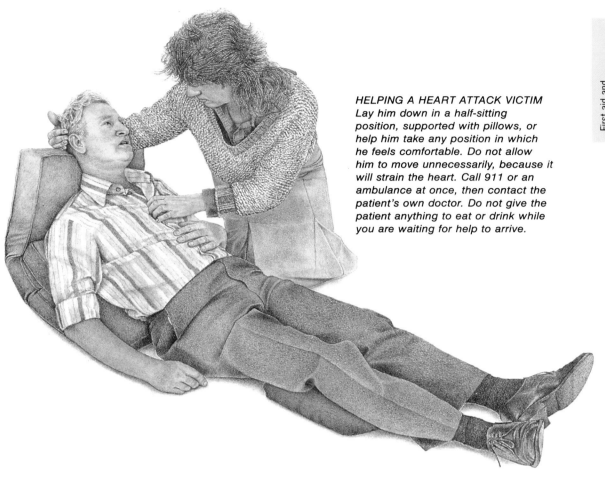

*HELPING A HEART ATTACK VICTIM
Lay him down in a half-sitting
position, supported with pillows, or
help him take any position in which
he feels comfortable. Do not allow
him to move unnecessarily, because it
will strain the heart. Call 911 or an
ambulance at once, then contact the
patient's own doctor. Do not give the
patient anything to eat or drink while
you are waiting for help to arrive.*

Severe, crushing pain in the chest, often spreading to one or both arms, the neck and the jaw, is the main symptom of a heart attack. It comes on suddenly and, unlike anginal pain, is not related to exertion. It does not pass off if the patient keeps still.

The patient may also become breathless and sweat profusely. He may suffer sudden giddiness, causing him to sit down or lean against something for support.

During the weeks before an attack, the patient is quite likely to have experienced unusual tiredness, shortness of breath and unaccustomed indigestion.

What you should do
• If the patient is conscious, put him in a half-sitting position, with head and shoulders supported with pillows, and knees bent.
• Call 911 or an ambulance immediately and make it clear that you suspect a heart attack. Then, if possible, contact the patient's own doctor, as there may be a history of heart disease.
• Loosen the patient's clothing around the neck, chest and waist to help circulation and ease his breathing.

• Do not give the patient anything to eat or drink.
• Do not allow him to move unnecessarily; it will put extra strain on the heart.
• If the patient becomes unconscious, put him in the recovery position (see page 136).

Preventing heart attacks
Most heart attacks are caused by a blood clot in one of the arteries supplying blood to the heart muscle. The process is known medically as coronary thrombosis.

The likelihood of coronary thrombosis is increased by smoking, obesity, diabetes, raised blood pressure, lack of exercise, faulty diet and a family history of heart attacks.

The following five rules will help you to avoid a heart attack:
• Stay within your ideal weight for height.
• If you smoke, give it up.
• Take regular exercise.
• Eat balanced meals, avoiding fatty cuts of beef, pork and lamb and high-fat dairy products. Eat only modest amounts of foods high in cholesterol – liver, kidney, eggs and shrimp.
• If you suffer from diabetes or high blood pressure, follow your doctor's advice carefully.

Heat exhaustion and heatstroke

People who exert themselves during a summer holiday in a hot climate, or long-distance runners on a warm day, may suffer from heat exhaustion, or from an even worse condition known as heatstroke.

Both conditions can lead to unconsciousness and they both require medical treatment.

The body can become overwhelmed by heat when its mechanism for keeping cool breaks down. Usually it cools itself in three ways:

• It produces sweat which evaporates and cools the skin – just as water that seeps through an unglazed jug will cool the remaining water when it evaporates off the outside.

• The capillaries of the skin enlarge and carry more blood to the surface, where it loses its heat. This produces the flushed look a hot person often has.

• Breathing increases, carrying surplus heat from the lungs.

The effects of heat exhaustion

Profuse sweating on a hot day leads to an excessive loss of moisture and salt, which is contained in sweat.

This brings on muscle cramps in the legs and body, and weakness – although the sweating prevents the body's temperature from rising. If the fluid and salt are not replaced, the condition will get worse and the victim will collapse.

Other symptoms of heat exhaustion are dizziness, headache and nausea. The temperature stays normal and the skin feels cold and moist. The face looks pale.

The breathing is fast and shallow, and the pulse is fast and weak.

The condition can be made worse if the sufferer has had a stomach upset with diarrhea or vomiting, causing even greater loss of fluid.

• To treat heat exhaustion, lay the victim in a cool place, preferably indoors, and give cold, salted water to drink.

• If the victim becomes unconscious, put him in the recovery position (see page 136) and get medical help.

TREATING HEAT EXHAUSTION

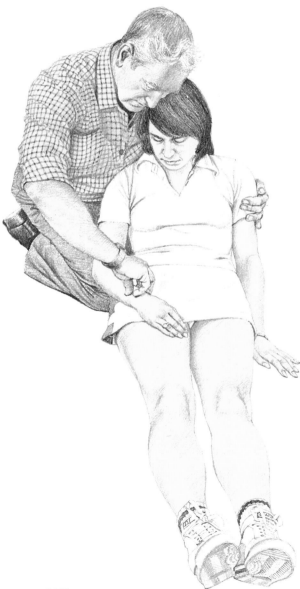

1 *Put the victim in a cool place, preferably indoors. Remove any heavy clothing. If she is suffering from heat exhaustion, her pulse will be fast and weak. Check her temperature; if it is higher than normal she may be suffering from heatstroke. If she becomes unconscious, put her in the recovery position (see page 136).*

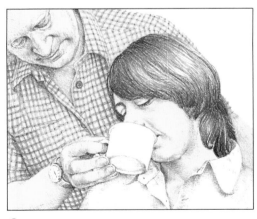

2 *If the victim is conscious, give her a cup of weakly salted water every 10 minutes. Use a quarter of a teaspoon of salt to each cup. Add fruit juice to improve the taste.*

Heatstroke: how to treat it

When humidity, as well as temperature, is very high, sweat is less able to cool the body as it cannot evaporate into the already moisture-laden air. It takes from three to six weeks to adjust to these conditions, and a person may suffer heatstroke before he has acclimatized.

Heatstroke may occur suddenly, with the body temperature rising to 104°F (40°C). The victim's skin feels hot and may be dry. He may complain of headache, dizziness and nausea. As the condition worsens, he may become confused and lapse into unconsciousness.

TREATING HEATSTROKE

Treatment for heatstroke must be given quickly or the victim may die. Babies and old people are particularly at risk.

• Move the sufferer to a cool place. Remove the clothing and cover the body with a wet sheet. Keep it wet with cold water, and fan the victim until the body temperature drops to 100°F (38°C).

• Call a doctor or ambulance as soon as possible. If the victim becomes unconscious, put him in the recovery position (see page 136), and continue the cooling treatment.

How to deal with prickly heat

An intensely irritating skin rash, which may develop in hot, humid weather, is known as prickly heat. It is caused by swelling of the skin cells because of excessive sweating, and mostly affects babies and fat people. Pimples or small blisters appear, particularly in the skin creases and where clothing has been tight.

There is no quick remedy, but some relief will be gained by wearing loose clothing and lying under a fan during the heat of the day. Have frequent baths in cool water, using little soap, and apply calamine lotion to the affected area.

It may be necessary to see a doctor if the irritation becomes too severe to bear, or if the sufferer becomes weak and lethargic.

The skin will rapidly return to normal when you return to a cool climate.

First aid and medical emergencies

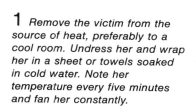

1 *Remove the victim from the source of heat, preferably to a cool room. Undress her and wrap her in a sheet or towels soaked in cold water. Note her temperature every five minutes and fan her constantly.*

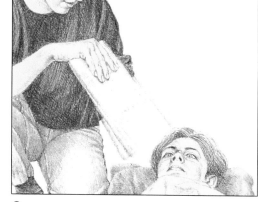

2 *When the victim's temperature is down to 100°F (38°C), replace the wet sheet with a dry one. Continue fanning. If her temperature rises again, restart the cooling treatment.*

Hiccups

Most attacks of hiccups are over in 10 to 20 minutes, but occasionally attacks can last for days, causing distress and interfering with sleep. Persistent hiccups suggest some abdominal disorder requiring medical treatment.

Most hiccups are caused by irritation of the diaphragm – a muscular partition which separates the chest cavity from the abdomen. This occurs when the sufferer has overfilled the stomach with a large amount of food or drink, especially hot drinks. The diaphragm then goes into repeated and involuntary spasms.

What can be done to stop hiccups

Carbon dioxide gas – one of the products of breathing – inhibits hiccups. Simply holding the breath several times will cause carbon dioxide to build up in the body, and the hiccups may stop without further treatment.

Breathing in and out of a paper bag works in the same way. But *do not* use a plastic bag. It can mould itself to the mouth and nose, and obstruct breathing altogether.

Most other household remedies work by making the sufferer hold his breath. Drinking water slowly, sucking ice or pulling out the tongue are all ways of building up carbon dioxide.

If the hiccups last more than a day, the sufferer should see a doctor, who may prescribe sedatives or arrange a supply of 5 percent carbon dioxide to be inhaled. The doctor may also examine the patient for kidney, liver, lung or abdominal disorders which could be causing the hiccups, although such disorders are rare.

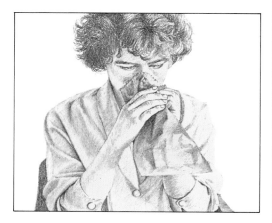

ONE WAY OF STOPPING HICCUPS
Breathing in and out of a paper bag builds up carbon dioxide in the body, which can bring the spasms of the diaphragm to a stop. But on no account use a plastic bag.

Hypothermia

If a baby in a cold room begins to look bright red, becomes lethargic and refuses food, it may have hypothermia, a serious condition in which the body's temperature drops below normal.

Unless the drop in temperature is reversed the baby may die in a few hours.

Old people are also at risk. At first they may complain of the cold. If these warnings go unnoticed or are ignored, the condition will grow worse until the victim becomes mentally confused and tired, with stiff muscles. Uncontrollable shivering may also occur or speech may be slurred.

Eventually the victim becomes unconscious, suffers brain damage and then dies.

(For hypothermia in outdoor conditions, see *Exposure: the silent killer*, page 281.)

How hypothermia sets in

Hypothermia begins when the body's temperature drops below about 95°F (35°C) from the normal level of 98.6°F (37°C).

With babies, the cause of hypothermia is usually a cold bedroom at night. Premature babies and babies who are suffering from illness are the most susceptible.

One problem in recognizing the condition is that the red color of the skin that develops may be mistaken for a healthy glow.

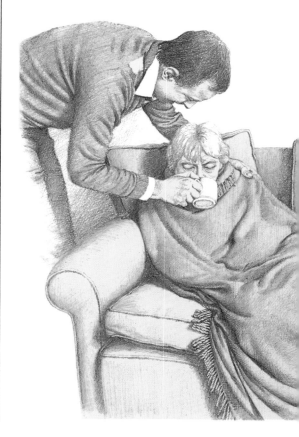

With old people, hypothermia usually results from inadequate food, clothing and heating in winter. Their resistance to cold will also be lessened if they are taking drugs or alcohol.

What you should do
If you suspect that someone is suffering from hypothermia, feel his or her skin. It will be abnormally cold to the touch if the condition has set in. You must take action to prevent the condition from getting worse, and you must call an ambulance or get the victim to hospital.
• If a blanket or rug is readily available, wrap it around the victim, covering the body but not the face.
• Lay him down. If he is unconscious, put him in the recovery position (see page 136).
• If possible, increase the temperature of the room, or move the victim to a warmer room.
• Call 911 and ask for an ambulance.
• While waiting for the ambulance, give the victim – if conscious – hot, sweet drinks such as milk or hot chocolate. Do not give alcohol.
• Do not massage the victim's limbs or suggest that he take exercise. This will only take blood away from the body's vital organs.
• If the ambulance is delayed, wrap a hot-water bottle in a towel or cloth and put it on the victim's trunk, not on the arms or legs.

Hysteria

A fit of hysterics is usually caused by an emotional upset or mental stress. The attack may resemble an epileptic seizure, but is more dramatized and is "staged" to gain sympathy and attention. It will continue as long as there is an audience.

In an adult, hysterics take longer to develop than an epileptic seizure and may vary from temporary loss of control, when the person shouts or screams, to a noisy display or arm waving, tearing at clothes and hair, and rolling on the ground in an apparent frenzy.

Although genuinely distressed, sufferers take care not to hurt themselves. They may, for example, "collapse" into a fairly safe position. They may also move weakly to suggest illness.

What you should do
• Be gentle but firm. Reassure and try to calm the person.
• Ask relatives and onlookers to leave the area.
• Do not slap a hysterical person on the face as it may cause psychological harm. In the case of a person with a weak heart, the shock could even be fatal.
• When the attack has subsided, suggest that the person see a doctor.

First aid and medical emergencies

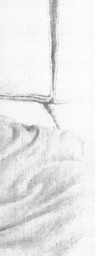

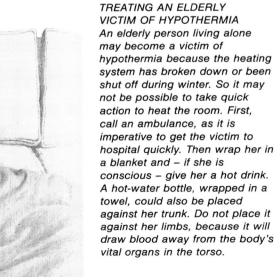

*TREATING AN ELDERLY
VICTIM OF HYPOTHERMIA
An elderly person living alone
may become a victim of
hypothermia because the heating
system has broken down or been
shut off during winter. So it may
not be possible to take quick
action to heat the room. First,
call an ambulance, as it is
imperative to get the victim to
hospital quickly. Then wrap her in
a blanket and – if she is
conscious – give her a hot drink.
A hot-water bottle, wrapped in a
towel, could also be placed
against her trunk. Do not place it
against her limbs, because it will
draw blood away from the body's
vital organs in the torso.*

Insect stings and bites

Stings and bites from bees, wasps and ants can be painful but are not usually dangerous. It is only an allergic reaction, or a sting or bite in the throat or mouth, that can endanger life.

If the victim has been stung by a bee, the sting may be embedded in the skin. Remove it by gently scraping the skin with a knife blade that has been sterilized in a flame. Let the knife cool for a moment before you use it.

Wasps and ants do not leave stings behind.

Dealing with an allergic reaction

A massive allergic reaction to a sting (or to a drug such as penicillin) is known as anaphylactic shock. It occurs within a few minutes – sometimes seconds – and the victim will become very weak and feel sick. His chest will feel tight and he will have difficulty breathing. He may be sneezing and his face may swell up, or he may lose consciousness and stop breathing.

• Call 911 and ask for an ambulance.
• Reassure the victim that help is on the way.
• Lay him on his back. Raise the feet on a cushion or folded coat. Keep his head low and turn it to one side in case he vomits.
• Keep the victim warm with a blanket or rug.
• Loosen tight clothing around the neck and waist to help with breathing.
• Do not give the victim anything to eat or drink. Do not allow him to smoke, either.
• If the victim becomes unconscious, or vomiting seems likely, or breathing becomes very difficult, put him in the recovery position (see page 136).

Stings to the mouth or throat

A sting to the mouth or throat can cause the throat to swell rapidly, blocking the airway.

• Give the victim an ice cube or some ice cream to suck, or cold water to drink, to lessen the swelling.
• If breathing stops, start artificial respiration immediately (see page 50).
• Call 911 and ask for an ambulance or take the victim at once to the emergency department of a hospital.

Blood-sucking ticks

Ticks are spiderlike creatures which live in woods or grassy areas. They cling to the skin of people and animals and their bodies swell up to hold the blood they feed on. If you live in an area infested with ticks, check your body several times daily and at bedtime, and remove ticks before their heads become embedded in the skin.

In some areas, tick bites can cause Rocky Mountain spotted fever, an infection that can be fatal if left untreated. Symptoms are high fever, severe headache and muscle aches. If you have any of these symptoms after a tick bite, consult a physician.

After removing a tick, wash the area with soap and water and apply antihistamine cream. At the first sign of infection, consult a doctor.

TREATING BEE, WASP OR ANT STINGS

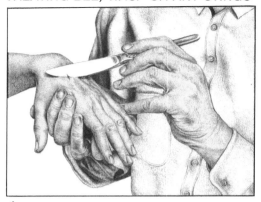

1 *Gently scrape a bee sting out with a sterilized knife. Do not press down on the sting: that will pump more poison into the skin. Wasps and ants do not leave stings behind.*

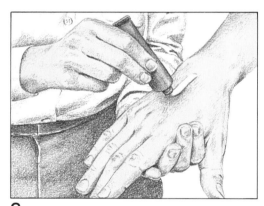

2 *Apply antihistamine cream to any sting. Or use a solution of 1 teaspoon of bicarbonate of soda in a tumbler of water for bee stings, a weak ammonia solution for wasps and ants.*

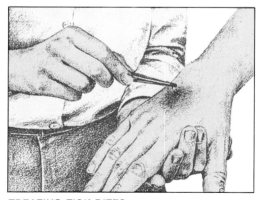

TREATING TICK BITES
Cover the tick with petroleum jelly or oil to close its breathing pores. If it does not fall off within 30 minutes, pull it out with tweezers, being careful not to crush it and thus release infected blood.

Measles

The most obvious symptom of measles is the rash of brownish-pink, slightly raised spots which starts behind the ears and spreads in blotches over the whole body.

But before the rash breaks out, a dry, irritating cough generally occurs and the patient develops a high temperature. The cough can occur up to four days before the rash starts. The eyes can also be sore and red, or "heavy," for a few days before the rash.

What you should do

• Put the patient – usually a child – to bed and give cool drinks to bring the temperature down. It does not matter if the child does not want to eat, as long as plenty of fluids are taken.
• Notify your doctor.
• Keep the child quiet and resting while there is a high temperature and illness. Many children prefer the room darkened because their eyes feel sore.
• If necessary, give temperature-reducing drugs, such as acetaminophen, in the recommended doses.
• The disease is likely to last five to seven days after the rash first appears.

Complications that can occur

Most victims of measles recover completely, but there can be serious complications affecting the ears, lungs and brain.

Consequently the doctor may check the child for otitis media (an ear infection which can cause severe earache and deafness), pneumonia and encephalitis (a rare disease of the brain which causes headache, confusion or unconsciousness, an aching neck and fever).

If one of these diseases occurs, a course of antibiotics will probably be prescribed. Because measles is caused by a virus, antibiotics are of no use against the measles itself.

Because of the serious complications of measles, attempts are being made to eradicate the disease by immunization. Children should be immunized between 12 and 18 months of age. Although the campaign has greatly reduced the number of cases and the complications, measles is still one of the commonest diseases in the world.

Someone who has had the disease cannot catch it a second time.

Miscarriage

At the first sign of a miscarriage, the woman should go to bed immediately. Rest is essential if the pregnancy is to be saved.

Three warning signs occur in succession if the miscarriage takes its full course.
• In the early stages, the commonest symptom is loss of blood from the vagina. If the embryo has not been dislodged, this stage is known medically as a "threatened abortion," and the pregnancy may still be saved.
• If the condition becomes worse, pains like small labor pains may come and go at regular intervals. This is a sign that the threatened miscarriage may have become inevitable.
• The bleeding may also increase at this stage.

What can be done

• Notify the doctor at the first signs and put the patient to bed.
• If the miscarriage passes into the inevitable stage, the doctor may send the patient to hospital.
• In hospital she may have an evacuation of the uterus, under anesthetic, to remove any placenta or membrane left behind, after the embryo has been lost.

How common are miscarriages?

Some medical studies have shown that about one-tenth of all pregnancies miscarry, but the figure may be higher. In many cases the woman never knows that she has been pregnant; the miscarriage occurs about four weeks after her last menstrual period, and so passes unrecognized. In other cases miscarriages may occur a week or so later, and she just thinks that she has had a late period.

Miscarriages may be nature's way of ending a pregnancy that is in some way likely to be unsatisfactory.

Avoiding a miscarriage

Once a woman has become aware that she is pregnant, she should avoid unnecessary fatigue and sporting activities, especially if there is a risk of injury.

If you have had a threatened abortion, or miscarriages in previous pregnancies, consult your doctor about any risks associated with sexual intercourse during pregnancy.

First aid and medical emergencies

Moving an injured person

Injured people should be moved only if they are in immediate danger, or if they have to be taken to where medical help is available. This may occur if you have to move a victim off a busy road, get him out of a burning house, or carry him to safety after a climbing accident.

Otherwise, leave the victim undisturbed and carry out first aid while someone else calls for an ambulance.

If moving is essential, take care not to injure yourself. Back injuries are easily suffered when moving heavy weights, so keep your backbone straight, your head up, and use the stronger parts of your body to do the lifting – the thigh muscles, the hip and the shoulder. Keep the weight as close as possible to your body.

If other people are on the scene, ask someone to help you. It is always easier for two people to lift a weight than one.

It is usually best for an accident victim to be taken to hospital in an ambulance, but if he is suffering from only minor injuries to the arms or hands, he can be taken in a car.

Moving a victim by yourself
If the person is only slightly injured and is able to stand, get him to put one arm around your shoulder. Supported in this way, he can be moved fairly easily. This is a useful method of moving a person with a sprained ankle.

An unconscious person can be dragged to safety on a coat or blanket. You can also hold him under the shoulders and drag him backward in a crouching or squatting position. Or you can tie his wrists together, put your head through the arms and crawl on all fours, dragging him with you. Any of these methods could be used to drag an unconscious person from a burning building or a gas-filled room.

When you have someone to help you
One of the simplest ways for two people to move a victim is to carry him on a chair, with one person holding the back of the chair and the other holding the front legs.

This is a useful way of carrying an injured person down a flight of stairs. But first make sure that the staircase and passage are clear of obstructions, or any hazards such as loose rugs or children's toys.

A disabled person in a wheelchair can be carried in a similar way. First, put the wheel-

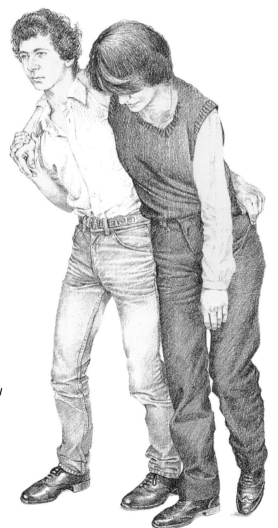

HELPING A CONSCIOUS PERSON
Stand close to the victim on the injured side, unless the wound is to the hand, arm or shoulder. In that case, support from the uninjured side. Put your arm around her waist and grip the clothing at the hip. Get her to put her arm around your neck and grasp her hand. Take her weight with your body and move forward with slow, short steps.

chair's brakes on, and get the victim to sit well back in the chair. Then stand to one side of the chair, with your helper on the other side facing you. Lift the chair together, holding the fixed parts. Do not hold the wheels, as they might turn, and be careful of the arm rests and side supports, as they might be removable.

A victim who cannot walk but can use his hands can be carried by two people using a "four-handed seat." The two helpers each grip their left wrist with their right hand, and then grip the other person's right wrist with their free hand. The victim puts an arm around each helper's neck and sits on the "seat." The two helpers stand up straight and start walking with the outside foot.

MOVING AN UNCONSCIOUS PERSON

1 *Use this method if you have a fairly long way to go or if the victim is heavy. Check the breathing but do not start artificial respiration until you are clear of danger. Place the victim on her back and cross her arms at the wrists.*

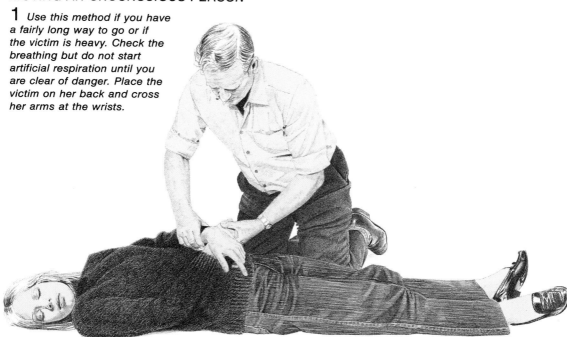

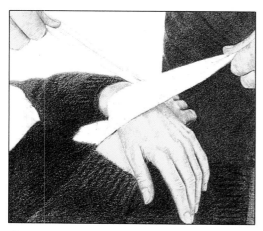

2 *Use a belt, scarf or bandage to tie the wrists together. Wind the material around the wrists tightly, but not so tightly as to impede circulation. Tie the ends with a reef knot, and check quickly with your fingers that the knot is completely secure.*

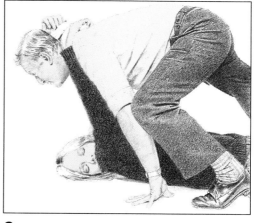

3 *Kneel astride the victim and slip your head through the wrists so they are resting on your shoulders at the base of your neck. Push yourself up into a crouch, and work forward to safety, using your arms to take the weight. Keep the victim's head off the ground.*

Making an improvised stretcher

Two people can move an injured person a long distance by making an improvised stretcher out of two or more coats with their sleeves turned inside out and a pair of poles, such as broom handles, pushed through the sleeves.

To get the person onto the stretcher, one of the stretcher-bearers should roll the victim gently onto the uninjured side. While he is doing that, the other bearer should put the open stretcher flat against the victim's back. Then the stretcher, with the victim on it, can be rolled back gently onto the ground.

If the victim is unconscious, put the open stretcher against his front so that he is carried in the recovery position (see page 136).

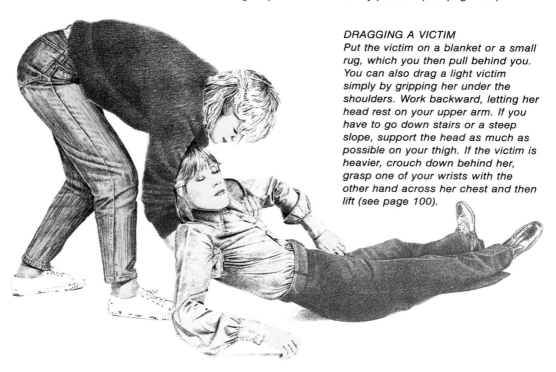

DRAGGING A VICTIM
Put the victim on a blanket or a small rug, which you then pull behind you. You can also drag a light victim simply by gripping her under the shoulders. Work backward, letting her head rest on your upper arm. If you have to go down stairs or a steep slope, support the head as much as possible on your thigh. If the victim is heavier, crouch down behind her, grasp one of your wrists with the other hand across her chest and then lift (see page 100).

CARRYING A CONSCIOUS PERSON ON A CHAIR

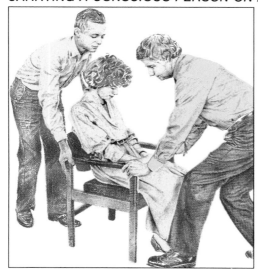

1 *Check that the chair is strong enough to take the weight. Sit the victim well back in it, and stand in front with the other helper behind. Tilt the chair backward as you lift it.*

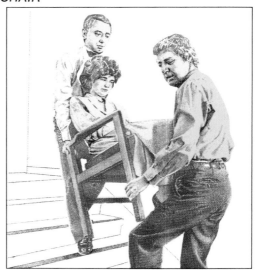

2 *Carry the chair with the victim facing forward, so that you go downstairs with the bearer at the front backing down. On wide stairs, the bearers can hold the sides instead.*

IMPROVISING A STRETCHER

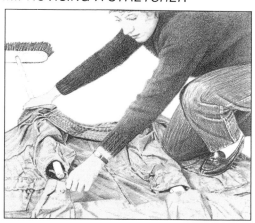

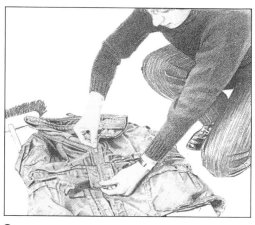

1 *Take two or three coats or jackets, and turn the sleeves inside out. Pass a strong pole through one of the sleeves of each jacket, and a second pole through the other sleeves.*

2 *Zip or button up the jackets to create the stretcher. If possible, get an uninjured person to lie on the stretcher first, and lift it to make sure that it can take the weight.*

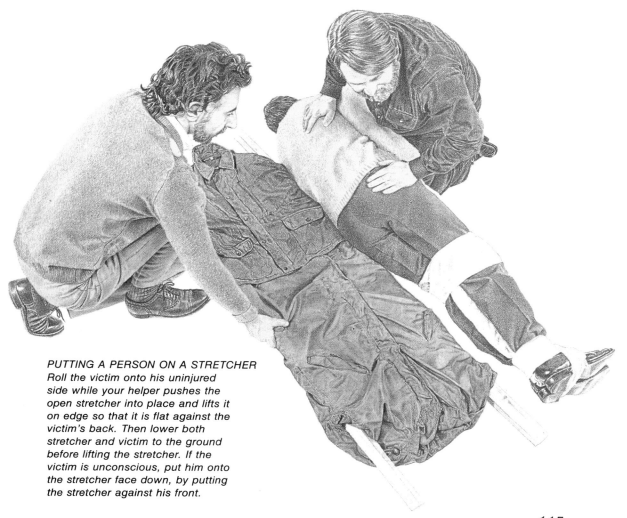

PUTTING A PERSON ON A STRETCHER
Roll the victim onto his uninjured side while your helper pushes the open stretcher into place and lifts it on edge so that it is flat against the victim's back. Then lower both stretcher and victim to the ground before lifting the stretcher. If the victim is unconscious, put him onto the stretcher face down, by putting the stretcher against his front.

Mumps

The most obvious sign of mumps is a large swelling on one side of the face. It is caused by a saliva-producing gland swelling up in front of the ear and over the angle of the jaw.

A day or two later the gland on the opposite side of the face may also swell. Other saliva-producing glands under the tongue and under the jaw may also be affected.

The patient may also suffer earache and pain when eating.

Mumps is a common infection, mostly affecting children over the age of two, and occurs in epidemics every three or four years. But it can also attack older people, and may cause inflammation of the testicles in men, inflammation of the ovaries in women, and inflammation of the pancreas in both sexes, producing pain in the abdomen.

What you should do
- Keep the patient at rest for a few days.
- If chewing is painful, offer soups and drinks.
- If a testicle is swollen or sore, support the scrotum with a pillow or bandage. A towel beneath the testicles, with the ends draped over the thighs, may help. Leave pajama trousers off and give a mild analgesic such as acetaminophen in recommended doses.

When you should call the doctor
- If the testicles are swollen or sore.
- If there is severe or persistent earache.
- If there is severe or persistent pain in the abdomen – the lower part of the trunk.
- If there is severe headache, with a stiff neck.
- If the patient finds light uncomfortable.

The doctor may examine the patient for an ear infection known as otitis media, for inflammation of the testicles (orchitis), or for inflammation of the fluid bathing the brain (meningitis) or, rarely, of the brain itself (encephalitis).

How long is the patient infectious?
Sufferers are infectious for about six days before the glands begin to swell, and remain infectious for a further ten days. As it is impossible to prevent spread of the disease in the symptomless period, there may be little point in isolating the patient once the disease has shown itself.

Someone who has already had the illness cannot catch it again.

Though mumps is not a serious disease, the complications that sometimes follow can be serious. For this reason, children should be vaccinated against mumps as part of their general immunization program. The vaccine is usually given between 12 and 15 months.

Nose injuries

The nose's function as an opening to the body and its prominent position on the face make it subject to a variety of problems.

Nosebleeds
Bleeding from the nose may be the result of blowing too hard, sneezing, picking, air-pressure changes or high blood pressure. Occasionally blood disorders may be the cause, and sometimes there may be no apparent cause for a nosebleed at all.

If blood mixed with a straw-colored fluid trickles from the nose of an unconscious person, suspect a fracture of the skull (see page 102).

For a normal nosebleed, sit in a chair with your head slightly forward and pinch the nostrils together for at least ten minutes.

Loosen any tight clothing around the neck.

Spit out any blood that goes down the back of the nose. It is preferable to spit it out as swallowed blood may make you feel sick, so have a bowl close by.

After ten minutes, release the nostrils gradually. If the bleeding has stopped, sit quietly for a while, and do not blow your nose for at least three hours.

If the bleeding starts up again, squeeze the nostrils for a further ten minutes.

If the bleeding still continues, see a doctor or go to the emergency department of your local hospital.

You should also see a doctor if you lose so much blood that you become pale or dizzy.

Broken nose
The bones at the bridge of the nose may be broken by an injury, often in a traffic accident. There is then a danger that a deformity of the nose may become permanent, as happens with some boxers.

The symptoms of a broken nose are:
- Severe pain.
- Irregular shape.
- Severe nosebleed.

If a broken nose is suspected, you should take the victim to a doctor or to the emergency department of your local hospital.

Bleeding can often be stopped with gauze packed into the nostrils.

If there is no deformity causing an obstruction of the nose, treatment is usually unnecessary, apart from an X ray. The fracture will take about two weeks to heal.

A deformed nose can be corrected by an operation under general anesthetic.

Foreign body in the nose
Small children often push objects, such as pebbles or beads, into their nostrils. A smooth object may stick harmlessly in the nose, but something jagged can easily cause damage to the inside of the nose and make it bleed.

You should suspect that something is lodged in the nose if:

• A child is playing with its nose.
• One nostril is obstructed, and possibly bleeding.
• The child complains of discomfort or pain in the nose.

Do not try to remove the object yourself; you may make the problem worse.

Take the child to your doctor or to the emergency department of your local hospital, where the object will be removed gently with forceps, or under a general anesthetic.

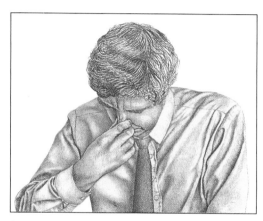

STOPPING A NOSEBLEED
Sit down with your head slightly forward to prevent blood running down into your throat. Hold the nostrils together for 10 minutes. If, after that, the bleeding continues, repeat for a further 10 minutes.

Poisoning

Many cases of poisoning occur when a person – often a child – drinks some household or garden chemical. A child may take bleach, cleaning fluid, laundry detergent, furniture polish, rat poison or paint stripper. Even adult gardeners have been known to accidentally drink insecticides and weed killers that they had made up in soft drink bottles.

Some plants are also dangerous: azaleas, mistletoe, dieffenbachia, rhododendrons, jimsonweed, daffodil bulbs and mushrooms have often caused poisoning.

The warning signs
A person who has taken poison is likely to show some of the following symptoms:
• Stomach pain.
• Retching or vomiting.
• Diarrhea.
• Delirium and convulsions.
• Burns around the mouth if the poison was corrosive, and severe pain in the mouth, throat and stomach.
• Difficulty in breathing.
• Unconsciousness.

What you should do
• If the victim is conscious, try to find out what he has swallowed. Remember that he may become unconscious at any time.
• Look around for any container or the remains of a poisonous plant that might be a clue.
• Call your nearest poison control center. The person on the line will tell you what to do and will send help if necessary. Be prepared to give the victim's age, to describe the poison (have the container with you when you call), and to say how much was taken and when. Follow the instructions you get exactly.
• If the victim is conscious, you may be told to do one of two things – dilute the poison with milk or water, or induce vomiting.
• If the victim is unconscious, place him in the recovery position (see page 136).
• If the victim's breathing stops, begin artificial respiration (see page 50). Take care not to get poison on your own mouth. Clean the victim's mouth, or use the mouth-to-nose technique.
• If the victim is being hospitalized, give the ambulance attendants anything that will help identify the poison – pill containers, for example – and a sample of vomit.

How to avoid poisoning
Many poisonous household substances may be drunk or eaten by an inquisitive toddler.

Apparently innocent things, including some detergents and cosmetics, can be poisonous. Paint remover, lighter fluid and turpentine are common household petroleum products which are very harmful when ingested.

Keep all dangerous chemicals out of the reach of small children, and never store unused weed killers and insecticides in soft drink bottles.

First aid and medical emergencies

Pulse and breathing

The pulse rate plays an important part in diagnosing some injuries which may have no very obvious symptoms.

A rapid or weak pulse is often associated with shock, internal bleeding and heat exhaustion. Occasionally, a rapid or irregular pulse, occurring while a person is at rest, may be a symptom of serious heart disorder.

A slow pulse can occur if the body cools down to an unnatural degree, as happens to a victim of hypothermia.

The pulse measures the rate at which the heart beats, and this varies throughout life. In a baby's first weeks it may beat 140 times a minute, but by the age of ten the rate will have dropped to an average of 90 a minute. A man, awake but at rest, has a pulse rate between 60 and 80 a minute, with an average of 72. A woman's average rate is slightly higher – 78 to 82 a minute.

An elderly person may have a rate of only 60 a minute, and a sleeping adult of either sex has a rate of 60 to 65.

In times of extreme activity the pulse rate of an adult can go up to 140 a minute.

Each pulse beat is caused by a wave of blood pressure driven along the arteries by the pumping action of the heart. The pulse is most easily detected at two places on the body – the inside of the wrist, just below the thumb joint, and in the hollow of the throat just below the angle of the jaw.

When you take a pulse, note whether it is fast or slow, strong or weak, regular or irregular. Accurate taking of the pulse requires practice, and may be difficult even then. Practice on yourself or a member of your family from time to time so that, if an emergency arises suddenly, you will be able to find the pulse in the wrist or throat without having to hunt for it.

The breathing rate

Respiration – the process of breathing – is closely linked to heartbeat. A person breathes to absorb oxygen from the air into the blood. The oxygen is then circulated to all parts of the

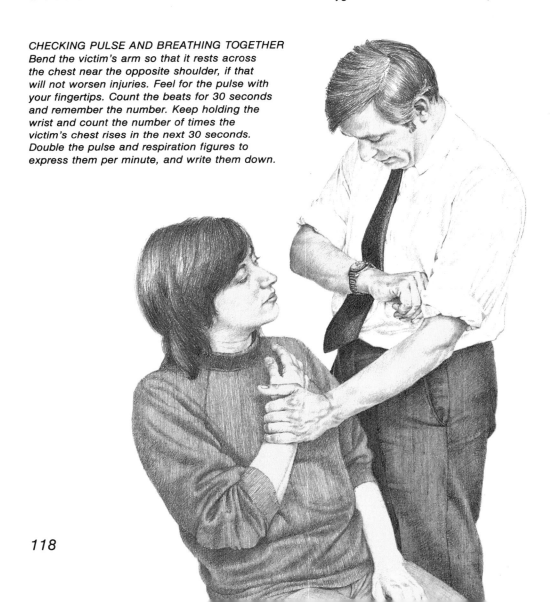

CHECKING PULSE AND BREATHING TOGETHER
Bend the victim's arm so that it rests across the chest near the opposite shoulder, if that will not worsen injuries. Feel for the pulse with your fingertips. Count the beats for 30 seconds and remember the number. Keep holding the wrist and count the number of times the victim's chest rises in the next 30 seconds. Double the pulse and respiration figures to express them per minute, and write them down.

Rabies

Rabies is a dangerous infectious disease caused by a virus carried by animals, particularly skunks, raccoons, foxes, bats, cattle, dogs and cats. It is also known as hydrophobia (meaning "fear of water"), because this fear is one of its symptoms.

The virus is transmitted to humans through the bite or scratch of an infected animal, and travels from the injured spot to the brain.

The nearer the bite is to the brain (on the face or neck, for example) the less far the virus has to travel and the quicker the treatment must be to prevent the disease.

The time between the bite and the onset of symptoms can range from ten days to more than a year, but is usually between 20 and 90 days. Before the symptoms begin, the bite usually heals but remains red and inflamed.

Once the symptoms have developed, treatment is ineffective and the patient usually dies within four days.

Rabies occurs in most parts of the world, except Britain, Scandinavia, Australia, Japan and Antarctica. In North America, it is rare for any person to develop a rabies infection. However, more than 25,000 persons are treated annually, because it is known or suspected that they were exposed to the virus.

What you should do
• See a doctor immediately if you are bitten by a wild animal or a wandering domestic animal. To be effective, treatment must begin before the symptoms appear. Depending on the circumstances, the doctor may give antirabies treatment immediately or, if the culprit has been captured, he may wait to see if the animal develops rabies symptoms.

• If possible, the animal should be captured (or its owner identified) so that the creature can be observed for symptoms of rabies. Call your local health authorities if you need help.

• If possible, isolate the animal, but take care not to endanger yourself or others. If it escapes, notify the police immediately.

Symptoms of rabies
• Fever, headache, sore throat and muscle pains are followed by pain or numbness at the site of the healed bite.

• One or two days later the patient becomes restless and agitated.

• Muscle spasms, stiffness of the neck and back, convulsions and areas of paralysis may also develop.

• Excess saliva and difficulty in swallowing produce foaming at the mouth.

• Painful throat spasms develop, with a reaction of terror on trying to swallow liquids.

body by the regular pumping action of the heart. Children breathe an average of 20 to 30 times a minute, and adults an average of 12 to 16 times a minute. This increases during exercise and when a person is injured or under stress.

When measuring the breathing rate, count only the number of times the chest rises. Many people unknowingly alter their breathing rate if they are aware it is being checked. So, if the victim is conscious, measure the rate, without telling him, while you hold his wrist.

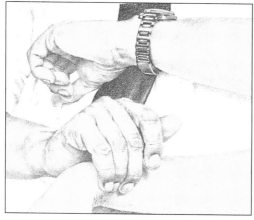

TAKING THE PULSE AT THE WRIST
The wrist pulse can be felt just below the base of the thumb, in the hollow between two bones. Place three fingers on the pulse and press slightly. Do not use your thumb as it has a pulse of its own. Count the beats for half a minute and double the number.

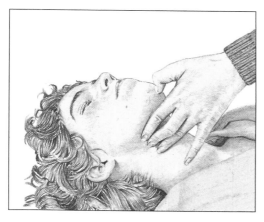

TAKING THE PULSE AT THE THROAT
The throat pulse can be felt in the hollow of the neck, to one side of the Adam's apple and below the angle of the jaw. Place three fingers on the pulse and press slightly. Count the beats for half a minute and double the number. Either side of the throat can be used.

Rib fractures

A hard blow to the chest, or a heavy fall, can fracture a rib, causing a sharp chest pain when the victim breathes deeply or coughs.

A victim who has only a simple rib fracture can be taken to hospital in a car, preferably in the back seat.

But there may be a serious chest injury if:
• The victim is unable to breathe properly, and seems to be suffocating.
• Red frothy blood comes from his mouth.
• He becomes restless and thirsty.

If the victim shows any of these symptoms, call an ambulance at once (see also *Chest injuries*, page 68).

Recognizing a simple rib fracture

A person with a simple rib fracture will feel extremely tender around the site of the injury. The area will swell. Pain will increase with movement, including deep breathing or coughing. And there may be a crackling sound from the ribs.

But he is not likely to feel ill and will have no difficulty in breathing, even though the breaths may be shallow to avoid pain.
• Treat a fractured rib by putting the arm on the injured side in an arm sling (see facing page), and then taking the victim to the emergency department of your local hospital.

Shock

Some injuries can cause the victim to become generally weak – or even unconscious – in a condition known as shock, or traumatic shock.

The condition arises because the blood supply, carrying oxygen to all parts of the body, slows down. This may be because the heartbeat has become weak – from extreme pain or distress, say – or because serious bleeding, vomiting, diarrhea or widespread burns have reduced the amount of body fluid, so that there is not enough blood to supply all the cells.

Shock may be immediate – as when someone receives bad news – or it may develop over two or three hours. And it can kill. It is not the same as the feeling of horror that occurs after an injury or other unpleasant experience, from which the victim may recover quickly.

The warning signs

Faced with the lack of adequate blood supply, the body reacts by concentrating the remaining supply on the vital organs – the heart, brain and kidneys. The less important areas, such as the muscles and skin, go without adequate blood, and the victim weakens and becomes pale.

The condition also produces other effects:
• Faintness and giddiness.
• A feeling of anxiousness and restlessness.
• Nausea and perhaps vomiting.
• Thirst.
• Sweating.
• Shallow, rapid breathing, with yawning and sighing.
• A weak pulse which is fast and may be irregular.

What you should do

• Lay the victim down with the head low, and treat any obvious injury or condition which may be causing the shock.
• Comfort and reassure the victim.
• Loosen clothing at the neck, chest and waist to assist breathing and blood circulation.
• Ask someone to call 911 for an ambulance.
• If possible, raise the legs on a folded coat or cushion to direct the blood to the brain.
• Keep the victim warm with a coat or blanket. But do not use a hot-water bottle, as it will bring the blood to the skin and away from the vital organs.
• If the victim complains of thirst, moisten his lips, but do not give him anything to drink or eat, as it may cause delay in giving an anesthetic in hospital.
• Do not move the victim unnecessarily. It will increase the shock.
• Do not allow the victim to smoke, as it may hinder breathing.
• If breathing becomes difficult, if the victim seems about to vomit, or if he becomes unconscious, put him in the recovery position (see page 136).
• If breathing stops, begin artificial respiration immediately (see page 50).

Slings

Once an injury to a hand, arm or chest has been treated, put a sling on the victim to give the damaged area support.

You can buy both ready-made slings and triangular bandages to make them at the drugstore. You can also make your own with any piece of material about 1 yd. sq. (1 m sq.), either cut or folded diagonally. Alternatively, there are a number of ways in which you can improvise a sling.

When to use an arm sling
For a wound on the arm, and for some rib injuries, a conventional arm sling is usually used. But it is effective only if the victim can stand or sit. It supports the forearm across the chest, with the hand slightly higher than the elbow and the fingers exposed.

When to use an elevation sling
A hand that must be raised to control bleeding

MAKING AN ARM SLING

1 *Get the victim to support the injured arm with his hand. Place an open triangular bandage between the chest and forearm, its point stretching well beyond the elbow. Take the upper end over the shoulder on the uninjured side, around the back of the neck to the front of the injured side.*

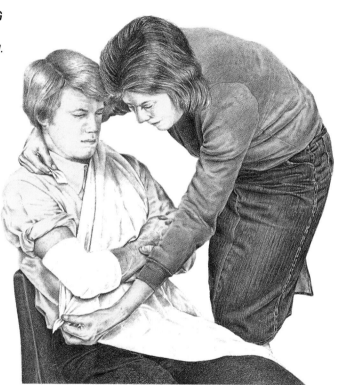

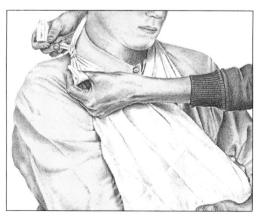

2 *Take the lower end of the bandage up over the hand and forearm and tie it in the hollow just above the collarbone. The tips of the fingers should just protrude from the sling.*

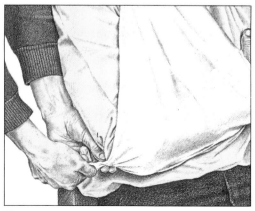

3 *Pin the point near the elbow, or twist and tuck it in. If the arm was bandaged before the sling went on, check that the nail beds are not turning blue. If they are, loosen the bandage.*

can be supported in an elevation sling. This sling is also used for complicated chest injuries or a broken collarbone. And it will support an arm for a victim who cannot stand or sit.

Improvising a sling

If no triangular bandage is available, and you cannot make one, there are several ways to improvise a sling. Good support can be given, for example, by turning up the bottom edge of the victim's jacket and pinning it firmly to the jacket at chest level. The arm will be well supported inside the fold.

Alternatively, suspend the injured arm from a belt, tie or scarf which is tied around the victim's neck.

The sleeve of the injured arm can be pinned to the front of the jacket, or the victim's hand can be pushed inside the fastened jacket at chest level, supported by a button or zipper.

IMPROVISING A SLING

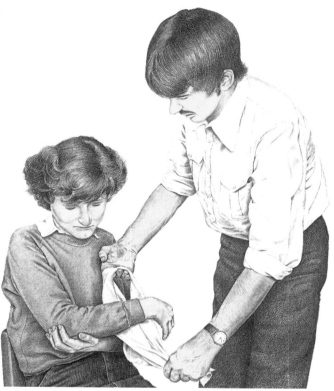

1 *If you do not have a triangular bandage, improvise a sling from a narrow scarf, tie or roll of gauze bandage. Wrap the strip of cloth once around the victim's wrist on the injured arm, or make a loop around the wrist.*

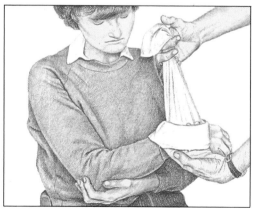

2 *Put one end of the sling over the victim's shoulder on the uninjured side. Then bring the other end across the chest and around the victim's neck to the uninjured shoulder.*

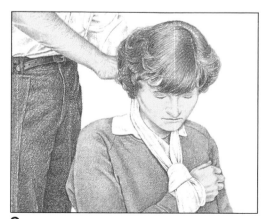

3 *Tie the ends in the hollow above the collarbone on the uninjured side. The hand should normally be just above elbow level, but at shoulder level for hand or forearm wounds.*

MAKING AN ELEVATION SLING

1 *Raise the injured arm – or the arm on the injured side, in the case of a chest injury – so that the hand rests on the opposite shoulder. If possible, get the victim to hold it in place while you make the sling.*

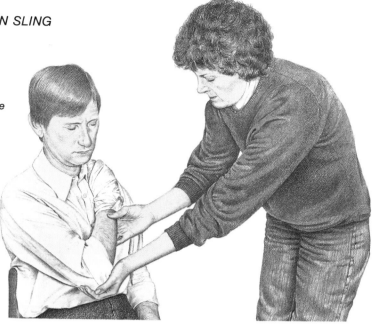

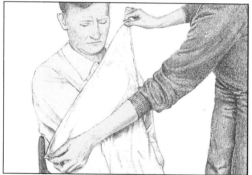

2 *Put one end of the base of the sling over the victim's shoulder on the uninjured side, with the point extended well beyond the elbow. The sling should then be hanging over the arm.*

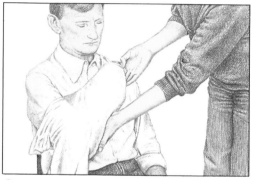

3 *Gently push the base of the sling under the hand, forearm and elbow of the injured arm, so that the lower end of the base is hanging free below the elbow.*

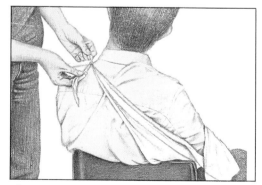

4 *Bring the lower end around the victim's back on the injured side. Join the two ends of the sling together at the shoulder on the uninjured side, and tie them together.*

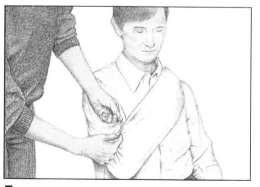

5 *Fold in the point and fasten it with a pin, or twist and tuck it in. If the arm has been bandaged, check that the nail beds are not turning blue. If they are, loosen the bandage.*

123

Slipped disc

A disc is a shock-absorbing layer between each of the vertebrae in the spine. A slipped disc is caused by the gradual degeneration and softening of these discs after the age of 25.

When a disc slips, its soft core protrudes from its fibrous casing and presses on one of the nerves leading from the spinal cord. This causes pain, which can be severe.

Warning signs

Most slipped discs occur in the lower back and the pain is usually felt there first. The pain may also spread down around the buttocks and hips and along one or both legs.

The pain often starts suddenly just after you have lifted something heavy or have straightened up after bending. But sometimes it comes on gradually or only becomes severe after several mild attacks.

The pain may be made worse by bending, getting up after sitting, coughing or straining. It is easier when lying flat, standing or walking.

The lower leg and the outer foot may also become numb.

What you should do

• Lie down on a firm flat bed which does not sag. If necessary, get somebody to put a wide board the full length of the bed under the mattress. Alternatively, have the mattress put directly on the floor. On no account try to move anything heavy yourself.

• Take analgesics, such as aspirin or acetaminophen, in recommended doses.

• A hot-water bottle or heat lamp applied to the painful area may give relief.

• If the pain is not relieved after a day or two of rest, call the doctor. The doctor may confirm the diagnosis with X rays, and perhaps arrange physiotherapy. Some cases may require immobilization in a plaster jacket or corset.

Manipulation may help but can be dangerous, and should be considered only after an X ray and discussion with the doctor.

Many mild attacks get better in a few days and never recur. About 75 percent of more severe attacks recur within five years, but may then get better.

Avoiding a slipped disc

The risk of a slipped disc can be reduced by keeping the back straight and bending at the knees when lifting, and holding the weight close to you. Particularly avoid lifting and twisting at the same time. These precautions are especially important to people who have already suffered a slipped disc.

Smoke inhalation

If you are trying to escape from a burning building, you will be concerned with getting out as quickly as possible. To do so, you must avoid suffocation by smoke.

Protect yourself by tying a towel or piece of thick cloth – preferably wet – around your nose and mouth. As you move through the building, keep low, and reduce the fire risk by closing windows and doors behind you (see *Fire rescue*, page 148).

If you are rescuing someone from a smoke-filled room, a child, say, or an aged parent, bear in mind that inhaled smoke can irritate the throat, causing it to contract in a sudden spasm and close the airway. So someone found in such circumstances may be unconscious and his breathing may have stopped.

Remember, too, that smoke from plastic foam can kill in a very short time.

What you should do

• Drag the victim away from the smoke (see page 113).

• Once clear of danger, if the victim is unconscious but breathing normally, put him in the recovery position (see page 136).

• If breathing has stopped or is very difficult, begin mouth-to-mouth resuscitation as soon as possible (see page 50).

• Get someone to call 911 and ask for an ambulance.

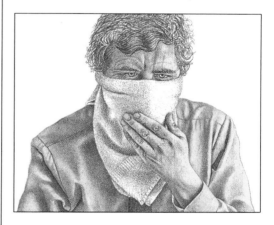

PROTECTING YOURSELF FROM SMOKE
Cover your mouth and nose with a piece of thick, wet cloth before entering a smoke-filled room. Keep close to the floor where the air should be clear, as hot, smoky air will rise.

Snakebite

North America's deadliest reptiles are coral snakes, which are prevalent from North Carolina to California. Most of the continent's venomous snakes, however, are pit vipers: rattlesnakes, copperheads and cottonmouths. Canada's three poisonous species – massasauga, prairie and timber rattlesnakes – are all rattlesnakes.

There are about 9,000 cases of poisonous snakebite a year in North America, nearly all of them in the United States. Mortality is low but there is a high incidence of crippling injuries to the affected limbs. All victims of snakebite should be treated in hospital.

Until reaching the hospital, the victim should remain still, keeping the area of the bite below the level of the heart.

Immobilize the bitten area with splints.

The victim should, if possible, be carried to an ambulance or car for the trip to hospital.

Kill the snake, if you can do so easily, and bring it to the hospital. If this is impossible, take note of its size, coloring and skin pattern. This way, hospital staff can identify the snake and decide if antivenin should be given.

Warning signs
• Sharp pain, bruising or swelling around the bite.
• One or two small puncture wounds.
• Blurry vision, nausea, vomiting, or diarrhea.
• Breathing difficulties, seizures or convulsions.

What you should do
• If medical help is more than two hours away, apply a constricting band 2 in. (5 cm) above the bite, or above the swelling if this has begun. Do not make the band too tight: you should be able to slip a finger underneath. Move the band as the swelling spreads, so that it stays 2 in. (5 cm) above the swelling. If there is no swelling, loosen the band every 15 to 30 minutes.
• Give the victim fluids to drink but no alcohol.
• If the victim becomes unconscious, but is breathing normally, put her in the recovery position (see page 136) until help arrives.
• If breathing stops, begin mouth-to-mouth respiration immediately (see page 50).
• If the victim is frightened and then becomes weak and pale, she may be suffering from shock. Treat as described on page 120.

Snakebite kits
The snakebite kits sold in drugstores and outdoor-equipment stores are strictly for situations where medical help cannot be reached. The kits, which contain instruments for incising and drawing venom from a bite, should be used only by those skilled in dealing with snakebite.

TREATING SNAKEBITE

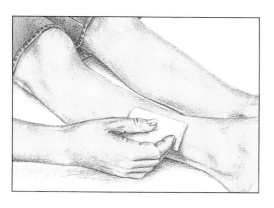

1 Rest the victim in a comfortable position, with the injured limb at, or below, heart level. Assure her that snakebites are seldom fatal, and that help is on the way. Treat for shock if necessary.

2 Remove venom from around the bite by washing it with water, then wiping outward from the wound. Do not raise the injured limb.

Splinters

Splinters of wood, metal or glass embedded in the skin can cause infection if they are not carefully, and cleanly, removed.

Do not try to remove a very large splinter, or one that is buried below the surface of the skin. In either case go to your doctor or to the emergency department of your local hospital.

Small, visible splinters can usually be removed with tweezers, but maintain hygienic conditions. If your hands are dirty, wash them before starting. Do not cough or sneeze on the wound, as germs may penetrate and infect it.

Sterilize the tweezers by passing the ends through a flame from a match or cigarette lighter. Let them cool for a few moments but do not wipe off any soot or touch the ends of the tweezers.

Do not probe to get to the splinter. If it is deeply embedded, get medical help. Otherwise you may only push the splinter farther in, making it even harder to remove.

THE RISK OF TETANUS

A piece of splinter left in a wound, or a dirty splinter even if it has been removed, may lead to tetanus. This is a dangerous infection which causes acute muscle contractions, particularly in the jaw, giving the disease its other name of lockjaw.

Tetanus bacteria live in soil and animal excrement and can invade the body through animal bites, burns and puncture wounds, such as those caused by nails or thorns. All road and agricultural accidents carry a risk of tetanus. So anyone who suffers such a wound and who has not had a tetanus inoculation in the past ten years should get a booster injection.

A person who contracts tetanus at first feels unwell and may have stiffness and pain in the jaw, difficulty in swallowing, raised temperature, headache and sweating.

Stiffness of other muscles may occur, in which case there may be painful arching of the back and drawing down of the neck. Sudden muscle contractions may be brought on by noise or by touching the patient.

If you suspect tetanus, take the patient to the emergency department of your local hospital immediately.

Immunization is the surest prevention for tetanus. Children are given three injections in their first six months, one at 18 months, another between 4 and 6 years, and one in the early teens (14 to 16 years).

REMOVING A SPLINTER

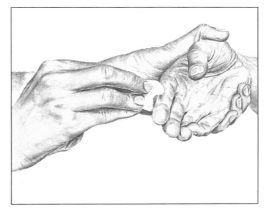

1 Wash the skin around the splinter with warm, soapy water. Wipe downward and outward from the wound to avoid carrying dirt to it. Pat the skin dry with a clean towel.

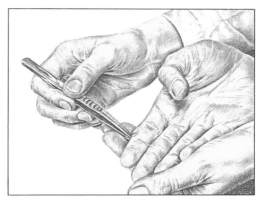

2 Sterilize a pair of tweezers, then pull out the splinter directly in line with the way it went in. A magnifying glass may help. If it will not come out, get medical help.

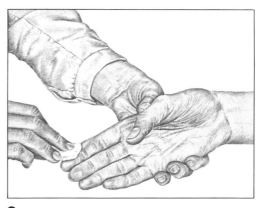

3 When the splinter has been removed, wash the wound with a mild antiseptic. Cover it with an adhesive bandage or sterile dressing. If it swells or becomes painful, see a doctor.

Splints

A person with a fractured bone should not be moved unless it is absolutely necessary (see page 112). But if the ambulance is delayed, or you have to take the person to hospital yourself, use splints to secure the fractured bone in the position you found it. The best way is to secure it to an uninjured part of the body with bandages – a technique known as body splinting. Never manipulate the fractured bone.

To immobilize an arm, put it in a sling and then bandage it against the chest. A broken leg can be bandaged to the other leg, provided that plenty of padding is put between the ankles and knees to prevent chafing.

If the injured person has to be carried to safety, the fractured limb can be given greater support with a rigid splint, such as a tightly rolled blanket, a walking stick or a plank.

Any splint must be long enough to extend well beyond the joints above and below the fracture.

Do not remove clothes to apply a splint, and if possible add extra padding between splint and limb to make the victim as comfortable as possible.

SECURING A FRACTURED ARM

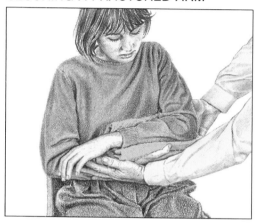

1 *If the arm will bend easily, place it across the chest and put some padding between the site of the fracture and the body. Do not bend the arm by force.*

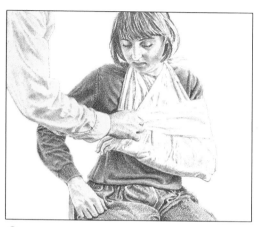

2 *Put on an arm sling (see page 121), and then strap the arm to the body with a piece of wide material around arm and chest. Tie off the strap on the uninjured side.*

SECURING AN ARM THAT WILL NOT BEND

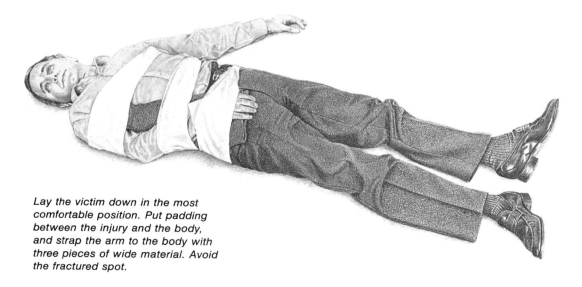

Lay the victim down in the most comfortable position. Put padding between the injury and the body, and strap the arm to the body with three pieces of wide material. Avoid the fractured spot.

First aid and medical emergencies

127

SPLINTING A FRACTURED ELBOW

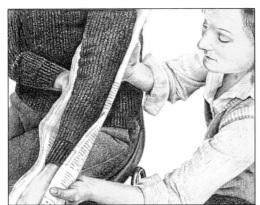

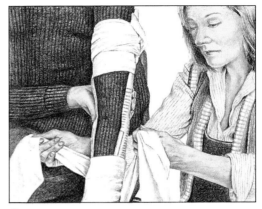

1 *If the elbow has been fractured, sit the victim down and keep the arm straight. Fold a newspaper and place it along the arm.*

2 *Get the victim to support the splint, and tie it in place with two bandages, one at the top of the splint and the other at the bottom.*

SECURING A FRACTURED LEG WITH BANDAGES

1 *A broken leg is most easily immobilized by bandaging it to the other leg. Move the uninjured leg to it, and put padding between the legs, especially at the knees and ankles.*

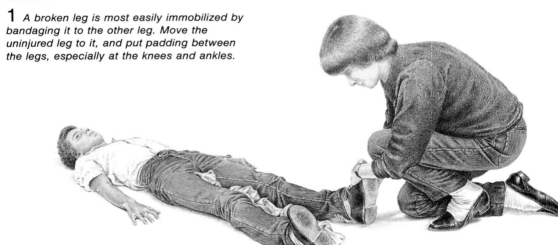

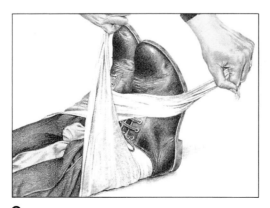

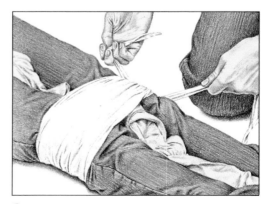

2 *Tie the feet together with a scarf or necktie in a figure eight. Knot it on the outer edge of the shoe on the uninjured leg.*

3 *Tie the knees together with a wide piece of material knotted on the uninjured side. Tie extra bandages above and below the fracture.*

128

A BLANKET SPLINT FOR A FRACTURED LEG

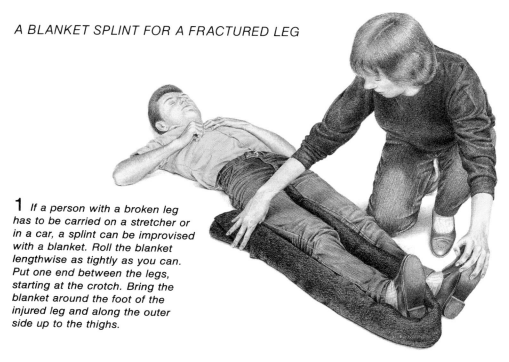

1 If a person with a broken leg has to be carried on a stretcher or in a car, a splint can be improvised with a blanket. Roll the blanket lengthwise as tightly as you can. Put one end between the legs, starting at the crotch. Bring the blanket around the foot of the injured leg and along the outer side up to the thighs.

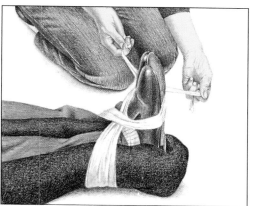

2 Tie the feet and ankles together with a bandage or other piece of material in a figure eight. Use a reef knot to tie it off.

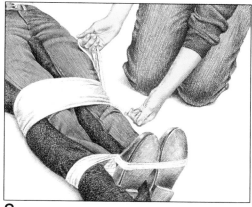

3 Tie a wide piece of material around the victim's knees, and knot the ends together on the uninjured side, again using a reef knot.

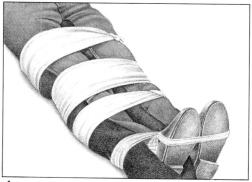

4 Tie a third and fourth bandage above and below the site of the fracture.

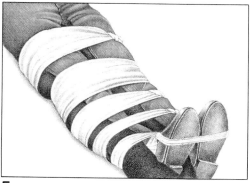

5 Tie a fifth bandage around the thigh or calf, avoiding the fracture.

Sports injuries

Two of the most common types of sports injuries are pulled muscles and sprained joints. The damage is similar in each case – tissue in the muscle or joint is torn and internal bleeding occurs, causing swelling and pain.

When one of these injuries occurs you should stop playing immediately, and rest. If you can use the injured part again in five minutes without pain, then it is safe to play on. But if the pain persists, you need treatment.

It is always possible that a bone has been broken (see page 98), in which case go to the emergency department of the local hospital. Suspect a broken bone if:

- The swollen part cannot be used.
- The swelling develops within minutes.
- The pain continues to be severe.

Treating a damaged muscle or joint

If the pain is not too severe and the swelling develops slowly it is usually safe to treat the injury without expert help.

- Put a cold compress on the injured area. Make the compress by putting ice cubes in a plastic bag and crushing them with a hammer or brick. Wrap the bag in a towel before applying it. Alternatively, use a cloth soaked in cold water and wrung out. The cold will cause the blood vessels to narrow and reduce bleeding.
- Bind the compress onto the injured part with a bandage and leave it for 20 to 30 minutes. The pressure also helps to close the blood vessels and slow the bleeding. But take care not to tie the bandage so tight as to cut off the circulation. If the person's fingers or toes become cold or tingle, loosen the bandage.
- At the same time, raise the injured area above the level of the heart for 30 minutes to an hour. This also slows the bleeding. Keep the limb raised as much as possible for the next 24 hours.
- If necessary, take aspirin or acetaminophen in recommended doses to reduce pain the first night after an injury. But painkillers should never be used so that you can go on playing. Pain is a valuable warning sign.
- When the injured area has been free of pain for at least ten days, light exercise can be started again.
- If recovery is very slow, or if the problem recurs frequently, see your doctor.

When muscles stiffen up

The reason why muscles stiffen up is not fully understood, but a probable cause is that many small tears occur in the muscles. Also, during exercise pressure builds up inside the blood vessels in the muscles. Some of the fluid in which the blood cells are carried seeps out into the muscle fibers and builds up the pressure there, causing stiffness.

The best treatment is gentle exercise – easy swimming, for example – which helps the fluid to be reabsorbed. Careful warming-up reduces stiffness, and so does "winding down." After hard exercise do not stop immediately; have a period of gentle exercise. Avoid wallowing in a hot bath after exercise. A quick shower and a brisk rubdown are much better.

Long-lasting injuries from overuse

Regular exercise often involves the repeated use of the same part of the body, and this can lead to the gradual development of painful injuries such as tennis elbow, golfer's shoulder and runner's knee.

To begin with, one part of the body aches toward the end of exercise. Then, as the damage increases, the pain lasts longer after exercise and may occur at other times, perhaps when in bed. This type of injury needs expert attention.

HOW DANGEROUS IS YOUR SPORT?

In North America the sporting activity that causes the most injuries is bicycling. But this statistic may reflect the level of participation rather than the danger associated with the sport.

Bicycling accidents usually produce broken bones and head injuries. Baseball and hockey also contribute to head injuries. Basketball and football injuries are usually to the knees; soccer injuries, to the arms. In squash, tennis and badminton, pulled muscles and sprains are the most common injuries, but eye injuries are also numerous in squash.

Most deaths in sport result from injuries to the head and spine – when the participant is thrown from a motorcycle or falls while rock climbing, for example.

The following list of 12 sports shows the rate of injuries in each one as a percentage of total sport injuries in North America requiring hospital treatment.

Bicycling (including bicycles, mopeds, all-terrain vehicles and minibikes)	29.0
Baseball	15.5
Basketball	12.0
Hockey	11.8
Football	9.6
Soccer	5.3
Ball games (including volleyball, rugby, lacrosse)	4.2
Swimming	3.5
Running (including jogging)	2.4
Tennis, badminton, squash, racquetball	2.3
Gymnastics (including aerobics)	1.8
Skiing	1.2

The first step is a period of rest, but if that does not help, see your doctor.

How to avoid sports injuries
Many sports injuries can be prevented altogether by proper training for the sport and warming-up immediately before a game.

Using the right shoes and equipment also cuts down the risk of injury. This is particularly important in sports such as skiing and rock climbing, but in almost every form of exercise problems can be reduced if you wear the right shoes – broad enough tennis shoes, for example, or jogging shoes with well-padded heels.

DO'S AND DON'TS ABOUT SPORTS INJURIES

An unconscious player

DO roll an unconscious player into the recovery position (page 136).

DON'T lay an unconscious person flat on his face.

DO remove foreign material (chewing gum, broken dentures, broken teeth, grass) from the mouth to prevent choking.

DON'T move an unconscious person with a suspected head or neck injury.

Damaged bones

DO support the injured area with padding, a splint or bandage.

DON'T attempt to manipulate a fractured bone or dislocation.

Injuries to the face

DO sit a player upright and press a cold pad to a black eye – which results from bleeding into the soft tissue around the eyeball.

DON'T waste time and money on applying a raw steak to a black eye. This is no more effective than using a cold pad.

DO treat a nosebleed by squeezing the soft part of the nose between finger and thumb and breathing through your mouth for 15 minutes.

DON'T continue with the treatment if the nosebleed lasts for more than 30 minutes. Either contact your doctor or go to a hospital.

DO splash water with your hand on your eye if you get dirt or mud in it.

DON'T add antiseptic to the water used on the affected eye.

Cuts and abrasions

DO thoroughly clean and disinfect an abrasion caused by the skin being scraped along a hard surface, such as the ground.

DON'T forget to protect yourself against tetanus (lockjaw) – which can arise from a simple scratch – with an antitetanus injection. Booster injections should be given every ten years.

DO see a doctor if particles of dirt remain in the abrasion after cleaning. A partly cleaned abrasion can result in an ugly scar – especially if the face is affected.

DON'T use old creams or harsh disinfectants on wounds; they can infect the cut or destroy tissues.

Caring for the feet

DO wash and carefully dry your feet immediately after sport to prevent athlete's foot – a fungus that affects sweaty skin.

DON'T soak your feet in very hot water.

Stiff muscles

DO take a quick warm shower or bath – followed by a cold shower or dip – to ease stiffness. Gentle exercise also helps.

DON'T wallow in hot water after sport or exercise.

DON'T sit around "resting."

Sprains and strains

Injuries to the joints and muscles – known as sprains and strains – are common and can be extremely painful.

A sprain occurs in a joint when a ligament – the flexible tissue that holds the bones together – is wrenched or torn. A strain occurs when a muscle is overstretched or torn.

Treatment for both injuries includes a cold compress, raising the injured limb and firm bandaging. All three techniques are aimed at restricting internal bleeding from the damaged tissues.

To make a cold compress, put some ice cubes into a plastic bag, knot the opening of the bag and crush the ice with a hammer or brick. Then wrap the bag of ice in a towel and apply it to the injury. Leave it in place for 20 to 30 minutes. If no ice is available, use a package of frozen peas, or soak a small towel or some other piece of cloth in cold water and squeeze out the excess, then wrap the towel around the injured area. Rewet the towel as necessary.

A cold compress works by chilling and constricting the blood vessels around the injury, thus limiting the swelling caused by internal bleeding. To be effective, though, the compress needs to be applied within about 30 minutes.

After about 30 minutes, most of the swelling will already have taken place and the compress will no longer be of much help. In these circumstances raise the limb and bandage it firmly for support instead.

TREATING A SPRAINED ANKLE

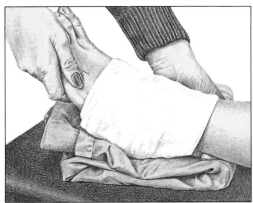

1 *Remove the shoe and raise the foot above the level of the heart. If the sprain has occurred within the past 15 to 30 minutes, apply a cold compress to the injured joint and bandage it in place for 20 to 30 minutes.*

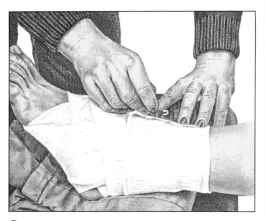

2 *After removing the compress, bandage the joint firmly. For an ankle joint, make one turn around the ankle, then go over the instep, under the foot, back across the instep and around the ankle again several times.*

TREATING A STRAINED MUSCLE

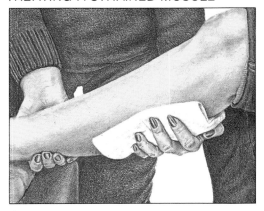

1 *Put the victim in the most comfortable position possible, with the injured limb above the level of the heart. Apply a cold compress to the strained muscle, and bandage it in place for 20 to 30 minutes.*

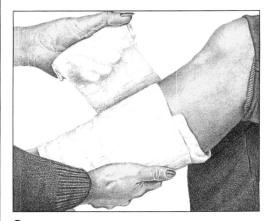

2 *Remove the compress and bandage the area firmly, but not so tightly as to stop circulation. The muscle may swell, causing pain if the bandage is too tight. Support a strained arm in an arm sling (see page 121).*

First aid and
medical emergencies

A sprained joint

The ankle is the joint most often affected by sprains, but the wrist, elbow, knee, hip and shoulder can also suffer.

A severe sprain can be extremely painful and is hard to distinguish from a fractured bone. If you are in any doubt, treat the injury as a fracture and get medical help (see *Fractures*, page 98, and *Splints*, page 127).

An ankle sprain occurs when a foot turns suddenly while walking or running – one of the reasons why boots (which help to support the ankle joints) are recommended for people walking in rough, stony country.

If a wrist, elbow or shoulder is sprained, support it in an arm sling after treatment with both a cold compress and firm bandaging (see *Bandages*, page 56, and *Slings*, page 121).

There are three main symptoms of sprains:
• Pain when moving the joint.
• Swelling of the joint, followed later by discoloration of the skin.
• Tenderness of the area over the torn ligament.

A strained muscle

A muscle may become overstretched or torn by sudden, unaccustomed exertion, perhaps when lifting a heavy weight. It can also be torn during a fall. If the injury occurs while playing sport it is known as a "pulled muscle," and usually affects the calf or thigh (see page 130).

The main symptoms are:
• Sudden, sharp pain in the muscle.
• Stiffness or cramp developing in the muscle.
• Swelling of the area.
• Possibly discoloration of the skin.

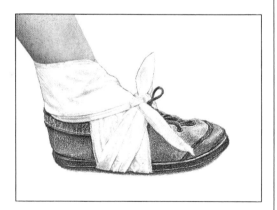

SUPPORTING AN ANKLE IN AN EMERGENCY
If you sprain an ankle during a country hike, leave your shoe and sock on, and bind a figure-eight bandage over the shoe or boot. This may give enough support to get you home.

Stab wounds

A nail sticking out of a piece of wood, or any other sharp object such as a bicycle spoke or needle, can cause a potentially serious wound.

On the surface the wound may look so small as not to be worth worrying about, but it may go deep into the flesh, carrying dirt or germs with it. If the wound becomes infected, the infection can spread to other parts of the body, causing serious illness and even death.

A stab wound can also cause serious internal injury to blood vessels and nerves.

Treat all stab wounds as serious. Stop any bleeding, dress the wound and take the victim to your doctor or to the emergency department of your local hospital.

If the object which caused the wound remains embedded in the flesh, do not try to remove it. It could be helping to plug the wound, and pulling it out could make the bleeding much worse. Instead, cover the object with a ring-pad (see page 58) or the bottom half of a paper cup, so that it will not be forced deeper by the dressing while the victim is being taken to hospital.

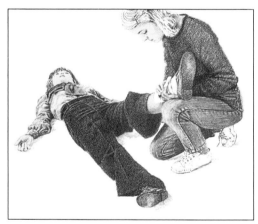

DEALING WITH A STAB WOUND
Stop any bleeding by pressing around the wound with a clean pad, or your bare hands. Do not try to remove any object embedded in the wound. Raise the injured area above the level of the heart to help stem the bleeding. Bandage the wound and get medical help.

Stroke

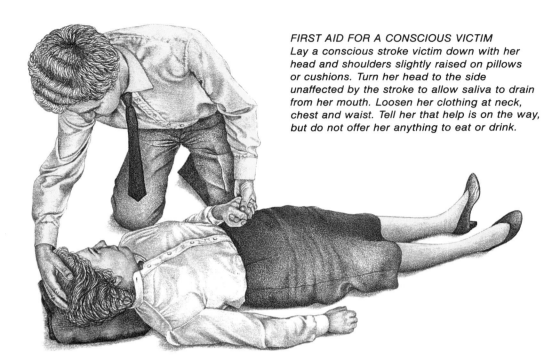

FIRST AID FOR A CONSCIOUS VICTIM
Lay a conscious stroke victim down with her head and shoulders slightly raised on pillows or cushions. Turn her head to the side unaffected by the stroke to allow saliva to drain from her mouth. Loosen her clothing at neck, chest and waist. Tell her that help is on the way, but do not offer her anything to eat or drink.

A person suffering a stroke may become weak or paralyzed down one side of the body, including the face, arm and leg.

Alternatively, the victim may have difficulty in speaking or swallowing, with only slight weakness in the limbs.

The victim may also suffer confusion, drowsiness and involuntary urination. The symptoms can resemble drunkenness.

A severe stroke will cause unconsciousness.

What you should do
• If the victim is conscious, lay her down, with head and shoulders slightly raised on pillows or cushions.
• Turn her head to one side to allow saliva to drain from the mouth.
• Call 911 and ask for an ambulance, then contact the patient's own doctor.
• Loosen clothing around the patient's neck, chest and waist to help blood circulation and breathing.
• Do not give her anything to eat or drink.
• If the patient becomes unconscious, put her in the recovery position (see page 136).

The aftereffects of a stroke
A person who suffers a stroke that paralyzes the right side of the body may also be unable to speak, write, read or understand speech, but if the paralysis is on the left, the person may lose the awareness of the left half of the body only.

Recovery from a stroke may be complete, with little risk of recurrence; but more usually – especially in elderly patients – the arm and, to

a lesser extent, the leg on the affected side of the body will remain disabled.

A massive stroke, particularly in an older patient, is grave; but if the patient survives the first month, a considerable amount of activity can often be restored.

The hospital will arrange a course of physiotherapy aimed at restoring the patient to as much activity as possible so that he or she can return home.

Relatives, with the help of their family doctor and hospital outpatient treatment, can make a large contribution to recovery. In the early days they can learn how to exercise the patient's affected limbs to prevent the muscles and joints from becoming stiff.

They can also help by speaking slowly or repeating things that seem not to be understood. They should listen carefully if speech is poor, and spend time talking to the patient, showing him photographs of friends and family, and encouraging him in his former interests.

Many areas have day hospitals which the patient can attend. This eases the burden on relatives while providing additional therapeutic help for the victim.

Hospital outpatient and social services personnel may be able to offer some help in obtaining special aids for use in the home. These aids include special beds, hoists, or walkers. Ask which aids are most appropriate for your situation.

To reduce the risk of further strokes, the patient should stop smoking, watch his weight and follow any treatment prescribed.

Sunburn

If sunburn is very severe and distressing, take the patient to a doctor who may prescribe a cream to give relief.

See a doctor also if the patient has a headache, nausea or a high temperature, because he may be suffering from heatstroke as well as sunburn (see page 106).

If the sunburn is out of all proportion to the time the skin was exposed to the sun, the patient may be suffering from a condition called photosensitivity, which can be brought on by some medicines. The patient should see his doctor, who may prescribe an alternative medicine.

Treating mild sunburn
The symptoms of sunburn can range from skin that turns pink and feels rather hot to skin that becomes red, swollen, blistered and extremely painful.

Reasonably mild sunburn can be treated at home without seeing a doctor.
• Keep the skin cool with calamine lotion or cold compresses. Make the compress by soaking a towel or other cloth in cold water and squeezing out the excess.
• Leave blistered skin exposed to the air.
• Take aspirin to relieve the pain. If you are allergic to aspirin, take acetaminophen instead.
• Avoid clothes that rub the sore area.
• Do not allow further exposure to the sun until the symptoms have disappeared.

How to avoid sunburn
Sunburn is caused by the ultraviolet rays of the sun. Fair-skinned people, who have little pigment in the skin, burn more easily than people with dark skin.
• To prevent sunburn, avoid overexposure to the sun on the first day of your vacation, particularly if you are fair skinned. Expose the skin for only 30 minutes the first day, increasing by 30 minutes each day until you have developed a suntan which will give protection. Remember that light cloud does not stop the sun's rays from burning.
• One half hour before going into the sun, apply a suntan lotion with an SPF (sun protection factor) appropriate to your type of skin. The higher the SPF number – they range from 2 to 15 – the more protection you get. Remember to reapply the lotion frequently, especially if you swim or exercise.
• Avoid tanning between 11 a.m. and 3 p.m., when the sun's ultraviolet rays are the strongest.
• Keep small children covered with a shirt during the first days of a vacation. Increase their exposure gradually.
• Remember that you can get burned without being aware it is happening. Sunburn only becomes apparent a few hours after exposure.
• Suntan lotions that do not have an SPF number will not protect you from sunburn. Use them only after you have been exposed to the sun for several days.

Tooth injuries

All injuries to the teeth should be checked as soon as possible by a dentist or hospital dental department. If there are serious injuries to the mouth, the immediate aim is to ensure that the victim can breathe properly.
• Clear broken teeth and blood from the mouth with your fingers.
• If the victim is conscious and has no other serious injuries, sit him in a chair with his head tilted forward over a bowl or basin.
• Call 911 and ask for an ambulance, or drive the victim to your local hospital. He should travel sitting up, leaning over the bowl.
• Never allow a person who is bleeding from the mouth to lie on his back, because he may choke on the blood.

When a tooth has been knocked out
If a tooth is knocked out completely, there may be profuse bleeding from the socket.
• Make a pad slightly larger than the socket from sterile gauze or other clean material. The pad should project slightly above the level of the surrounding teeth.
• Get the victim to put it over the socket and bite on it firmly, spitting out any blood that leaks through.
• If the bleeding still does not stop, call your dentist and ask for emergency treatment, or go to the emergency department of your local hospital.

Saving a knocked-out tooth
It is sometimes possible to save a tooth that has been knocked out of its socket.

The roots must be kept moist, so wrap the tooth in a piece of sterile gauze or clean cloth, dampen it, and place it in a container over ice for the trip to the hospital or dentist.

If you get toothache
If you develop toothache at night or during a weekend when you cannot contact your dentist, check the *Yellow Pages* for dentists offering emergency service. However, the fees for such services can be high. Alternatively, ask a druggist or the emergency department of a hospital for the name of a dentist who can help.
• While you are waiting for a dentist, relieve the pain with analgesics such as aspirin in recommended doses.
• Try also holding in your mouth a mouthful of ice-cold water or a mouthful of hot, salty water (one teaspoon of salt in a glass of water). Hold the water in your mouth for at least five minutes, spitting it out and renewing it as necessary, and repeat the treatment every 2 to 3 hours.

First aid and medical emergencies

Unconsciousness

A person who has become unconscious is in danger of choking to death if left lying face up.

Vomit, blood or saliva may block the top of the windpipe, or the base of the tongue may slide back over the windpipe.

Normal reflexes do not work properly when people become unconscious. So they may not cough or turn over if something blocks their airway, as they would do automatically if they were asleep.

If an unconscious person is breathing normally, put her in the recovery position. This is a lifesaving technique and, in most circumstances, it takes priority over other treatment. The exception is when a victim has back or neck injuries. In that case, she should not be moved at all (see page 55).

If the victim is particularly heavy, it may be necessary to get someone else to help you by pushing while you pull.

If an unconscious person has to be carried on a stretcher, or if she is in a confined space, a modified version of the recovery position is used. In this case a rolled blanket is used to prop up one side of the patient's body, rather than a bent arm and leg.

If the unconscious person is not breathing, you must begin artificial respiration immediately (see page 50). In any case get someone to call 911 and ask for an ambulance or, if nobody is

IS THE VICTIM BREATHING?

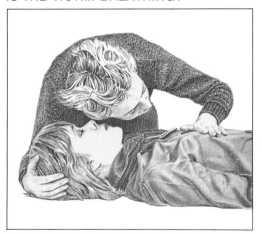

1 Tilt the victim's head back to open the airway. Put your ear to her nose and mouth, and listen for breathing. Watch the chest, or rest your hand on it to feel its rise and fall.

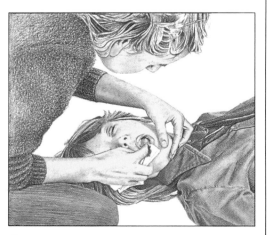

2 If the victim is not breathing, start artificial respiration (see page 50). If she is breathing, clear the mouth of foreign matter. Use a tissue to wipe blood from around the mouth.

THE RECOVERY POSITION

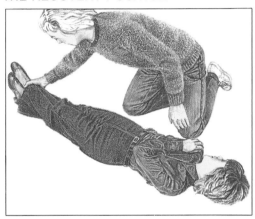

1 Kneel beside the victim and turn her head toward you. Tuck the near arm under the body, keeping it straight. Put the other arm across the chest, and the far ankle over the near ankle.

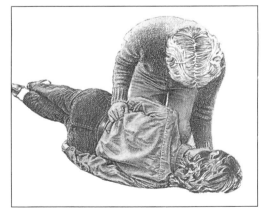

2 Grip the clothing at the far hip and turn the victim onto her front by pulling quickly toward you. Cushion her head with one hand as you do so, and support her body with your knees as she rolls over.

available, do it yourself at the first opportunity. Anyone who has been unconscious, even for a short time, should receive immediate medical treatment.

Handle any serious wound gently while positioning the victim. Once in the recovery position, she can be helped by having clothing at the neck, chest and waist loosened. Injuries can be treated while you wait for expert help to arrive.

Whatever the circumstances, do not leave an unconscious person alone at any time, and do not give her anything to eat or drink, even if she regains consciousness (see also *What to do if someone collapses*, page 199).

Three stages of unconsciousness

Unconsciousness is not always total insensibility. There are three stages, and a person may go through all three or remain in one. The three stages are:

• Drowsiness, in which the victim is easily roused for a few moments, but then passes back into a sleeplike state. She may be able to give reasonably coherent answers to questions you ask her about her condition.

• Stupor, in which the victim does not react to questions easily or does so incoherently, giving the impression of being drunk.

• Coma, in which the victim cannot be roused at all, and is motionless and silent.

First aid and
medical emergencies

WHILE YOU WAIT FOR HELP

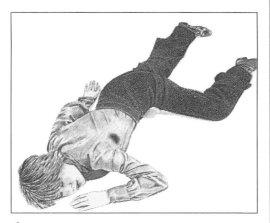

3 *Tilt the victim's chin backward to straighten the throat. This will keep the airway open, preventing the tongue from slipping back into the throat, and so will allow her to go on breathing freely.*

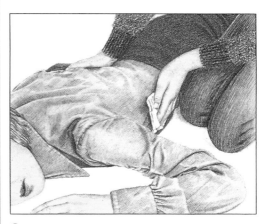

1 *Once the victim is safely in the recovery position, loosen any tight clothing at the neck, chest and waist to assist breathing and blood circulation. Provide fresh air by opening a window or door.*

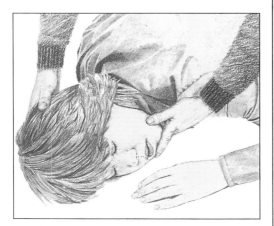

4 *Bend the arm nearest to you to prop up the upper body. Bend the leg nearest to you to prop up the lower body. Pull the other arm out from under the body to prevent her from rolling over onto her back. Do not leave her alone.*

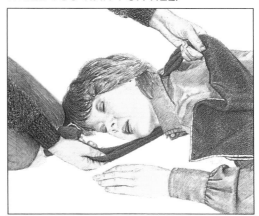

2 *Check for any other injuries and stop any bleeding (see page 60). See if the victim is wearing a Medic-Alert bracelet. If so, she should have a card identifying her illness and perhaps instructions for emergencies.*

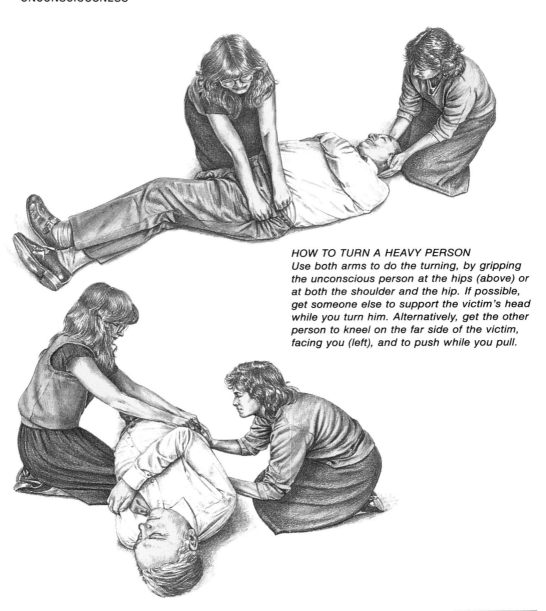

HOW TO TURN A HEAVY PERSON
Use both arms to do the turning, by gripping the unconscious person at the hips (above) or at both the shoulder and the hip. If possible, get someone else to support the victim's head while you turn him. Alternatively, get the other person to kneel on the far side of the victim, facing you (left), and to push while you pull.

SUPPORTING AN UNCONSCIOUS PERSON ON A STRETCHER

Use a modified version of the recovery position if you are carrying an unconscious person on a stretcher or if she is in some other confined space. Put a rolled blanket or coat under the side toward which the victim is facing.

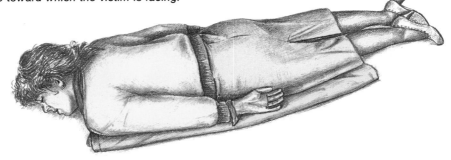

Vertigo

An unpleasant feeling of giddiness, as though the patient's head is moving when it is actually still, usually has a cause related to the ear.

The giddiness may be accompanied by nausea and some loss of hearing, and also by flickering of the eyes – a condition called nystagmus.

Vertigo can arise from several different medical conditions.

• An injury to the head.
• Ménière's disease and labyrinthitis, two ailments that disturb the hearing and also the balance of the inner ear.
• High blood pressure.
• A blockage of the blood vessels leading to the brain.
• Travel sickness.

What you should do
The patient should lie down quietly and rest until the attack ends. The length of an attack can range from seconds to hours.

Consult a doctor if:
• The attacks recur.
• There is severe vomiting.
• Deafness develops.

The doctor may prescribe drugs to relieve the symptoms, but even without treatment a person with recurring vertigo may recover spontaneously after several months.

Some elderly people suffer from vertigo without a treatable cause being found.

Positional vertigo, which is felt when the head is in certain positions, may continue to occur.

Whooping cough

A child who has a cold with a runny nose and bouts of excessive coughing may be in the early stages of whooping cough.

As the disease develops the cough will become worse, mainly at night. A few days after the cold begins, the "whoop" will start – a sudden noisy intake of breath at the end of a coughing spasm. Vomiting may also occur after the coughing.

What you should do
Whooping cough is a serious disease that can lead to pneumonia and to severe dehydration if fluid loss from the vomiting is not controlled. So notify your doctor as soon as you suspect that a child has the disease.

The doctor may prescribe antibiotics for the patient and also for other children in the family. These do not cure whooping cough, but may prevent it from spreading to other people. In severe cases the patient will be sent to hospital for treatment.

While nursing the patient at home, provide extra drinks to make up for fluid lost by vomiting.

Do not expose the patient to cigarette smoke – it will make the cough worse.

Whooping cough may last for a period ranging from three weeks to as long as four months.

How to prevent whooping cough
The disease is caused by bacteria which are spread by droplets in the air breathed out by an infected child.

Because whooping cough is more dangerous than the risks of immunization, all children should have a course of five injections (usually with diphtheria and tetanus vaccine) at 2, 4, 6 and 18 months, and between 4 and 6 years.

Because of a rare chance of brain damage, however, immunization may be risky under a number of circumstances:
• If the child has epileptic seizures.
• If there is a history of epilepsy in brothers, sisters or parents.
• If the child has a disorder of the nervous system or is known to have suffered brain damage at birth.
• If there is a feverish illness at the time of the proposed injection.
• If there has been a severe reaction to a previous dose of the vaccine.

In all these cases – or if you are in any doubt – consult your doctor before the child is immunized.

First aid and medical emergencies

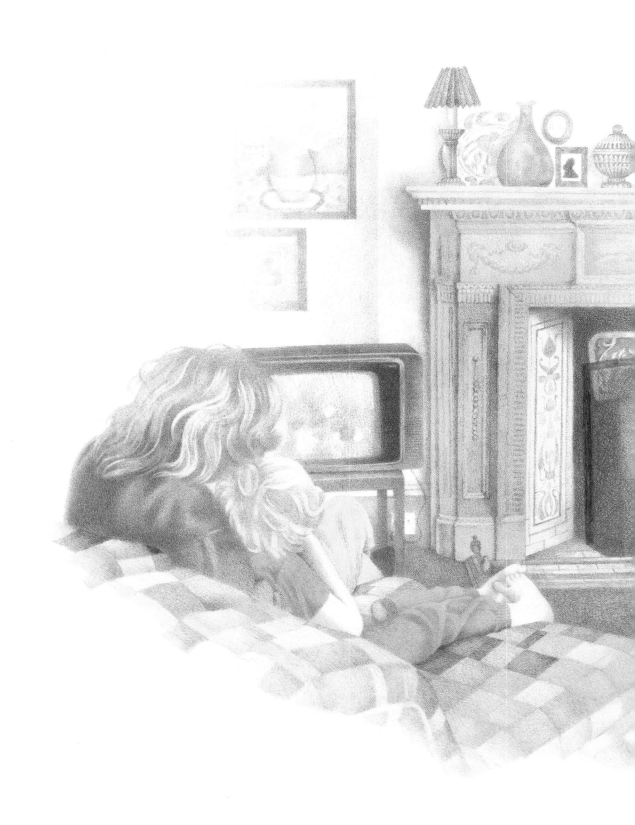

In the home and at work

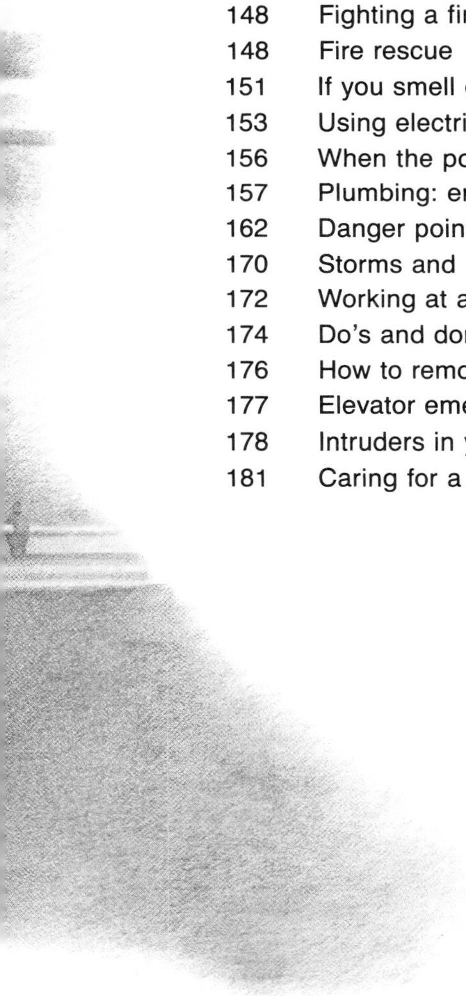

142   If you are trapped in a blazing house

148   Fighting a fire

148   Fire rescue

151   If you smell gas or suspect a leak

153   Using electricity safely

156   When the power supply fails

157   Plumbing: emergency repairs

162   Danger points – room by room

170   Storms and high winds

172   Working at a height

174   Do's and don'ts of using tools

176   How to remove stains

177   Elevator emergency

178   Intruders in your home

181   Caring for a sick or injured animal

If you are trapped in a blazing house

Once a fire takes hold, there is only one completely safe place to be – outside. If you are trapped inside, getting out is the priority.

Planning an escape route

If a fire should occur in your home, you have a better chance of escaping quickly if you have worked out the best route from each room beforehand. If you have not done this, take a moment to decide the best way out, unless this is obvious.

• If you cannot get down the stairs, for instance, consider which upstairs room is the easiest to get out of. Which has the largest windows? Which window is closest to the ground, and which has the clearest drop and the softest ground beneath it? Are there any balconies or garage roofs which might make it easier to reach the ground safely?

• Consider, too, which windows can be opened. It is more difficult to climb out through a window you have had to break, and it is more difficult to break a double-glazed window than a single-glazed one.

How to get out

• Try to find a safe way past the blaze to a ground floor door or window. Firemen follow three cardinal rules when they move through a burning building: test all doors; close doors and windows; and stay low.

• Feel each door before opening it. Do not open it if it is hot, or if smoke is seeping around the edges. In a large or unfamiliar building, you can test doors quickly by touching the knob briefly with the back of your hand. The metal knob conducts heat faster than the paneling.

• Use the back of the hand for safety – heat on the back will make you jerk it away instinctively.

• If the door is cool, stand behind it, open it a crack and glance out before deciding whether to go through. Put your foot against the back of the door to prevent it being opened by pressure from hot gases. If there are flames beyond, flinging the door wide could create a draft and cause a lethal surge in the fire's intensity.

• Close doors behind you and also close any open windows, if possible. This will help to slow the spread of fire. Open doors and windows feed air to the flames and allow them an easier passage from room to room.

• Stay low. Smoke fills a room from the ceiling down. Near the floor the air should be easier to breathe, and it should be easier to see.

When you have got out

• Once you have got outside and are safely clear of the building, check that everyone is accounted for. Stop anyone going back into the building to rescue possessions.

• Send someone to a neighbor's house or a phone booth to dial 911 or the fire department, if that has not been done already.

• Remember when calling to give the exact

MOVING SAFELY FROM ROOM TO ROOM

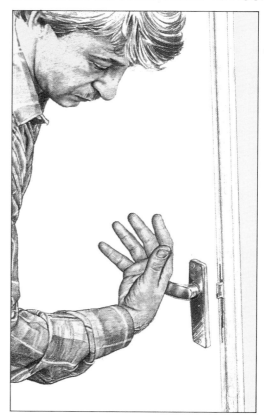

1 *As you move through rooms on your way out, test each door for heat by touching the handle or knob briefly. Use the back of the hand for safety – heat on the back will make you jerk it away instinctively, and avoid burns.*

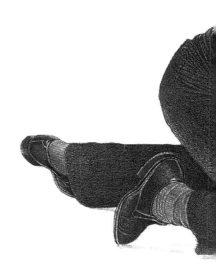

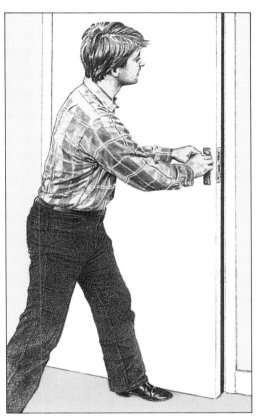

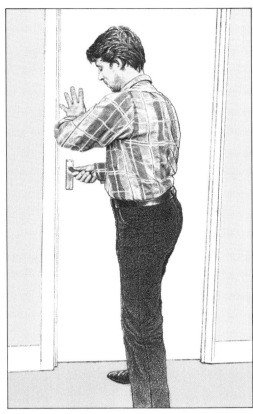

In the home and at work

2 *Stand behind the door and brace your foot against the bottom before opening it a crack to peep out into the next room. Your foot will stop the door being forced wide open by the pressure of any hot gases on the other side.*

3 *Once through the door, take the time to close it firmly behind you. This will help to slow the spread of fire, fumes and smoke. Open doors (or windows) create drafts that feed air to the flames, intensifying the blaze.*

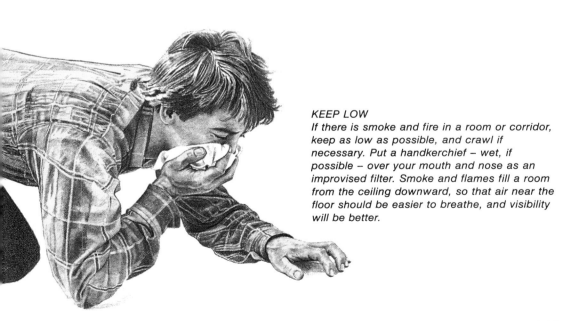

KEEP LOW
If there is smoke and fire in a room or corridor, keep as low as possible, and crawl if necessary. Put a handkerchief – wet, if possible – over your mouth and nose as an improvised filter. Smoke and flames fill a room from the ceiling downward, so that air near the floor should be easier to breathe, and visibility will be better.

address and nearest cross street – in a moment of stress it is easy to forget such vital details, and that could delay the arrival of help.

If the exit is blocked

• Try to reach a window or balcony. Open the window. If there is a balcony get onto it and close the window behind you.

• If you are on the ground floor, jump out.

• If you are not on the ground floor and the drop is not too far and onto soft ground – a flowerbed, for example – hang out of the window with fully outstretched arms to lessen the distance you have to fall. It may be safer to risk a sprain or a broken bone than to wait for rescue by the fire department.

• Just before you drop, let go with one hand and use that arm and your legs to push yourself away from the wall as you fall.

• Do not jump out of an upstairs window except as a last resort. Instead, use anything to hand – knotted sheets, for example – to reach the ground or at least get closer to it before dropping. Anchor the rope to a solid piece of furniture inside the room.

• If you have to break a window to get out, use a chair or kick it out. If you have to use your hands, wrap something around your fist to protect it, or use an elbow if you are wearing something with sleeves.

• Knock out jagged pieces of glass around the edge, or throw a blanket or clothing over them, before climbing through.

• If there is no safe way down, shut the door of the room, open the window, hang out a sheet to signal for help, then wave and shout to attract attention.

• Try to keep the blaze out of the room while waiting for help.

• Douse the walls and door between you and the flames with water. This will delay or prevent the spread of fire.

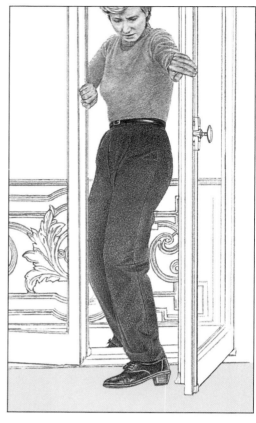

GET OUT ONTO A BALCONY
If you are trapped by fire on an upstairs floor and you can get out onto a balcony, do so. Close the door into the room before you go. Once outside, shut the balcony door firmly behind you and shout for help. Try to remain calm while you are waiting to be rescued.

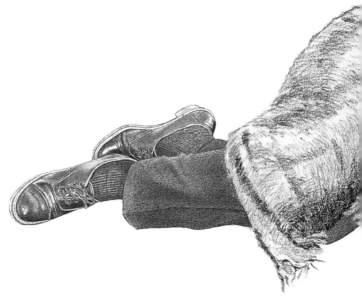

WHEN YOU ARE TRAPPED IN AN UPSTAIRS ROOM

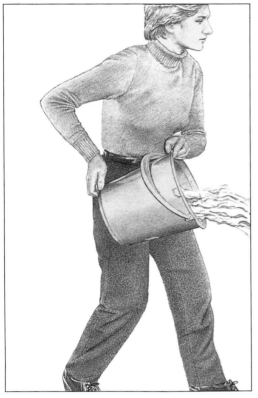

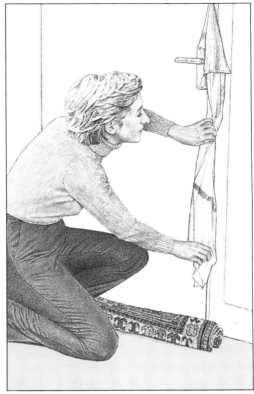

1 *If you cannot get onto a balcony, try to keep the blaze out of the room. If you can reach a faucet, douse the walls and door with buckets of water. If you do not have a bucket, use a saucepan, vase or any large container.*

2 *Stop smoke and fumes from entering the room by stuffing the cracks between the door and door frame with cloths – curtains, if necessary. Wet them first, if possible, and put a rolled-up carpet or blanket against the bottom.*

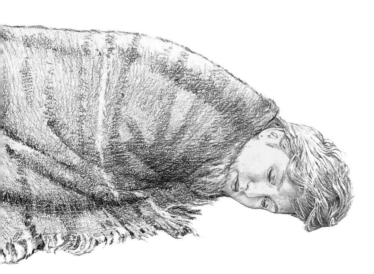

IF YOUR CLOTHES
CATCH FIRE
Do not panic and run if your clothes catch fire. You will only fan the flames. Stop, drop to the floor at once, and put your hands on your head to keep your hair from igniting. Smother the flames by rolling slowly – not quickly – over and over. Wrap yourself in a blanket or carpet, if you can.

• Stuff cloths – wet, if possible – into the ventilation outlets and the cracks around the door to stop smoke and fumes getting in. Smoke is a far bigger killer than the flames themselves – for every two people burned to death in fires, five lose their lives through being asphyxiated by smoke or toxic fumes.

Escaping from a high-rise building

Just as you should plan in advance your escape route from a house fire, you should also know what to do to escape a fire in a high-rise building or hotel.

• Never use an elevator in a fire – you could be trapped if the power fails, or the doors could open on the floor that is ablaze, killing all inside.

• In many hotels a fire escape map is displayed in each room or corridor. Make a point of studying it when you arrive – there may not be time in an emergency.

• Make a mental picture of the halls and stairs between your room and the exit.

• Try the stairway door – if it is locked, have it opened.

• If a fire starts, make your way out as quickly as possible, testing each door before opening it, and closing it behind you. Main doors made of fire-resistant materials can take 45 minutes or longer to burn through, and make excellent fire shields.

• Always take your key with you, in case you are forced back into your room.

• As you go, alert others by banging on doors and shouting "Fire!" Set off a fire alarm if there is one.

• If the stairway is blocked by flames or smoke, do not try to run through. Return to your room, or try to reach a floor which is not affected by the blaze. If necessary, walk up to the roof, then stand on the windward side of the building, with any smoke or flames being blown away from you, until firemen reach you.

• If you get trapped in your room and are too high to shout for help, wave a sheet, pillowcase or towel from the window to attract attention on the ground.

• If there is a telephone in your room, use it to call for help – the line may be open even if the fire has cut off the building's power supply.

When clothing catches fire

Clothing set ablaze through standing too near an unguarded fire or radiant heater is a common cause of serious burns – especially to children.

• Act instantly to smother the flames.

• If the clothing is your own, cross your arms over your chest, so that your hands touch your shoulders. This helps to keep the flames away from your face.

• Drop to the floor and roll over and over slowly.

• If possible, wrap yourself in a rug, wool blanket, coat or heavy drapes.

• If someone else's clothing is alight, get the victim onto the floor – trip him if necessary.

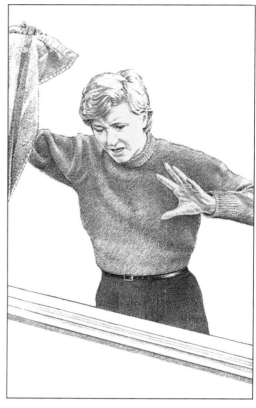

SIGNALING FOR HELP
If you are trapped in a high-rise building too far from the ground for your voice to be heard, attract attention by waving something from the window. Use the largest and most brightly colored piece of cloth you can find – a towel, say, a sheet, a rug or a curtain. Keep waving it until you are spotted by someone on the ground. You are unlikely to have to wait long for rescue. High-rise buildings are almost always in densely populated areas where a fire is likely to be noticed quickly and a fire department is probably within a few minutes' drive.

• Smother the fire with a rug, wool blanket, coat or heavy drapes.

• Throw water over the victim to help to cool him as well as extinguish the flames. Avoid using a fire extinguisher because it will not cool him, and any chemicals in it could cause difficulties when the burns are treated.

• When the fire is out, do not try to pull clothing away from the victim's skin.

• Call for medical help (dial 911) and treat the victim for shock (see page 120).

Using a rope ladder

In a house, storing a rope ladder on an upper floor is a useful precaution. You can buy a rope ladder at a safety equipment store.

Ideally it should have built-in supports so that

it stands away from the wall in use, leaving room for hands and toes.

A traditional rope ladder is difficult to use if you try to climb up or down it as you would a rigid ladder – facing the rungs.

Used that way, the ladder will hug the wall of the building unless there is someone at the bottom to hold it away.

However, if it is the only type available, there is a simple, effective technique used by sailors and mountaineers.

- Climb down the *side* rope of the ladder, placing one foot across the rung at the front of the ladder, and the other foot across the next rung at the back, splaying your feet with your toes pointing outward.
- Your shoulder and hip will hold the ladder away from the wall, allowing plenty of room for hands and feet to grip.

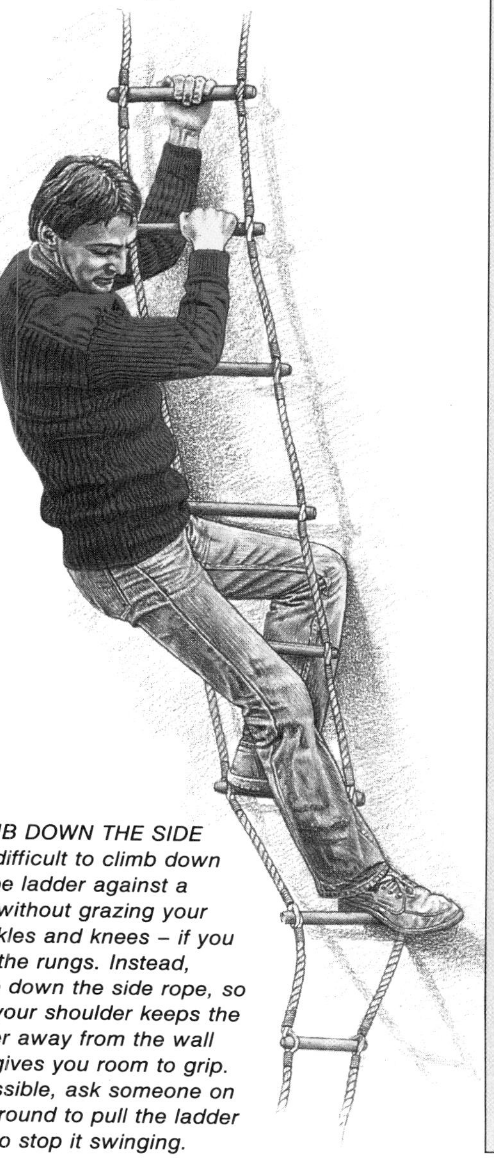

CLIMB DOWN THE SIDE
It is difficult to climb down a rope ladder against a wall without grazing your knuckles and knees – if you face the rungs. Instead, climb down the side rope, so that your shoulder keeps the ladder away from the wall and gives you room to grip. If possible, ask someone on the ground to pull the ladder taut to stop it swinging.

FIRE IN THE HOME: THE SOURCES OF DANGER

Every year in North America, more than 600,000 homes – single-family dwellings, duplexes, apartments and mobile homes – are damaged or destroyed by fires that are started by accident.

Each year more than 4,500 people die in fires in the home, and another 19,750 are burned – many seriously.

About 80 percent of all accidental fires can be traced to one of the following sources: heating and cooking equipment, electrical systems, smoking materials, matches and lighters, candles, tapers and open flames.

HEATING EQUIPMENT causes more than 195,000 blazes a year – about a third of all domestic fires in North America. Potential hazards include: central-heating systems (furnaces, boilers, etc.); water and space heaters; portable electric and kerosene heaters; chimneys and fireplaces. Chimneys – even those serving central-heating systems – catch fire if soot collects in them over long periods. And fire in them can, if unchecked, spread to the rest of the house. Have your chimney cleaned once a year.

COOKING EQUIPMENT is another major cause of domestic fires – nearly 123,000, or more than 20 percent of the total – and the fires are often started by blazing deep fat fryers and frying pans. But stoves, ovens, microwave ovens, electric kettles and cooking appliances, such as toasters and waffle irons, are also involved in household fires.

ELECTRICAL SYSTEMS are the source of some 55,000 accidental fires a year. The blazes are often set off by faulty wiring, incorrect fuses, and overloaded sockets.

SMOKING MATERIALS include cigars, cigarettes, pipes, matches and lighters, which start about 50,000 fires a year. Particularly dangerous is the fire started by a cigarette left on an upholstered armchair or sofa. It can roll down the back or side of the seat and the upholstery can smolder slowly, giving off poisonous fumes while the people in the house are asleep.

MATCHES and lighters (used for other purposes than smoking) start about 33,000 blazes a year. Often they are left too close to fires or are lit by children who are playing with them.

CANDLES, tapers and open flames from blowtorches and welding equipment cause around 30,000 fires each year.

Fighting a fire

If a fire breaks out, make sure that nobody is in danger. Only then should you even consider trying to put out a small fire. If the fire is large, fierce or spreading, get out and call 911 or the firemen.
• Stand back from the fire and out of the smoke.
• Stand on the side of the fire near your escape route so that you cannot be cut off.
• Never drag burning objects away from a fire.
• Work from the outside of the fire toward the center. Use water, sand or a fire extinguisher (see page 150).

These guidelines apply to all fires. Steps for dealing with specific fires are given below.

Deep fat fryers
Fires in deep fat fryers start when cooking oil gets too hot and bursts into flame. If smoke is rising from the fryer, the oil is about to ignite.
• Turn off the heat immediately.
• Do not move the fryer.
• Do not use water on the flames.
• Smother the flames with the lid of the fryer.
• Hold the lid in front of you to shield your face as you place it over the deep fryer.
• Once the fire is out, keep the fryer covered for about 30 minutes. Otherwise it might reignite.
• If the fire is uncontrollable, close all windows and doors, leave the house and call the fire department.

Electric blanket
• Unplug the blanket. But do not lift off the bedclothes – this will let air in and may turn a smoldering bed into a blaze.
• Call the fire department.
• Drench the bed with water.

Furniture
Furnishings upholstered with synthetic materials burn quickly, giving off smoke and toxic fumes.
• Do not try to put out the fire.
• Get everybody out of the room immediately.
• Close the door.
• Call the fire department – even if the fire appears to be out.
• Do not take smoldering or burning furniture outside. The fresh air could cause it to flare up.

Television sets or computers
Parts in older TV sets can overheat. As a result, a fire can start even if a set is off. A burning set gives off fierce flames and toxic fumes, and the tube behind the screen can explode. The same risks also apply to computers. TV and computer fires should be handled in the same way.
• If you smell burning rubber or plastic, or you see smoke, unplug the set and call a repairman.
• If smoke or flames begin to pour out, unplug the set or cut the power.
• Call the fire department.
• Do not throw water on a TV set or computer, or use a fire extinguisher of any kind.
• Keep away from the set until the fire is out.

Fire rescue

Entering a burning building to rescue someone calls for specialized knowledge and equipment and is highly dangerous for the inexperienced. Safety experts say it should always be left to the fire department.

If, however, you are escaping from a burning building where you have to rescue someone – a child, for example, or an elderly or disabled person – who has been trapped or overcome by smoke, there are just two priorities: do not endanger your own life; and act quickly. Get the victim outside as fast as possible, regardless of his or her injuries.
• Tie a wet handkerchief over your mouth and nose. This will keep out the smoke, although it cannot protect you from poisonous fumes.
• If you have a blanket or coat at hand, carry it with you or drape it around your shoulders. It

HOW TO DO A FIREMAN'S LIFT

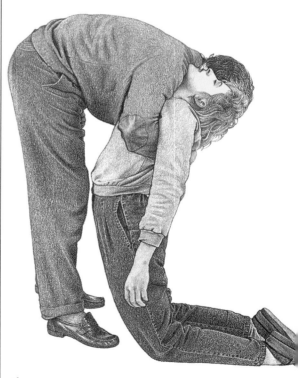

1 *Get the victim onto her feet. If she is unconscious, lay her face down with her head at your feet. With your arms under her armpits, raise her to her knees, then to her feet.*

may be useful for wrapping up the victim or for protecting both of you from heat.

• As you go through the building, test each door before you go through it by touching the knob with the back of your hand. If the knob is hot, do not enter the room.

• Do not go forward if there is any danger of your escape route being cut off.

• If the door is cool, hold the handle firmly when opening it so that the door cannot be sucked wide open by any hot gases inside. If it opens outward, stand behind it and put your foot against the back to stop it bursting open.

• Take several deep breaths. Open the door a crack and wait for any hot air to be released, then go in (see *If you are trapped in a blazing house*, page 142).

• Keep low to the floor if you enter a smoke-filled room. If necessary, crawl along the floor until you reach the victim.

• Once you find the victim, drag or carry her to safety as quickly as possible. Do not give first aid until you are both out of danger (see *Moving an injured person*, page 112).

Fireman's lift

If you have to negotiate stairs or manage many doors, you may find it easier to carry a victim with the fireman's lift shown below, which leaves you with one hand free, than to drag her.

• Get the victim onto her feet, facing you.

• Then put her across your shoulder.

• If you have to go down stairs while you are carrying someone in a fireman's lift, look down them first to see if there are any hazards, then go down backward.

In the home and at work

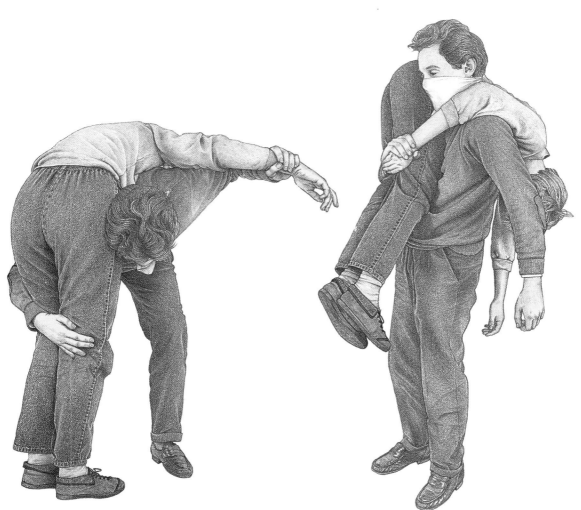

2 *Once she is on her feet, hold her right wrist with your left hand. Bend down, with knees bent, and put your head beside her right hip. Let her fall across your right shoulder.*

3 *Stand up carefully, keeping your back as straight as possible. Transfer her right wrist to your right hand, so leaving your left hand free to open doors and hold banisters.*

PROTECTING YOUR HOME AGAINST FIRE

• Do not smoke in bed.

• Provide deep ashtrays in all rooms where people might smoke.

• Keep matches well away from children.

• Do not light matches in closets.

• Do not run electric cords or wires under rugs, or string them around a room on hooks or nails. Check for any frayed cords.

• Unplug electric appliances such as TV sets and heaters when they are not in use. This is safer than just switching them off.

• Before leaving the house or going to bed, close all doors and windows in empty rooms.

• Never overfill deep fat fryers. Oil and fat expand when heated, and they could overflow onto the burner and catch fire.

• Keep furniture, curtains and bedding well away from open fires and electric heaters.

• Surround open fires with a fireguard. The guard should cover the entire fireplace.

• Do not put a mirror over the fireplace. It encourages people to get too close to the fire.

• Do not use candles or matches to check gas leaks. Call the gas company.

Fire extinguishers

The most useful piece of home fire fighting equipment is a portable fire extinguisher. It should be used to put out a small fire, but not a big one. Install the extinguishers near potential fire hazards.

Fire extinguishers are divided into classes A, B, C and D. Class A extinguishers hold water or water-based liquids, and classes B, C and D contain chemicals. Each class is used to put out fires involving specific materials.

CLASS A Use on wood, paper, cloth and trash. Do not use a class A extinguisher on electrical fires if the apparatus is switched on, or on flammable liquids such as gasoline, oil or cooking fat. Do not use on a TV fire, even if the set is switched off.

CLASS B Use on fuel oil, gas, paint, tar, cooking oil, solvents and other flammable liquids. Do not use water on this type of fire. This will cause the fire to spread explosively.

CLASS C Use on wiring, fuse boxes, conductors and other electric equipment. Switch off the current to convert this fire into a class A or B fire. Do not throw water on an electric fire. It can give a fatal shock.

CLASS D Use on metals such as aluminum, magnesium, potassium, sodium and zinc.

Match your fire extinguisher to potential fire hazards. For example, buy a BC type for possible cooking or electric fires, or an A for upholstered furniture. The ABC type is the best general-purpose fire extinguisher for the home.

The number preceding the A or B rating (for example, 1-A or 5-B) indicates the size of a standard test fire that the extinguisher can put out. The higher the number, the more fire the extinguisher puts out. If you are in doubt about what size of extinguisher to buy, choose one larger than you think you might need.

Learn how to use a fire extinguisher in advance. Crouch to keep clear of smoke, and move the extinguisher from side to side with a sweeping movement. Aim it at the base of the flames and work in from the edge.

Keep fire extinguishers regularly maintained. The supplier will be able to advise you on how often your extinguisher needs checking. Make sure that your extinguishers and fire detectors (see below) carry the label of a recognized national laboratory such as Underwriters' Laboratories or Factory Mutual.

Fire detectors

There are three kinds of fire detector. *Heat or thermal detectors* are suitable for closets or storage rooms, where heat can build up. *Flame detectors* are used in areas where fire might be expected to appear – for example, an open flame near flammable liquids. *Smoke detectors* give the earliest warning and are the most suitable for home use.

Two types of smoke detector are available. The *photoelectric model* has a light beam that spots smoke coming through its openings. When the smoke breaks the light beam, the detector sounds its alarm. The *ionization model* has a tiny amount of shielded radioactive material that breaks down air into charged atoms, resulting in a weak flow of electric current. Smoke disrupts the flow and sets off the alarm.

Each model has specific advantages. The photoelectric model responds quickly to smoke from smoldering fires. The ionization model is best at detecting fast-burning fires. Experts recommend that you have at least one of each model in your home. Both models are powered by batteries or by house current and can be installed easily.

The best locations for smoke detectors are near bedrooms and living areas. Do not place them near air currents from vents or radiators, dead-air corners or the end of halls. For maximum protection, install smoke detectors in the center of the ceiling in every room. Test detectors monthly and clean them yearly.

If you smell gas or suspect a leak

Natural gas is not poisonous, but it can be extremely dangerous when there are certain levels of it in the atmosphere. For example, it becomes explosive whenever it forms 5 to 15 percent of the gases in the air. It has no color, taste or smell of its own. But a smell is added deliberately, before the gas is piped to homes, to alert householders to leaks.

• If you get a strong odor of gas, put out cigarettes or any naked flames – a candle, say – at once.

• Alert others and get everyone out of the house.

• Do not turn any switch or electric appliance either on *or* off. Operating a switch in either direction is likely to cause a spark which could ignite the gas.

• Do not operate anything that might produce a spark or flame – a cigarette lighter, a flashlight, lamp, or telephone.

• Leave the doors and windows open as you exit to let the gas escape and to ventilate the house.

• Call the gas company from a phone outside the house. If you do not have the number, call 911 or the operator.

• Stay out of the house until the leak has been found and fixed, and the smell of gas cleared completely.

• Do not attempt to repair any appliances or pipes, or allow anyone else to do so. Repairs should be left to gas company employees or qualified gas fitters or plumbers.

When the gas has cleared
Simple gas escape repairs are usually carried out by the gas company without any charge to the customer. Moreover, it is unlikely that you will be charged for repairs to parts of the system

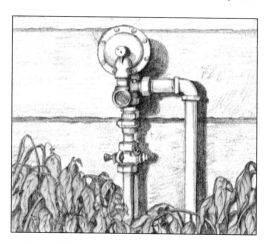

HOW TO SPOT AN OUTDOOR GAS LEAK
If you smell natural gas outdoors, look for signs of its escape route. Dead or wilting plants and dry soil near the base of a gas meter at the side of a house may be indications of a gas leak.

belonging to the gas company – that is, on the supply side of the gas meter in your home.

• Once the gas company has repaired the leak, make sure that all gas appliances are turned off.

• Then relight any pilot lights, unless the gas company already did this at the time the leak was fixed.

If the gas supply fails
The gas supply may be affected by problems outside the home – a burst gas main, say, or a sharp drop in pressure.

• If the gas pressure does drop sharply (so that the flames on a stove or heater become much smaller than usual), or the supply stops altogether so that the flames go out, turn off all gas appliances, and call the gas company immediately.

• Do not attempt to use the supply again until someone from the gas company has advised you that it is safe to do so.

If you think the meter is faulty
If you suspect that your gas meter is at fault – if, for example, it appears to be running when no gas is being used – ask your gas company to test it. Most gas companies make no charge for the test.

If you smell gas outside
Proceed as you would if you detected the smell of gas indoors.

• Put out any cigarettes or open flames.

• Do not switch on your car's ignition. Any spark could ignite the gas.

• Get out of the immediate area and call the local gas company or 911.

• Before you leave the area, you may notice some evidence of the outside leak. When you phone the gas company, describe any detail that might help its technicians to pinpoint and to correct the problem.

• Be aware of the signs of outdoor gas leaks. Look for signs of excavation and construction in the immediate area. Gas leaks sometimes occur when underground pipelines are disturbed by these activities.

• Underground gas leaks slowly dry out the soil by depriving it of water. A patch of dead or wilted vegetation in a grassy area or near an outdoor gas meter may indicate an underground gas leak.

• After rain, underground gas may bubble to the surface.

• During winter, ice or pavement covering the ground may impede an underground gas leak, causing the gas to escape at a site remote from the leak.

Living safely with gas
• Do not allow children to play near a gas appliance.

• Never use your gas oven or stove to heat your kitchen.

USING BOTTLED GAS

Bottled gas – the fuel sold in canisters for use by campers, in trailers, on boats, in heated greenhouses, for barbecues, and in the home – is propane, also called liquefied petroleum gas (LPG).

• Unlike natural gas, propane is heavier than air. For this reason, canisters should always be stored outside, above ground level and away from drains if they are to be left for any length of time. This applies whether they are full or empty.

• Keep the canister upright, with the valve uppermost, whether it is in use or not.

• If a canister has to be left in a confined space – a trailer or boat, say – ventilate the area thoroughly before turning it on, before lighting any naked flame (even a cigarette) and before switching on any electrical equipment (because a spark could ignite leaked gas and cause an explosion).

• In particular, make sure that you ventilate thoroughly the bottom of the space – the bilges on a boat, say, or a cellar – to get rid of any gas that has collected there.

• Check gas hoses regularly for leaks by rubbing soapy water over them. Any leaks will be marked by erupting bubbles. Never use a naked flame to check for leaks.

• If you find any leaks, or if the hose is becoming worn, replace it. Do not try to repair it.

• When fitting connections, tighten them with a wrench. Finger pressure is not enough to ensure a gastight seal.

• Change canisters well away from any open flame or intense heat, preferably outdoors.

• Open the valve slowly when you want to turn the gas on.

• Ventilate any room where gas-burning appliances are in use.

• Call the gas company immediately to check any appliance that ignites slowly or makes unusual noises.

• Avoid using your vacuum cleaner too close to a gas flame or burner.

• Do not clean gas appliances with flammable liquids. If you use a flammable cleaner on a gas water heater, the appliance could light suddenly and ignite the fumes.

• Do not keep aerosol cans or bottles of combustible material near gas appliances. The containers could explode if they are exposed to the fluctuating temperatures of an appliance such as a gas stove.

• Never try to defeat or to tamper with the safety devices on gas appliances.

• Never block vents in a room where there are gas appliances. If a gas appliance is deprived of fresh air while burning, it can give off carbon dioxide fumes (see below).

• If you are moving from one house to another, get the gas company to cut off your gas supply before you go.

• Leave the instructions for gas appliances you are not taking with you, for whoever is moving in.

Avoiding explosions

Gas explosions at home can happen because people have interfered with appliances – either deliberately (such as by tampering with the gas meter), or by accident, or when attempting a repair that they were not competent to carry out properly.

• Many accidents caused by faulty gas appliances involve secondhand equipment. If you buy such equipment, get it installed properly by a gas fitter.

• Make sure that all gas appliances are serviced regularly – furnaces, water heaters, vented and unvented space heaters at least once a year, and other gas appliances at least once every two years.

• If you know, or are warned, that a gas appliance or installation in your home is faulty, you must get it repaired. Failure to do so is dangerous to lives and property.

Danger signs of carbon dioxide

Watch out for the danger signs that fumes of carbon monoxide – a poisonous gas which is given off when gas burns at low oxygen levels – are present in a room where there is a gas appliance.

• Carbon dioxide is given off when a chimney flue or a vented space heater becomes blocked, cutting off the necessary air supply. With an unvented heater, this could occur if the room is not properly ventilated.

• Danger signs of poor ventilation are staining, soot or discoloration around the burner, and the appliance may burn with a yellow or orange flame.

• If you notice any of these danger signs, or if sitting in the room gives you a headache or makes you feel sick, weak or tired, turn off the appliance at once and get it checked.

• If a person is overcome by carbon monoxide fumes, get the victim into the fresh air at once and call for emergency help. If the victim isn't breathing, start mouth-to-mouth resuscitation. (See *Gas poisoning*, page 100.)

Using electricity safely

The two major electrical hazards are shocks and fire. Any electrical wire gets warm in use. The thinner the wire or the greater the amount of current it is carrying, the hotter it gets. Fuses and circuit breakers are designed to cut off the power long before this heat builds up to the point where insulation could melt or a fire could start.

By following the guidelines suggested here, you can minimize the risks of suffering an electric shock (for details of first aid treatment, see page 93). Moreover, you can also save yourself from being plunged into darkness by a blown fuse or tripped circuit breaker.

How to avoid electric shocks
Serious electric shock occurs when a current flows through the body – say, from one hand to the other, or from the hand to the feet. The combination of electricity and water presents one of the greatest risks of shock. Never touch electric appliances or equipment while your hands are wet or while wearing wet shoes, while standing barefoot on damp ground or concrete, or dangling your foot in the water from a dock or a boat. Your best protection against shock is provided by dry shoes, dry floors, rubber boots and gloves.
• Do not touch your home's main electrical service panel when water is present. If the floor is damp, stand on a dry board. If the wiring is wet, have an electrician or the power company turn off the electricity. In an emergency, use a dry wood pole to turn off the main switches.
• If an appliance shocks, unplug it immediately. Do not use it again until the cause of the shock has been found and eliminated.
• Do not poke into an electric appliance, such as a toaster or heater, with a fork, a knife or any other metal object.
• Do not immerse any part of an electric appliance in water unless the manufacturer says that it can be immersed.
• Switch off the main switch before checking lamp cords and before cleaning them with a damp cloth. Water seeping into a worn or frayed cord could give you a shock.
• Even though power is off, there may still be a shock hazard. Some devices – for example, television sets, computers, air conditioners – have components that store charge. Discharge them before you work on them.
• To avoid the risk of shock, have electric outlets equipped with GFCIs (ground fault circuit interrupters), which detect electric leakage and cut off the power before harm occurs. Many areas insist on the installation of GFCIs in bathrooms, kitchens, and outdoors in all new housing.

Plugs
When replacing a plug because it is damaged or a wire has come loose, always check that each wire goes to the correct terminal. Electric cords generally contain two or three separate wires. There is usually a live (black) and a neutral (white) wire, and often a ground wire (green or bare metal). The white wire should be connected to the chrome screw; the black, to the brass screw; and the ground, to the green or hexagonal screw.
• Never put wires directly into an outlet – always fit a plug.
• Always unplug appliances after use or before working on them or making any adjustments.
• When unplugging an appliance, remove the plug at the outlet. Never disconnect by yanking the cord; you could pull the wires loose.
• When using a portable appliance with a detachable cord, connect the cord to the appliance before putting the plug at the other end of the cord into an outlet. Disconnect the plug at the outlet before you disconnect the plug at the appliance.
• Check plugs and cords regularly on appliances such as toasters, which are moved often or get hot. Also check cords and plugs on appliances in constant use, such as refrigerators, freezers, and dishwashers.
• Fit rubber plugs to appliances that get hard wear; they chip and crack less than plastic plugs.
• Plugs that fit loosely in wall outlets make poor contact and may fall out. Replace the outlets.
• Do not use multi-outlet taps as regular practice. Have extra outlets installed if necessary.
• If you use a multi-outlet tap, you risk overloading a circuit. For example, a toaster and an iron together on the same outlet take 18 amperes – which is too much for a standard 15-ampere outlet.

Extension and power cords
Inadequate extension and power cords can cause a major fire in the home. For example, you should never connect a 1,400-watt portable heater to an 18-gauge extension cord because the cord will overheat. The fuse or circuit breaker controlling the circuit will not cut off the power because it only protects the house wiring.
• If an electrical cord becomes worn, discard it and replace it with a new one.
• Always replace an appliance cord with the manufacturer's equivalent or a recommended replacement.
• Keep the lengths of extension cords to a minimum.
• Use a grounding type, three-wire extension if the appliance has a three-prong plug.
• Choose extension cords with at least the same gauge as the power cord of your appliance. If you are not sure of the gauge, use the following chart as a guide.

For 120-volt appliances:	Use:
Up to 6 amp. (0–720 watts)	18-gauge cord
6–9 amp. (720–1,080 watts)	16-gauge cord
9–14 amp. (1,080–1,680 watts)	14-gauge cord
14–18 amp. (1,680–2,160 watts)	12-gauge cord

In the home and at work

153

• Never run an extension cord under a rug or inside an enclosed space.

• Use an orange or yellow cord on electric appliances such as lawn mowers, which are used outdoors. An orange or yellow cord is easier to see than a black one.

• Never wrap a cord around an iron or any electric heating appliance while it is still warm after use.

• When storing an electric appliance, do not wrap the cord around sharp edges that could cut or fray it.

• If the power cord of your washer does not reach the outlet, move the outlet or install a longer cord. Do not use an extension cord with a washer. If water touches the connection between the extension and power cords, you could be electrocuted.

• When using an extension cord fitted to a reel, pull out the entire length when it is in use. Wire warms up when current passes through it – the smaller the wire or the larger the appliance, the more heat is generated. If the wire is left on the reel, the heat cannot escape so easily, and it can build up to a point where the insulation melts, causing a short circuit.

• Rub electric cords with a bar of strong laundry soap to prevent pets from chewing them.

• Never join wires by twisting them together and insulating them with tape.

• Have a certified electrician check the wiring of your home every five years. If your home is over 20 years old and has never been rewired, it undoubtedly needs improvements in its wiring system.

• If you decide to do the rewiring of your home yourself, remember that the job calls for skill, care, and, ultimately, checking by an inspection authority.

Fuses and circuit breakers

Electricity from the power company enters your home through the main switch, but the distribution is controlled from a service panel – either a fuse box or a circuit breaker panel. The panel is usually located in the basement or the garage.

From the service panel the electricity flows through the house on separate circuits. Each of these household circuits is controlled by a fuse or circuit breaker. If too much current flows through the circuit, the fuse blows or the circuit breaker trips, cutting off the current. Overloading a circuit with too many appliances is the commonest cause of blown fuses and tripped circuit breakers.

• Before replacing a fuse or resetting a circuit breaker, find and correct the cause of the problem.

• If overloading is the problem, disconnect some of the appliances before you change a fuse or reset a circuit breaker.

• Turn off the main switch or circuit breaker, or remove the main fuse holder. If the basement floor is damp, make sure you are standing on a dry surface or use a broom handle to trip off the main switch.

• Remove the blown fuse by turning it counter-clockwise.

• A close look at the fuse may reveal why it has blown. A clear fuse window with a broken metal strip inside is the sign of an overloaded circuit. A blackened fuse window usually indicates a short circuit.

• Always remember to replace a blown fuse with another one of the same amperage. Using a higher capacity fuse can cause overheating and may start a fire.

• If your service panel has circuit breakers, which are designed to turn themselves off automatically when the circuit becomes overloaded, there is no need to repair or replace anything. Switch off some of the appliances on the circuit, then reset the circuit breaker by turning it first to the *off* position and then to the *on* position.

• If a fuse blows repeatedly, or if a circuit breaker will not stay on when you reset it, call an electrician for help.

Volts, watts and amperes

Most households receive 120/240 volts of electrical power. Smaller appliances operate on 120-volt current; heavy-duty appliances, such as electric stoves and clothes dryers, require 240 volts.

The box on the opposite page shows the wattage and amperage ratings of individual appliances. Wattage is the total amount of electricity used by an appliance. Amperage is the current or rate at which electricity is delivered to an appliance.

Wattage is found by multiplying volts by amperes. For example, an air conditioner using 120 volts and 11 amperes would be rated 1,320 watts. In most cases, you do not need to use this formula, because the wattage rating is listed on the nameplate of the appliance.

The standard 120-volt household circuit has a capacity of 15 amperes. In other words, the total number of appliances on one circuit should not exceed 15 amperes. For this reason, you risk overloading when you have too many appliances on the same circuit.

There is a simple solution, however. Before you increase the demands on a circuit, check the total load by adding up the amperage for each appliance (see box). For example, a 1,050-watt iron (9 amperes) and a 300-watt television (2.5 amperes) will – if they are together – use 11.5 amperes, safely inside the capacity of the standard household circuit.

The amperages given in the box are approximate and may vary considerably from one model to another. To get a more precise amperage figure, divide the number of watts used by an appliance by the number of volts in the system.

APPLIANCES: WATTAGE AND AMPERAGE RATINGS

Appliance	Watts	Amperes (120 volts)	Amperes (240 volts)
Air conditioner (central)	5,000	—	21
(room size, small)	800	6.5	—
(room size, medium)	1,300	11	5.5
(room size, large)	1,600	13.5	17
Blender	Up to 1,000	1–8	—
Broiler	1,500	12.5	—
Can opener	150	1.2	—
Coffee maker	500–1,000	4–8	—
Dishwasher	1,000–1,500	8.5–12.5	—
Dryer	4,000–8,000	—	16.5–34
Electric blanket	200	1.5	—
Fan (portable)	250	2	—
Freezer (frost-free)	350–500	3–4	—
(standard)	250–400	2–3.5	—
Frying pan (electric)	1,100	9	—
Furnace (oil) fan and controls	750–1,600	6.5–13.5	—
Garbage disposal	400–900	3.5–7.5	—
Hair dryer	350–1,400	3–11.5	—
Heater, portable electric	1,250 and up	10 and up	—
Hotplate (each burner)	750	6	—
Iron	1,050	9	—
Microwave oven	600	5	—
Mixer	150	1	—
Refrigerator (frost-free)	300–450	2.5–4	—
(standard)	250–350	2–3	—
Rotisserie	1,400	11.5	—
Sander (hand-held)	750	6	—
Saw (bench)	1,300–1,600	11–13.5	—
Sewing machine	100	1	—
Stereo phonograph	300	2.5	—
Stove (oven)	4,000–8,000	—	16.5–34
(top)	4,000–5,000	—	16.5–21
Sump pump	300	2.5	—
Sunlamp	400	3.5	—
Television (black and white)	250	2	—
(color)	300	2.5	—
Toaster	1,100	9	—
Vacuum cleaner	720–1,300	6–11	—
Washing machine	1,500	12.5	—
Water heater	2,000–5,000	—	8.5–21

In the home and at work

When the power supply fails

Power failures are always unexpected and never pleasant. When they occur at the height of winter, or during a heat wave, they cause maximum inconvenience and discomfort.

But it is possible to minimize the inconvenience, and the risk of accidents during a failure, by taking a few simple precautions.

• Switch off all electrical appliances except those that are normally on all the time, such as clocks, refrigerators and central-heating thermostats. When the power is restored after the failure, there will be an initial surge of current and, if a lot of appliances are on, the surge may be great enough to blow a fuse. More important, appliances such as heaters could become fire hazards if they are left on and forgotten, and the power comes back on late at night.

• As an extra precaution, make a point of unplugging the appliances at the outlets. Move the cords out of the way as well so that nobody can trip over them in the dark.

• Leave at least one light switched on so that you know when power is restored.

• Avoid opening a freezer, even a chest type. Food will generally keep safely for at least 12 hours with the power off. The fuller the freezer, the longer it will stay cold – up to 48 hours in safety, for instance, for a completely full freezer that is left unopened.

• Pack blankets and crumpled newspaper under and around the freezer's base to prevent heat rising into the appliance.

• No special action is needed for central heating – most systems are electrically controlled and will just not operate during a power failure.

• Use hot water carefully during a power failure. Although the water should stay hot for some time if the tank is well insulated, cold water is fed into the tank every time you draw off some of the hot.

• Use thermos bottles to store spare water for hot drinks.

• If the failure is unexpected, telephone your local utility company to tell them the power is off – it helps the company to identify an affected area quickly. The telephone has its own power supply and will not be affected by the failure.

When power is restored

• Reset electric clocks and timers, including the timed thermostat, after the power failure.

• Remove any insulation that you have put around the base of your refrigerator or freezer. Make sure, particularly, that you uncover the vent or grille at the back through which surplus heat is discharged.

• Check the contents of your freezer. If any food has an unusual color or odor, throw it out. Never refreeze ice cream or precooked food that has thawed. Uncooked food that still has ice crystals or has been kept below 45°F (7°C) for less than two days can be refrozen.

• After checking the freezer, do not reopen it for several hours after a long power failure,

to give time for the temperature inside to be lowered to a safe level again.

• If further failures are expected, set freezer and refrigerator controls to maximum to extend the time that food will stay safely frozen.

Preparing for a power shutdown

Often there is some warning – either through a notice from the local utility or via newspapers, radio and TV – of a temporary power shutdown. If there is, try to be ready for the stoppage well ahead of time.

• Keep a small flashlight by your bed, and a large battery-powered lantern in the kitchen.

• Fit these lamps with long-life batteries, and check them regularly.

• If you have to use candles, keep them away from anything that might catch fire, such as curtains. Stand candles in holders that cannot be easily knocked over.

• Try to set up alternative heating in at least one room: for example, a wood-burning stove.

• In an all-electric house, consider buying a camping stove for emergency cooking and heating during power failures.

• About 24 hours before the power goes off, set freezer and fridge controls to maximum – the colder they are, the longer the food will keep.

• Check to see if your homeowner's insurance covers the loss of the contents of your freezer in case of a power failure. If not, ask your agent if you can have protection against loss included in your policy.

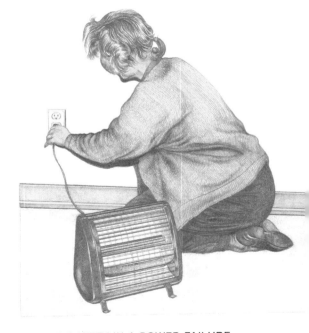

HEATER SAFETY IN A POWER FAILURE
If your power supply fails, turn off all electric heaters. Pull all the plugs out at the outlets. Then tidy the cords away so that you cannot trip over them in the dark.

Plumbing: emergency repairs

A flood in the home – from a blocked drain or a burst pipe – can be controlled or stopped before it does serious damage without waiting for a plumber to arrive. But taking effective action calls for a cool head, speed and some preparation. It is therefore important to think ahead.

You need to know where to find the main water valve for the house and the shutoff valves

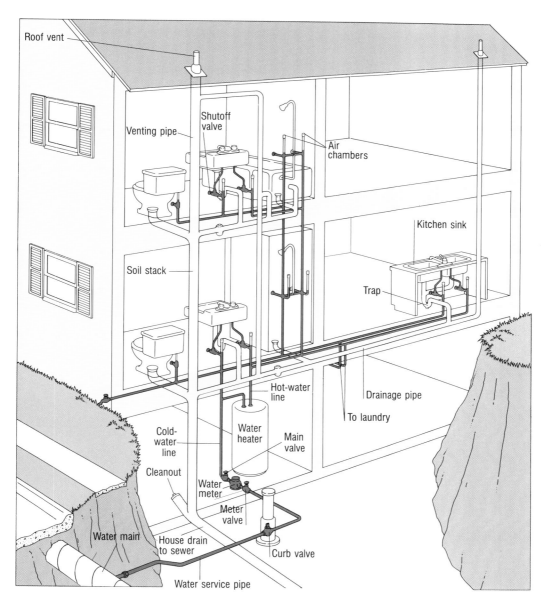

HOW THE WATER PIPES ARE LAID OUT IN A TWO-STORY HOUSE

Water enters the house from a public main through a service pipe. It flows through an outside curb valve, then a meter valve, a water meter, and finally a main valve. After the service pipe enters the house, it branches into the cold-water line and a pipe to a water heater or boiler. From the heater, the hot-water line runs to faucets and appliances that require hot water. Fixtures other than tubs and showers should be equipped with shutoff valves on both the cold- and hot-water lines.

The drainage pipes carry water from appliances, sinks and tubs, and waste from toilets, to the soil stack, then the house drain, and into the public sewer. Most fixtures have traps – usually curved pipes – filled with water, which acts as a seal to keep sewage gases from entering the house from drainage and waste pipes. The venting pipes are tied into the drainage and waste pipes to form the DWV (drain-waste-vent) system. They allow the escape of gases and the entry of air to equalize pressures within the system.

157

HOW TO DEAL WITH A LEAK

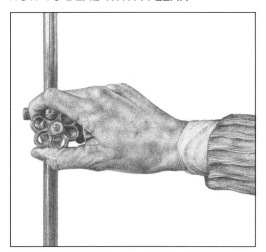

1 *If necessary, shut off all the water at the main valve, which is in the basement near the water meter. Turn on the faucets on the lower floor to empty all the pipes.*

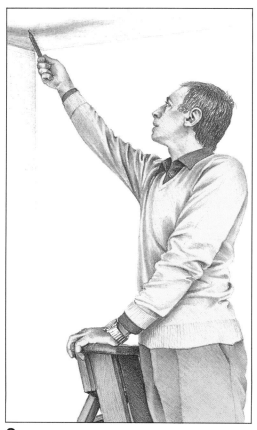

2 *If the leaking water has collected above a ceiling, forming a bulge in the plaster, put a bucket or any container below the bulge, and pierce the bulge with a large screwdriver.*

for each fixture inside the house. If you do not know, find them and note their position in case an emergency arises. You will find the shutoff valves under or near plumbing fixtures. The main water valve is usually in the basement near the water meter. Once you have identified these valves, it might be helpful to label each one so that you can be sure of identifying them quickly in case of an emergency.

If any valves are stuck, free them with a penetrating lubricant. Check them regularly.

Never leave any faucet or valve full on for too long – it can easily become jammed. Once you have opened it fully, turn it back about half a turn and leave it in that position.

Emergency repairs will also be quicker and simpler if you keep the following items in the house: duct or pipe repair tape; electrical tape; fiberglass tape; plumber's tape (used to seal threaded pipe joints); epoxy adhesive; a drain plunger; and a tin of radiator seal.

If water leaks through a ceiling

If water starts to drip through a ceiling, the most probable cause (other than a leaking roof) is a burst pipe.

• The priority is to reduce the amount of water coming through the ceiling as quickly as possible to stop flooding. Do not waste time at this stage looking for the cause.

• Turn off the main valve, which is usually in the basement near the water meter.

• Turn on the faucets on the lower floor of the house to drain the pipes. Leave the faucets on until the water stops running.

If you see a distinct bulge in the ceiling at the site of the leak, it means that a pool of water has collected over the spot.

• To stop the weight of water bringing down the

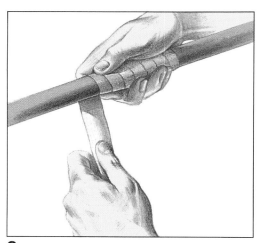

3 *Track down the source of the leak. When you find it, wait until the dripping stops and the pipe is dry, then bind the hole with duct or pipe repair tape. Call a plumber.*

ceiling, puncture the center of the bulge with a large screwdriver and let the water drain out into a bucket or any other available container.

• Once water stops flowing from the ceiling, find the source of the leak. If you suspect it is through the roof, inspect the attic, but step only on the joists. If the floor is not boarded, you could put your foot through the plaster ceiling and injure yourself seriously.

• If the leak is small and manageable, bind the puncture temporarily with duct or electrical tape. You will then be able to turn the water on. If you cannot repair the leak, leave the water off.

• Call a plumber (consult the *Yellow Pages* of a telephone directory) to make permanent repairs.

• If the leak is through a hole in the roof, make a temporary repair with a sheet of plastic (see *Storms and high winds*, page 170).

If a pipe freezes and bursts

Water expands when it freezes, and if the water is trapped inside a pipe, the expansion can be strong enough to burst the pipe.

If you find a burst and frozen pipe, aim to make a temporary repair *before* it thaws out and the leak causes damage. Before starting any temporary repairs, shut off the main water valve to prevent water from gushing out as soon as the pipe is thawed.

• Bind the damaged section of pipe with duct tape, following the maker's instructions on the packet. Properly used, duct tape will withstand water pressure.

• Alternatively, repair the break by wrapping fiberglass tape around it several times to form a seal.

• Once the seal is in place, thaw out the pipe with gentle heat – use a hand-held dryer or a heat lamp. Open the nearest faucet on the frozen pipe and work back from the faucet to the frozen area. The open faucet reduces the steam and water pressure within the pipe.

• Have the pipe repaired later by a plumber.

• If the damaged pipe has already thawed and water is pouring out, try to cut off the water supply to the pipe.

• Turn off the nearest shutoff valve, if there is one, or run the faucets that are fed by the pipe to reduce water pressure inside.

• When the leak stops or slows, bind the damaged section with duct tape or repair the damage with fiberglass tape and epoxy adhesive.

• If the damage is extensive, it may be necessary to turn off the water supply to the house completely by shutting off the main valve. Wrap the pipe with a towel to confine the water and lead it into a bucket. Call a plumber.

If a joint leaks

If a pipe leaks at a joint, the repair needed depends on the type of joint. There are two types: compression and soldered joints.

• Compression joints, where the pipes are threaded and held together by nuts, can be made watertight by tightening the nut slightly with a wrench.

• Alternatively, shut off the water supply to the pipes, unscrew the nuts and wrap the threaded areas with several turns of plumber's tape. Then reassemble the joint.

• Soldered joints, where the pipes are sealed by a sleeve of metal soldered to them, may have to be remade by a plumber.

• On either type of joint you can also make a temporary repair.

• Turn off the nearest shutoff valve and run faucets to reduce the water pressure inside.

• Bind the joint with duct tape or seal it with epoxy adhesive or silicone sealant.

If a radiator leaks

A large leak from a radiator can often be fixed by draining the radiator and plugging the hole with epoxy adhesive. But a pinhole leak which allows water to weep out slowly is best dealt with by a liquid radiator sealant.

• Add the sealant to the expansion tank near the boiler. You can recognize it from the instructions given on the sealant.

• Again following the instructions, open the shutoff valve near the boiler so that water in the expansion tank flows into the system. The seal will then find its own way to the leak, on the same principle as the sealants used to mend car radiators.

• Either type of leak often means that the radiator is heavily corroded inside – and that other radiators in the system are also affected. So the only long-term answer is to drain the whole central-heating system and install a corrosion inhibitor. Consult a central-heating firm (local ones will be listed in the *Yellow Pages*).

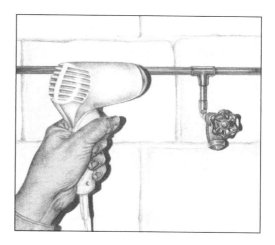

HOW TO THAW A FROZEN PIPE
Thaw a pipe with a hand-held hair dryer. Open the faucet nearest the frozen area and work back toward the frozen area. With the faucet open you can see when the ice has melted.

If a central-heating pipe leaks
• If possible, put a container under the leak to catch as much of the water as possible.
• Switch off the electricity to the boiler or disconnect the gas or oil supply. Shut off the water supply to the tank.
• Attach a garden hose to the drain cock, which is usually beside the boiler.
• Run the hose to a nearby sink or floor drain. Open the drain cock with a wrench or pliers, and let the water run out of the central-heating circuit until water stops flowing from the leak. When the leak stops, close the drain cock.
• Once the tank is empty, wipe off the excess water around your tank, and close the drain cock again.
• Call a plumber as soon as possible. Do not switch on any current or reconnect the gas or oil supply until all the repairs are done.

How to stop a toilet tank dripping
If a toilet tank drips water, particularly in hot, humid weather, the problem is probably condensation – not a leak.
   Moisture in the air is condensing on the cold outer surface of the tank and dripping onto the floor, or trickling down the flush pipe between tank and toilet.
• The best long-term cure is to keep the bathroom dry and to insulate the toilet tank. You can line the inside of the tank with a ready-made liner or insulating rubber foam.

If water leaks under the bath
The commonest sources of bath leaks are the overflow outlet and the plughole. Older bathtubs have exposed pipes that are easy to reach if there is a leak. Modern bathtubs have concealed and usually inaccessible pipes, which should be fixed by a plumber.
• With an older bathtub, try replacing the rubber gasket between the drain pipe and bath.
• Alternatively, try tightening the securing nut on the plughole joint very slightly – overtightening can make the leak worse.

If a sink overflows
Floods in bathrooms, kitchens and basements are most often caused by leaving the plug in a sink with a faucet running.
• If the overflow outlet is blocked, fill the sink so that the outlet is underwater, then try to force out the obstruction with a drain plunger.
• Alternatively, push a straightened wire hanger or a small auger down the outlet and try to clear the blockage.
• Once the water starts to drain away, flush more water down the outlet – with a liquid drain cleaner if necessary – to clear any remaining debris.

If a drain or pipe is blocked
• Turn off any faucets that drain into the blocked section.
• Feel with your hand at the upper opening of the drain or waste pipe, and clear any obstructions you find. Outside drains, for example, can become choked with fallen leaves, silt and other debris.
• On a waste pipe from a sink or basin, if there is no obvious obstruction, seal the overflow outlet with a wet rag and use a drain plunger to try to force the blockage free.
• Once the water starts to flow again, flush more

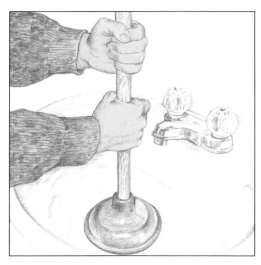

HOW TO CLEAR A BLOCKED SINK DRAIN
Partly fill the sink, and use a drain plunger to free the blockage. Stuff a wet cloth in the overflow outlet if necessary to stop water spurting out of it while you pump the plunger.

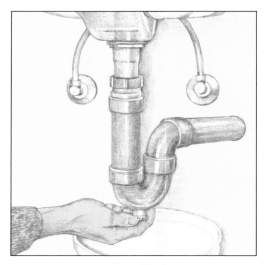

HOW TO CLEAN OUT A TRAP
If plunging does not work on a blocked sink or basin, put a bucket under the trap. Undo the trap valve, or take the whole trap apart and clean it out thoroughly by hand.

IF WATER REACHES ELECTRICAL WIRING

Water conducts electricity so there is a danger of shocks, short circuits and fire if water from a leak runs along the wiring. If there is a risk of this happening, switch off the electricity. The switch is usually near the service panel. Alternatively, switch off the appropriate circuit at the service panel.

If any wiring or electrical components have become wet, make sure they are thoroughly dry before switching on again.

If water from a leak is dirty – as a result of flooding, say – it can leave grime on the wiring and other electrical equipment components. If you turn on the equipment, you risk damaging it. Clean off grime and flush it away with fresh water *before* leaving the wiring and other components to dry. Call an electrician if the equipment cannot be cleaned completely.

---

water through to clear any remaining debris.
• If plunging fails on a kitchen sink or basin, put a bucket under the trap, disconnect the trap and clean it out. On modern plastic fittings, finger pressure may be enough to unscrew the trap. If you use a wrench, be gentle with it.
• If none of these methods works, it means that the obstruction is lodged farther along the pipe.
• Shift the obstruction with a plumber's snake or sink auger – a stiff but flexible wire – if the pipe itself is blocked. If the drain is blocked, use a closet (toilet) auger or an electrically operated auger. Both items of equipment can usually be rented from tool rental shops.
• If this does not work, or if you cannot get hold of the equipment, call a plumber.

If the toilet will not flush properly
• If water keeps flowing after the tank fills, lift the float ball. If the flow stops, bend the float arm down so that, after a flush, the refill water stops ¾ in. (2 cm) below the top of the overflow tub. If this fails, check the float ball and replace it if it is cracked or water-filled.
• If water keeps flowing into the toilet bowl but the tank does not refill, the flush valve (at the bottom of the tank) is leaking. Shut off the water supply and flush the toilet to empty the tank. If the stopper ball does not sit squarely on the flush valve, straighten the lift wires or chain. Replace a worn-out stopper ball with a new one or with a rubber flapper.
• If the fault is in some other part of the flushing mechanism, call a plumber. But you can go on using the toilet until the plumber comes. Pour a

bucket of water into the toilet bowl – not the tank – after each use. This will flush the bowl.

If a toilet or drain is blocked
• Do not use or flush a toilet if the bowl or sewage pipe beyond is blocked. You could create a health hazard if the sewage overflows, and you will make the job of clearing it difficult.
• Try to clear the blockage with a large drain plunger. Place the plunger over the drain hole and pump up and down about a dozen times. If this fails to work, give it another try an hour later.
• If plunging does not work, aim the bent end of a closet (toilet) auger into the drain hole. Crank the handle and move the auger up the trap toward the obstruction. Try to hook the blockage and pull it down, or break it up. When broken up, the debris can be flushed away.
• If you fail to unclog the toilet, try to find if the blockage is in the drain pipe.
• Remove the cleanout plugs on the drain pipe. If water runs out of the cleanout, it means the blockage is farther down the pipe. If no water runs out of the cleanout, it means that the blockage is farther up the pipe.
• When you find the area of the blockage, explore the drain with a long stick. You may be able to dislodge the obstruction.
• If you cannot reach or shift the blockage, consider borrowing or renting a set of drain augers or a plumber's snake (both are usually available from tool rental shops).
• Once the backed-up water begins to flow again, flush hot water or a chemical drain cleaner through the pipes to clear away any remaining debris. If you cannot clear the blockage yourself, call a plumber.

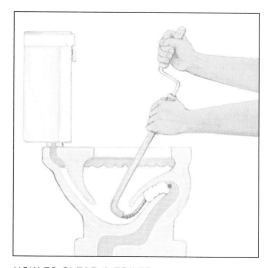

HOW TO CLEAR A TOILET
If a clog is difficult to dislodge, use a toilet auger. Aim the bend of the auger into the trap area, turn the crank, and keep moving the auger up the trap to hook the blockage.

Danger points – room by room

Your own home can be the most dangerous place on earth if you fail to take proper precautions. More accidents happen there than anywhere else. Each year in North America, around 23,000 people are killed in accidents at home and another 24 million are hurt badly enough to seek some form of medical treatment.

Most accidents happen in the evenings or on weekends when people are usually at home. Inside the house, the kitchen is the most dangerous area for nonfatal accidents. But the bedroom is the scene of the commonest fatal accidents – falls, fires, poisonings, and suffocations. There are more domestic accidents in summer than in winter. And almost all other household accidents happen in the yard or the garden.

Although your home has many danger spots, there is much you can do to make it safer, and so reduce the risks to yourself and your family. A room-by-room check of the potential hazards shown on these pages could prevent a hazard becoming a tragedy. Special additional precautions are needed if there are young children or elderly people in the house.

There are also safety devices on the market, such as fire extinguishers and smoke detectors that can be installed easily. For example, smoke detectors will warn of a fire before it gets out of control, giving valuable time in which to fight the blaze or to escape.

Kitchen

There are more potential hazards – sharp knives, hot flames, scalding liquids, slippery surfaces, dangerous liquids – in the kitchen than elsewhere in the house. The most frequent kitchen injuries are cuts and burns. For example, about 150,000 North Americans are treated in emergency wards each year for injuries involving kitchen knives. Falls and poisonings are among the other serious accidents that occur in the kitchen. Haste and carelessness are usually given as the reasons for these accidents.

• Ensure kitchen shelving is easy to reach, or have a stepladder to reach high shelves.
• Store dangerous liquids, such as bleach and disinfectant, well out of reach of children and preferably in a locked cupboard. Do not keep dangerous liquids in food containers or store them with food.
• Keep knives out of reach of children.
• Turn pan handles away from the edge of the stove when cooking. That way no one can tip a pot and spill its scalding contents.
• If there is a toddler in the house, do not use a tablecloth which hangs over the edge of the table. He might pull it, and whatever is on it, onto his head.
• Never leave deep fat fryers or frying pans unattended, and do not fill them more than a third full with fat or oil.
• When using a deep fat fryer or frying pan, have the lid handy to smother any fire. A large plate or chopping board will do as long as it is larger than the top of the fryer or pan. Never move a pot of burning fat. Never douse the

---

USING A MICROWAVE OVEN SAFELY

Microwave ovens are built to meet government standards for safety. Here is a checklist to help make sure that you use your oven safely.

• Never try to operate a microwave oven with the door open. You risk exposure to harmful microwave energy.
• Frequently inspect your oven's interior, door and seals.
• Do not allow food residues to build up inside your oven. Remove dirt and any cleaning film from the door seals. Use a mild detergent and water – no abrasives, scouring pads or steel wool.
• If your oven suddenly begins to take longer than usual to cook food, the oven door may be damaged. If this is so, get a properly qualified serviceman to check and adjust it.
• Have your oven tested regularly for microwave leakage, particularly if it is an old or secondhand model.
• Do not stand in front of your oven when it is operating.
• If there is a fire in your microwave, keep the door closed and unplug the unit. Do not attempt to put out the fire. Keep the door closed until the blaze is extinguished.
• Cooking food on a dish containing metal produces sparks and flashes in the microwave. Remove the dish and transfer the food to one that is safe for a microwave.
• While microwaves do not heat up glass dishes, the hot food in the dish can. Use pot holders to remove food from the oven.

flames with water (see *Fighting a fire*, page 148).
• Consider using french fries that can be oven cooked to remove the need for deep fat frying.
• If a grease fire starts in the oven, close the oven door and turn off the heat.
• When using a pressure cooker, follow the manufacturer's instructions about how much water to put in, and time the cooking carefully so that the cooker does not boil dry.
• Wipe up any grease that spills on the floor immediately. Glue down the edges of any floor tiles that lift, to stop people tripping over them.
• Never use thin or wet pot holders.
• Make sure that all burners in a gas oven are lit before closing the door. If you have turned the heat right down, close the door slowly so as not to blow the flame out.
• Do not hang cloths or plastic bags above gas burners.
• Store matches in a fireproof container out of reach of children.

• Do not set burners so high that the flames come up the sides of cooking pans. The extra heat is wasted, and the flames may melt the handles or make them painfully hot.
• Store plastic shopping and garbage bags away from young children. A bag pulled over the head in play can suffocate.
• Keep cupboard and cabinet doors closed whenever possible. Their sharp corners can be dangerous, particularly if they are near eye level.
• Lock potential hiding places for young children such as the freezer, broom cupboard, washing machine or tumble drier. A toddler could get trapped inside.
• Put a baby's bouncing chair on the floor – never on a countertop or table. It may shift as the baby bounces, and topple off the edge.
• Always unplug the cord from the outlet before you disconnect it from the appliance.
• Check your user's manual to see if all or only part of an electric appliance can be washed.

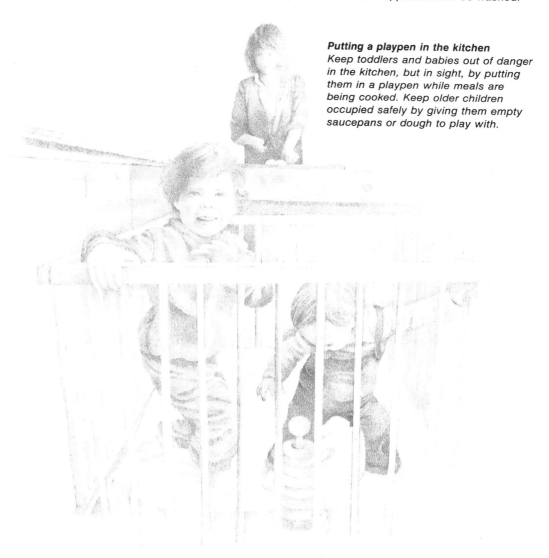

Putting a playpen in the kitchen
Keep toddlers and babies out of danger in the kitchen, but in sight, by putting them in a playpen while meals are being cooked. Keep older children occupied safely by giving them empty saucepans or dough to play with.

• If a live cord falls into water, turn off the power and unplug it before pulling it out of the water. If you put your hands in the water while the power is still on, you could receive a severe electric shock.

• If a plug or cord becomes wet, turn off the power and dry the plug thoroughly before attempting to use it.

• Turn the iron off if you are called away when ironing. When you have finished with it, leave it to cool out of reach of young children.

Bathroom

Many danger spots are present in the bathroom. Soapy surfaces and scalding water in bathtubs and showers can cause slips, falls and burns. Electrical switches and appliances can shock or electrocute anyone who is wet or in the tub. Each year 220,000 North Americans suffer non-fatal injuries in the bathroom, and more than 200 drownings occur in tubs and showers.

• If your bath or the base of your shower is smooth, use an internal bath mat which grips with suction cups. This will prevent you slipping.

• Fit a grab handle on the wall above the bath.

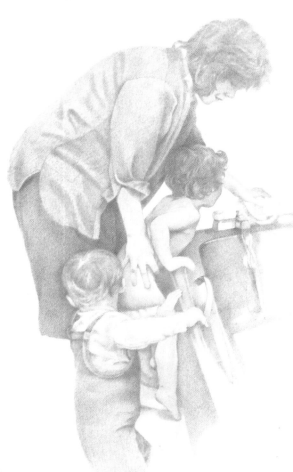

THE CURE THAT KILLED
Drinking water is a valuable on-the-spot first aid treatment for anyone who swallows a poisonous substance of any kind – a household cleaner, for instance, such as bleach. The water helps to dilute the poison and thus lessen its effects. The patient should drink as much water as he comfortably can without making himself sick. For an average adult, this may be 2-4 pints (about 1-2 litres). For a child, it could be less than 1 pint (about half a litre).

Drunk quickly in very large quantities, however, water can itself be poisonous.

In October 1982, a 40-year-old housewife from London, England, accidentally swallowed some bleach that had been left in a cup to remove a stain. A hospital she rang advised her by telephone to drink water to minimize any risk, but in panic she took the remedy too far.

She drank water in enormous quantities, gulping it from a plastic bucket. "She literally drank gallons," a coroner later reported, "and, despite making herself sick, continued to drink."

Eventually the woman had a seizure, collapsed and died from brain damage caused by water intoxication. At the inquest, doctors reported that the bleach had done her no harm at all.

This is useful for older people or for anyone who feels dizzy when getting up from a hot bath.

• If you have a shower unit, fit a thermostat to it to guard against scalding. Or consider buying a shower head which has a thermostat built in for the purpose.

Cold water before hot
Always run the cold water into a bath first, then add the hot, in case a child falls in accidentally. Children can die from being scalded in very hot baths.

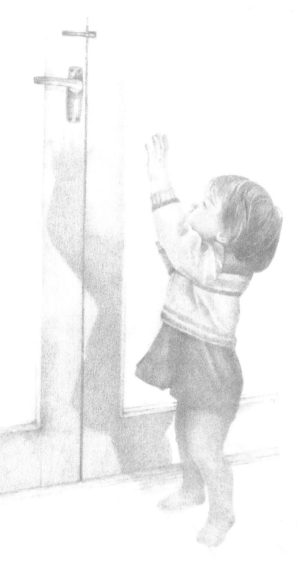

• Unplug all electrical appliances not in use. If possible, choose battery-operated ones, which have lower voltages.
• Mop up water that spills on the floor to avoid the risk of you – or someone else – slipping on it. For the same reason, if you use a bath mat on the floor, make sure it has a nonslip backing.
• Never leave young children alone in the bath. If you have to leave the room, take them with you, wrapped in a towel to keep them warm.
• If you put a bolt on the inside of your bathroom or toilet door, fit it high enough so that young children cannot reach it and lock themselves in. Remove the keys for the same reason.
• Never mix bleach or any bleach-based cleaner with other toilet cleaners. The mixture can give off a poisonous gas.
• Store medicines well out of reach of children in a cabinet that can be locked.
• Do not transfer medicines from child-proof containers to ordinary ones.
• Dispose of old medicines safely. Either flush them down the toilet, or return them to the drugstore. Do not throw them away with the household rubbish.

Living and dining rooms
Falls and fire hazards are the commonest accidents in the living room or dining room. Among the causes of falls are: clutter on the floor; loose or worn rugs and carpets; trailing electrical or telephone wires; and inconveniently placed furniture. Poor wiring, heat buildup from lamps and TVs, and burning cigarettes and

Put door handles out of reach
Fit handles high up to stop toddlers letting themselves out of the house or into a cupboard. As an extra precaution, add a bolt higher up from the handle.

• Many electric codes specify the installation of ground fault circuit interrupters (GFCIs) in new bathrooms. GFCIs can detect electric leakages and cut off the power well before you can be hurt. Consider installing GFCIs if you intend to remodel your bathroom.
• To avoid electric shock in the bathroom, never touch any electric appliance while your hands are wet or you are standing on a wet floor.
• Put electric appliances for personal care – hair dryers, shavers, and toothbrushes – where they cannot fall into the tub, shower or toilet.

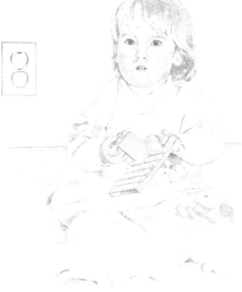

Cover electric outlets
Fit plastic safety plugs to electric outlets when they are not in use, to cover up the holes and stop children electrocuting themselves.

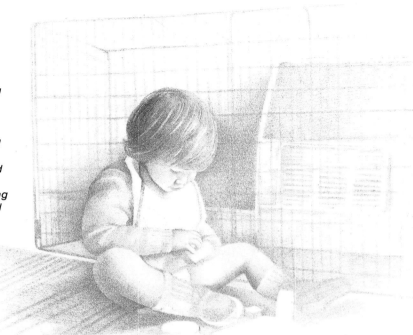

**Fix a fire screen
around every fire**
*Sturdy screens should be
fixed around all radiant
electric and gas fires, and
around open fires, and
attached to the wall with
fastenings that a child
cannot undo. They should
cover the whole fireplace,
not just the fire, and stand
far enough away from the
fire to stop a child reaching
it with bits of paper poked
through the wire.*

other smoker's materials are frequently the causes of fires in these rooms.
• Make sure that the electrical outlets are not overloaded. If there are not enough outlets for your appliances, have extra outlets installed.
• Check that cords for lamps and other appliances do not trail across the floor where people could trip over them.
• Do not run cords under the carpet – they may overheat and you will not be able to see if they become worn.
• Fix rugs to the floor. Repair worn rugs or carpets. Use nonslip polish on wooden floors.
• To avoid slips and falls, wear shoes or slippers with nonskid treads; never go around in your stocking feet.
• Do not balance cigarette-laden ashtrays on the arms of chairs and sofas. If hot cigarette ash falls on the covering, it may burn through the fabric and, worse, it might ignite the foam padding. Much modern upholstered furniture contains foam plastic that gives off toxic fumes and dense smoke if it catches fire. The smoke and fumes, which can kill, are more dangerous than the fire.
• Before going out or to bed, make sure that cigarettes are out and that fires are damped down or contained behind a fire screen.

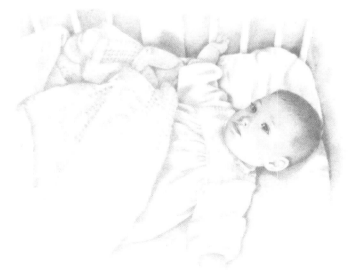

No pillows for a baby
*Babies under 12 months old
should never be given a
pillow. Because they cannot
easily turn over, they could
suffocate on it. For the same
reason, dress babies and
toddlers in blanket sleepers;
avoid wrapping them in too
many blankets and covers.*

Bedroom

Falls are one of the commonest fatal accidents that occur in the bedroom. The elderly and the very young are at greatest risk. Older people can injure themselves in falls while getting in and out of bed, dressing themselves, or making the bed. Babies can fall while attempting to climb over crib rails. Other fatal accidents occurring in the bedroom include fires, poisonings, and suffocations.

• Moving about in the dark can be dangerous: keep a small flashlight, fitted with long-life batteries, by your bedside. Make sure that there are no trailing cords or furniture to trip over.

• For the same reason, consider having a telephone jack installed beside your bed, and plugging your phone in there at night. This is particularly valuable for elderly people who – if they become ill or have an accident – may not be able to reach the phone downstairs.

• Do not smoke in bed.

• Have your electric blanket checked for safety every year, and check its cord for brittleness and cracks every few months.

• Make sure that the bulb in your bedside light is within the wattage range of the shade – too powerful a bulb can overheat the shade and create a fire hazard.

• Do not cover a shade with cloth or paper to cut down the brightness – this too can be a fire risk. Use a weaker bulb or a darker shade, or fit a dimmer switch.

• Fit safety locks to windows in rooms for children. Do not position furniture that a child could climb on under a window.

Attic

If the attic is unfloored, tread only on the joists – the ceiling between the joists will not bear the lightest foot.

• Make sure that the joists are strong enough if you plan to make any regular use of the attic – for storage, for example. A rough rule is to measure the unsupported length of the joists in feet, halve it and add 1, and that gives you the depth in inches the joists should be. A joist across a span of 12 ft. (3.65 m) needs to be at least 7 in. (17.5 cm) deep if it is to be used in this way. If in doubt, get professional advice from an architect or a reliable local builder.

• If you plan to make extensive use of your attic, bear in mind that you must have adequate ventilation and light, and the floor may need to be strengthened. Check your local building regulations before making any changes.

• Use either a properly fitted attic ladder or extending steps to gain access to the attic. Do not try to jump up from the top of a ladder.

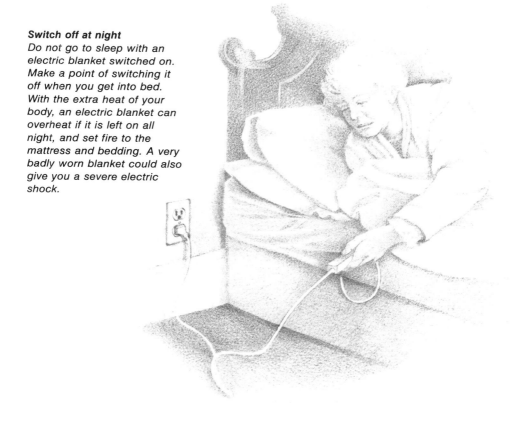

Switch off at night
Do not go to sleep with an electric blanket switched on. Make a point of switching it off when you get into bed. With the extra heat of your body, an electric blanket can overheat if it is left on all night, and set fire to the mattress and bedding. A very badly worn blanket could also give you a severe electric shock.

Stairs and landings

Falls from stairs are particularly dangerous to the elderly and to children less than 5 years old.

• Stair and landing carpets should be in good condition and firmly fastened – people may trip on loose or worn carpet.

• There should be at least one firm, continuous handrail on the staircase. If there are old people in the house, fit one on each side. Ensure that stairs are well lit, with two-way switches so that lights can be put on from either floor.

• Replace horizontal rails on an open staircase or landing with vertical balusters (close together so that a child cannot stick his head through them) or board the rails over.

• Consider fitting boards to the back of each step on an open-riser staircase so that the gap is too narrow for a child to put his head through.

• Fit safety gates at the top and bottom of the staircase to prevent toddlers falling down the stairs or climbing them without supervision.

• Never put or leave loose objects on the stairs

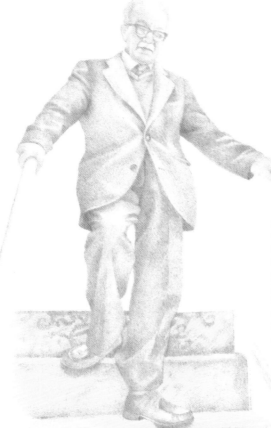

– if you walk on them you will almost certainly stumble, and may fall.

• Do not put a glass door at the bottom of a staircase – anyone falling into it could break it and suffer cuts on top of other injuries.

Doors

• When the house is unoccupied, or at night, keep all internal doors closed. In the event of fire breaking out, this will help to slow the flames.

• Fit safety locks on external doors so that young children cannot run outside.

• Glass doors should be fitted with safety glass – either toughened or laminated. Ordinary glass can shatter into lethal shards.

• If the glass in a door is clear, stick colored tape or decals onto the glass so that it is clearly visible when the door is closed. Alternatively, a wood or metal bar fixed across a glass door can serve the same purpose.

Outside the house

About one in four of all home deaths and non-fatal injuries occurs just outside the home: in the yard, the garden, or the garage, and on the porch or outside steps.

• Install lighting near entrances, around the garage, and along walks and driveways, to reduce the risk of falls and deter intruders.

• Keep walkways in good repair. Ensure that there are no holes or no loose or uneven stones on which people may trip.

• Do not leave tools such as rakes lying about.

Making stairs safe

Old people should have two firm, continuous handrails to help them on the stairs. Keep the stairs well lit; dark areas can cause an elderly person to misjudge a step – and fall. The very young are also at risk on stairs. Every year, thousands of children are injured on them – and some die. To cut this risk, fit safety gates top and bottom. Teach toddlers to climb down backward, on all fours.

• If you have young children, enclose or cover any garden pond or rain barrel. A child can drown in even a very shallow pool.

• Do not let a child use a lawn mower. If you are using a mower, keep children away.

• You may need a permit if you intend to have a barbecue in your yard. Check your local regulations first.

• Never light a barbecue with gasoline or kerosene; it could ignite explosively. Keep a barbecue fire under control.

• If children are likely to play in your garden, check that there are no poisonous trees or plants such as laburnum, deadly nightshade, yew, privet and mountain laurel. The berries of all these plants can be dangerous to children.

• Tell children not to eat any part of a wild or cultivated plant without permission. Even food plants such as potatoes and rhubarb have leaves that are dangerous when eaten.

• Keep garden gates locked or bolted high up so that young children cannot open them and run out into the street.

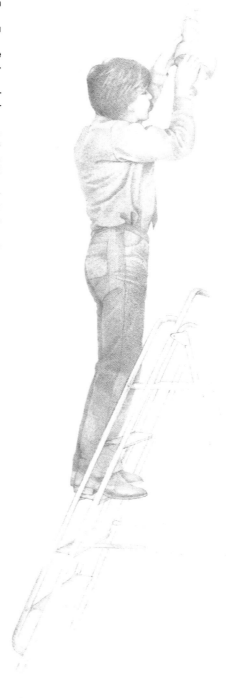

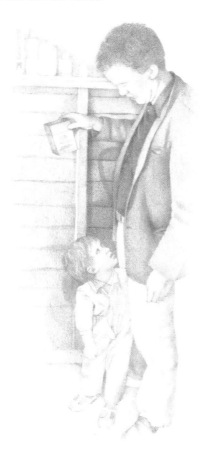

Where to store poisonous substances
Many household products, including turpentine, some glues, and oven cleaners, are poisonous. Lock them away out of reach of children. Do not leave them under the sink.

Take steps to be safe
Use a stepladder if you have to climb when working around the house. Even to change a bulb, take the time to set up a ladder. Do not be tempted to take shortcuts by standing on a chair or stool. They are less stable than a stepladder, and you have nothing to hold onto if you lose your balance.

Storms and high winds

Strong winds – even those well below hurricane force – can cause considerable damage, ripping shingles or tiles from roofs, dislodging chimneys and tearing down power cables and telephone wires. However, most well-constructed houses in good repair suffer little damage until winds reach speeds of about 47 mph (75 km/h).

Preparing for a storm
• Move indoors anything outside – for example, patio furniture, garden tools or toys – that might be blown about and damaged in the storm. This includes children's swings and slides, unless they are securely fixed.
• Move garbage cans into the garage. Make sure cold frame lids and greenhouse windows are securely fastened.
• Close windows and doors tightly, especially those on the side facing the wind. If the windows have external shutters, close them.
• If the storm is likely to be particularly severe, consider reinforcing the inside of windows with boards or heavy furniture (see *How to stay safe in a hurricane,* page 306).
• Put candles, matches and flashlights close at hand in case the electricity is cut off. If you have camping equipment – a stove, for example, or a battery-powered lamp – get it out and keep it handy.
• Have buckets ready in case the roof starts to leak, and plywood, hammer and nails to shore up any window that is blown in.
• If you are expecting a thunderstorm, unplug electrical appliances where possible, including floor or table lamps. If you have a roof antenna, unplug it at the wall socket if there is one or else at the back of the TV set (see *Safety during a thunderstorm,* page 278).
• If your home is prone to flooding in heavy rain, improvise sandbags – strong plastic bags, for instance, filled with any sand, soil or gravel at

hand. Use the bags to line the bottoms of doors and low windows (see *What to do if you are caught in a flood,* page 309).

If a window is blown in
Wind and rain can wreak havoc in a room with a broken window.
• Move valuable objects, and anything else that can be shifted, to another room.
• Block the window with boards, plywood or heavy furniture.
• Do not touch any electrical switches or appliances if you are wet or standing in water or on a damp surface.

If shingles or tiles are blown off the roof
• Do not go outside to inspect the damage to the roof until the storm has passed or eased considerably. More shingles or tiles may come spinning off the roof onto you.
• If water starts coming through the roof, try to move the furniture from the rooms likely to be flooded.
• Put buckets or large bowls underneath all the drips.
• If you can gain access to the attic, beneath the leaking area, place the buckets directly there.
• Set the buckets on the joists or on boards across the joists – not on the ceiling itself. Otherwise, the weight of the water or the water splashing over the edge of the buckets may weaken the plaster and bring part of the ceiling down.

If the roof leaks from the outside
If a leak through the ceiling becomes apparent during heavy rain, it is probably coming through from outside.
• Before you try to find the leak in the roof, reduce the risk of ceiling damage. If you discover that there is a large blister forming on

---

HOW TO AVOID STORM DAMAGE

• Check that gutters and drains are kept clear of leaves and debris.
• Have a builder check shingles, TV antennas and chimney pointing regularly. Make sure that all the windows and doors fit properly, and that the catches and locks are not loose.
• If your house is in an exposed position, consider having a lightning conductor fitted to the roof.
• If there are any large old trees in your garden that could fall on the house during a storm, have them looked over by a tree surgeon.

• Cut back any branches on trees or shrubs that might flap violently against windows during a storm.
• Check that neighbors' trees are safe, too. If any appear to be dangerous, report their condition to the owner in writing. This precaution will strengthen your position later if a tree does fall on your property and you want to claim compensation from the neighbor or his insurance company.
• After a storm, check around the house for any signs of damage – loose or fallen shingles, for instance – and get them repaired as soon as possible.

the ceiling, this is the point where the leaking water is collecting. Carefully poke a few holes in this blister with a large screwdriver or a nail. Use a bucket or large bowl to catch the water that is released (see *If water leaks through a ceiling*, page 158).

• Your next priority is to go into the attic and look for the source of the leak. Using a flashlight, try to track the path the water has taken to its highest point. It is important to remember that the point on the ceiling from which the water drips is unlikely to be directly below the point in the roof where the water is getting in.

• If the rafters in your attic are visible, you may find the hole in the roof quickly. Use your flashlight to examine the underside of the roof directly above the wet spot. If the roof at this point is dry, keep looking higher up. You will probably find water running along the rafters and the roof beam and then dropping to the attic floorboards or joists.

• You can fix a hole in the roof temporarily by sealing it with caulking compound. Work the caulking compound well into and around the hole. This should keep the water out during the storm and until you are ready to make a permanent repair.

• If there is insulation between the rafters on the underside of the roof, remove the batts – one at a time – until you uncover the leak.

• Examine the insulation batts for dampness or discoloration – signs that there is a leak nearby in the roof.

• Once you have located a hole in the roof, circle it with crayon so that you will know where it is when the storm has passed. Then push a nail or a piece of wire through the hole. This will help you – or a roofing specialist or builder – find the exact location of the hole on the outside of the roof.

If a chimney pot is blown off

Rubble and shingles may come down the chimney if a chimney pot is blown off during a storm. The falling chimney pot will probably damage the roof as well on its way down, letting water into the attic.

• Put out any fires caused by the scattering of coals in the fireplace.

• Prevent debris from pouring down the chimney onto the carpet by blocking the fireplace with boards or the fire screen.

• When the debris has stopped falling, seal the base of the chimney with cardboard, bits of wood and newspaper to keep out the rain. Make sure that there are no burning embers in the fireplace before you do this.

• Do the same in other rooms with fireplaces served by the same chimney. There may be other pots on the stack that have been weakened by the storm.

• Check in the attic for leaks.

• Call a builder to repair the chimney after the storm ends.

COPING WITH THE COLD

Falling on hard ice or snow can be extremely dangerous, particularly for the elderly (because their bones are brittle) and for young children (who have less strength in their necks and so are more likely to injure their heads).

It is possible, though, to cut the risk of falling by adopting some of the techniques used by skiers and mountaineers.

• Wear shoes or boots with a deep tread to improve your grip.

• On the sidewalk or flat ground, walk with your legs more apart than usual and with smaller steps.

• If possible, avoid walking on icy patches. But if you cannot avoid a patch of ice, try to find something – a guardrail, for example – for support.

• On slopes, walk with your toes pointing inward. On each step, stamp your foot down firmly and at a slight angle so that the outside edge of your shoe digs into the snow and forms a small step.

• On steep downward slopes, bend your knees to improve your grip.

Protection for the elderly

Elderly people need to keep warm in winter to avoid hypothermia (a potentially fatal loss of body heat). Unfortunately, the ability to sense a drop in body temperature declines with age. As a result, many elderly people who are unaware of the cold can become ill with pneumonia and flu – both diseases to which the body is more vulnerable in the cold.

By following the precautions suggested here, the elderly can protect themselves at home against the effects of cold:

• Wear several layers of clothing. Several thin layers are warmer than one thick one.

• If your bedroom gets cold at night, wear gloves and socks – and a nightcap.

• Hang a thermometer on the wall, and keep an eye on it. The ideal temperature in the living room is 70°F (21°C).

• Stick kitchen foil, shiny side out, to the wall behind radiators to reflect heat into the room. Fix small shelves above radiators to push warm air toward the centre of the room.

• Hang a heavy curtain inside the front door to make the hall warmer.

• As a substitute for double glazing, attach clear plastic sheeting to the inside of windows. Fix it with masking tape or a wooden frame. Make sure the sheeting is easily detachable in case of fire.

In the home and at work

Working at a height

At least 129,000 accidents a year in North American homes involve ladders or scaffolding.

The safest way to work at a height in any situation – up a ladder, say, or in a tree – is to follow the "three holds" principle used by mountaineers and rock climbers. Always make sure that you have at least three secure holds: two footholds and one handhold, or one foothold and two handholds. Do not leave any of the holds until your free hand or foot is secure on a hold to replace it.

• Check ladders or steps before use for cracked or rotten rungs or loose joints. If a stepladder or extension ladder has ropes, make sure they are in good condition.

• Varnish wooden ladders to protect them, but do not paint them. Paint could conceal developing cracks or weak spots in the wood.

• When you use a ladder, set it up so that its base is between a quarter and one-third of its height away from the object it rests against. The base of a 20 ft. (6 m) ladder should be 5-7 ft. (1.5–2 m) away from the wall or tree it is propped on. Any closer, and you risk pulling the ladder over backward when you climb it; any farther, and you risk the base sliding outward.

• On soft ground, rest the foot of the ladder on a wide board. Nail a batten firmly to the board to stop the ladder slipping off.

• On hard ground, lay something heavy – bricks or a bag of cement – against the foot. If possible, have someone hold the foot of the ladder steady as well.

• Make sure the top of the ladder is at least three rungs higher than the highest point you want to reach, so that the top is always within reach of your hands.

• Open a stepladder fully and lock its braces. Climb no higher than the second step from the top. Standing on the top may cause an accident.

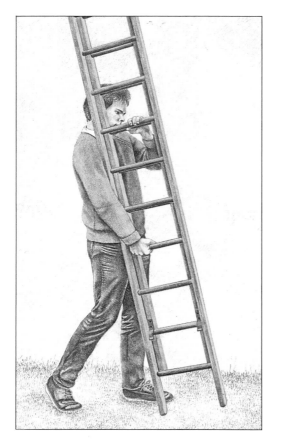

THE SAFE WAY TO CARRY A LADDER
Carry a ladder vertically to avoid accidentally hitting anyone behind you. Bend your knees slightly and, with one hand, grip the rung just below waist level. With the other hand, grip the rung at eye level. Rest the ladder against your shoulder and straighten up. Keep the ladder steady with the upper hand.

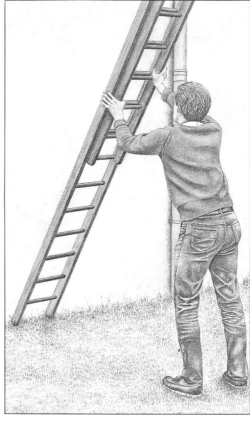

HOW TO RAISE AN EXTENDED LADDER
Extend the ladder while it is still on the ground and wedge its foot against the wall. Lift the top over your head and push the ladder up by moving forward and working your hands down it. When the top is against the wall, pull the bottom out until it is at least a quarter of the ladder's length away from the wall.

THREE WAYS TO STEADY A LADDER

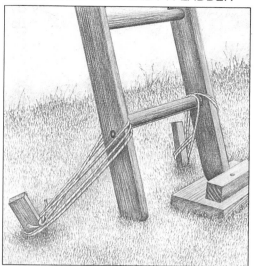

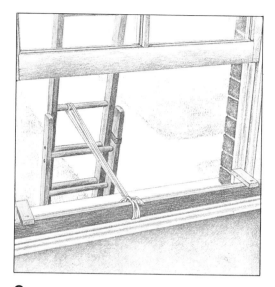

1 *Secure the foot of a ladder by tying it to stakes, which are embedded in the ground. On uneven ground, level the ladder up by putting a wide board with a batten nailed to it under one side of the ladder. On soft ground, put the board under both sides.*

2 *Another way to hold a ladder steady is to anchor it by passing some rope around one of the rungs and tying it to a wooden batten secured behind a window frame. Nail pieces of wood to the wooden batten to stop the ladder sliding sideways.*

• Never lean an extension ladder against a gutter. It is unsafe and could break the gutter.
• When climbing up or down any ladder, always face the ladder and use both hands.
• Do not climb a ladder while carrying a heavy load in one hand. Tie the load to a rope, carry the end of the rope up the ladder, then haul the load up once you are in position.
• Do not lean to the side of a ladder to reach the work – when painting a wall, for example. Keep your hips within the span of the ladder's side rails. Move the ladder to suit the work.
• For work requiring a lot of sideways movement, such as replacing gutters or pointing brickwork, rent a scaffold platform, or make your own platform by suspending one or two planks between two stepladders.
• When setting up your own platform, place the planks across the rungs rather than at the tops of the stepladders.
• Lash the planks both to the rungs and to one side of the ladders to stop them shifting around either lengthways or sideways.
• If the planks have not been used for some time, test each one's strength at ground level first by putting a large block under each end and standing in the middle. Jump up and down on the plank. If it sags worryingly or creaks, do not use it.

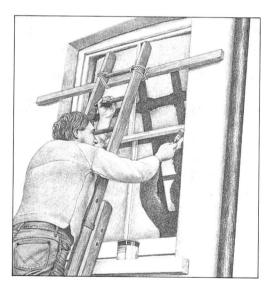

3 *If you have to lean a ladder against a window, lash a strong wooden batten, longer than the window is wide, to the top of the ladder. When you put the ladder up, rest batten on the wall on either side of the window.*

In the home
and at work

Do's and don'ts of using tools

Tools are safe as long as they are used and stored correctly, and kept in good condition and well out of the reach of children.

Yet more than 630,000 people have to get hospital treatment every year in North America as a result of accidents involving the use of tools. About 360,000 of these accidents are caused by home workshop equipment. Another 270,000 involve the use of yard and garden equipment.

Of these accidents, more than 130,000 involve or are caused by power saws in the home workshop and chain saws in the yard and garden. About 120,000 involve the use of hand tools such as screwdrivers, knives, pliers and hammers in the home workshop.

Anyone who plans to use tools, especially power tools, in the home should make a point of becoming familiar beforehand with the positions of concealed water pipes and electric cables. The effort required to draw up a detailed plan is much less than the risk involved in cutting a wire accidentally or the trouble of repairing a hidden pipe.

Hand tools

• Keep sharp-edged tools sheathed and out of the reach of children when not in use, preferably under lock and key.
• Keep tools sharp – blunt tools are dangerous because they require more force to use and thus are more likely to slip.
• Protect the sharp ends of tools such as chisels and bradawls when carrying them in a toolbox. Cover them with fitted plastic covers, wrap them with several layers of cloth or push old bottle corks onto the blades or points.
• Similarly, cover the blades of saws, axes and similar tools when carrying them about.
• Make sure hammerheads are firmly attached to their handles. If necessary, replace the wedges.
• The metal head of a cold chisel roughens when the tool is struck, and sharp fragments may fly off in use. Grind or file these rough edges away regularly.
• Make sure that the material you are working on – a piece of wood or metal, say – is firmly held in a vise or by clamps so that both hands are free to manipulate the tools.
• In the garden, never leave a rake or fork lying down with the prongs up. If you step on the prongs the handle can fly up and strike you in the face.
• Keep sharp-edged garden tools such as clippers, garden and pruning shears, saws, and billhooks well away from your fingers and legs while in use.

Power tools

• Keep power tools unplugged except when in use, so that they cannot be started accidentally.
• For the same reason, unplug power tools before changing accessories, cleaning, adjusting or lubricating.

• With gasoline-powered tools, remove the wire from the spark plug before working on them to prevent the motor starting up by accident. Otherwise, a lawn mower, for example, may spring into life when the blades are turned by hand.
• Wear protective goggles when sparks or chips are liable to fly – when using a grinding wheel, say, or an electric saw. Wear them too when working on bricks or concrete with a cold chisel or a hammer drill.
• Tie back long hair and avoid wearing loose clothing – both may catch in revolving machinery.
• Do not defeat the manufacturers' instructions to keep power tools safe by, for example, tying back the guard on a circular saw.
• Do not use electric tools outdoors in the rain – the damp may cause current leakage and give you a severe shock.
• Use heavy-insulated orange or yellow extension cords for outdoor work. Plug the cord into the power outlet only after the cord has been

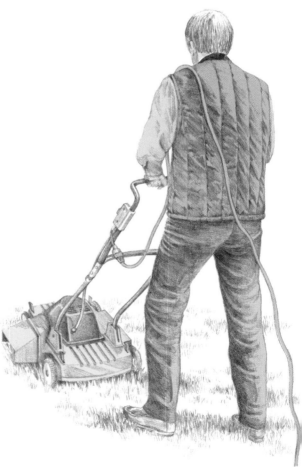

USING AN ELECTRIC LAWN MOWER
Hang the cord for the mower over one shoulder to keep it behind you, and make sure there is nothing it could catch on. If you are on a slope, mow across it – not up and down.

attached to the power tool. For the same reason, unplug the cord at the outlet first when the work is finished. Check cords and plugs regularly for signs of wear or cracked insulation.

• Never tape loose plugs and extension cords together, indoors or out – they may pull apart and are not safe. Use plugs and cords that fit well and are waterproof.

• When using an electric hedge trimmer or lawn mower, keep the cord behind you. Make sure the cord has a clear run so that it does not become snagged while you are working.

• Push a mower away from you – never pull it – and mow across slopes, not up them. That way there is less risk of the mower running over your foot.

• When using mowers and grass trimmers, always wear sturdy shoes. If possible wear goggles when using trimmers – they can throw up small stones and dust.

• Remember that the blade of an electric lawn mower continues spinning for several seconds after the power is switched off. Unplug it before clearing debris from around the blade.

• Consider installing a ground fault circuit interrupter (GFCI) on all your outdoor outlets. The GFCI cuts off the power if there is current leakage or other shock hazard, before it can harm you. Many electric codes require GFCIs in all newly installed outdoor outlets.

• Look for the term "double insulation" or a symbol showing two squares, one inside the other, when buying power tools. Both mean that the tool is doubly insulated and needs no grounding.

Using a chain saw

• Apply the saw to the top of the work you are cutting. Do not cut from underneath – unless you are cutting a piece of wood supported at both ends. Otherwise the weight of the wood will tend to close the cut, gripping the saw.

• Cut using the part of the saw closest to the motor end. If you use the tip, you may lose control of the saw.

• Do not carry the saw about with the engine running, even if the blade is disengaged.

• Keep the chain at the correct tension, or it may fly off and cause a serious accident.

• Sharpen the teeth frequently, preferably every time you use the saw. Blunt teeth may make you use too much pressure.

• Before refilling the tank of a gasoline-powered saw, make sure the engine is cold, or gasoline spilled onto it may ignite.

• If you have a can of gasoline with you, keep it well away from the saw. The exhaust will occasionally emit sparks.

• Wear sensible clothing: thick trousers or slacks and sturdy shoes (preferably with reinforced toe caps), and no loose sleeves. Wear goggles to protect your eyes against chips and sawdust.

• Always work in a clear area, so that there are no twigs or branches to catch the blade or the trigger. Hold the saw with both hands.

• If you have an assistant, make sure he or she keeps at least 10 yd. (9 m) away, out of range of any flying chips.

• Always disconnect the spark plug or the electric cord before cleaning or adjusting the saw. Have the saw serviced regularly and the cutting chain checked for signs of wear.

Getting tools from tool rental shops

Specialized power tools – such as jackhammers, cultivators, and belt sanders – can be rented by the day from tool rental shops. This is a convenient way of getting the use of expensive tools that you need only occasionally. But do not forget that many of these tools are potentially dangerous.

Do not even attempt to use them unless you know exactly how to handle them. Get the rental shop to give you clear instructions and preferably a demonstration, too.

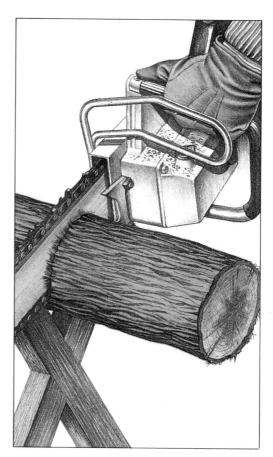

HOW TO USE A CHAIN SAW
Saw from the top downward to cut the unsupported end off a log. Cut with the part of the blade closest to the motor. That way it is easier to hold the saw steady.

In the home and at work

How to remove stains

The best way to remove a stain depends on what has been spilled and what it has been spilled on. But one rule applies to any stain anywhere: try to deal with it quickly, before it dries. Once dry, most stains become more difficult to remove.

Remember, too, that many stain-removing agents are poisonous, flammable or both (see chart, this page).

Read carefully any instructions on commercial preparations. Never store them in unmarked bottles, and keep them out of the reach of children. Work out of doors if possible, or in a well-ventilated place.

• The first step in treating a stain is to blot, lightly scrape or vacuum the material in order to clear as much of the stain as possible before further treatment.

• For grease stains, shake on plenty of talcum powder, powdered starch or a similar absorbent agent. When the worst of the grease has been absorbed, brush clear.

RAPID GUIDE TO STAIN REMOVAL

KEY TO CHART
1 Flammable
2 Equal parts with warm water
3 1 part peroxide (20 volume strength) to 4 parts cold water
4 Harmful vapor
5 1 tablespoon to 2 cups water

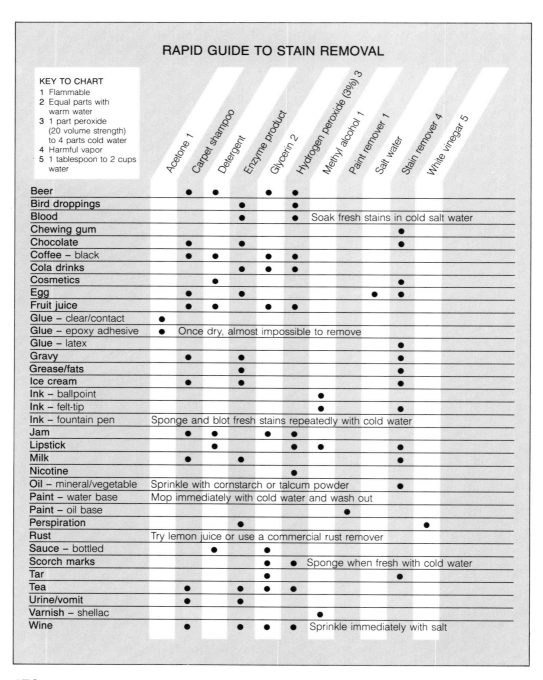

	Acetone 1	Carpet shampoo	Detergent	Enzyme product	Glycerin 2	Hydrogen peroxide (3%) 3	Methyl alcohol 1	Paint remover 1	Salt water	Stain remover 4	White vinegar 5
Beer	●	●		●	●						
Bird droppings			●			●					
Blood			●			●	Soak fresh stains in cold salt water				
Chewing gum										●	
Chocolate	●		●							●	
Coffee – black	●	●		●	●						
Cola drinks			●	●	●						
Cosmetics		●								●	
Egg	●		●						●	●	
Fruit juice	●	●		●	●						
Glue – clear/contact	●										
Glue – epoxy adhesive	●	Once dry, almost impossible to remove									
Glue – latex										●	
Gravy		●	●							●	
Grease/fats			●							●	
Ice cream	●		●							●	
Ink – ballpoint							●				
Ink – felt-tip							●			●	
Ink – fountain pen	Sponge and blot fresh stains repeatedly with cold water										
Jam	●	●		●	●						
Lipstick		●			●		●			●	
Milk	●		●							●	
Nicotine						●					
Oil – mineral/vegetable	Sprinkle with cornstarch or talcum powder									●	
Paint – water base	Mop immediately with cold water and wash out										
Paint – oil base								●			
Perspiration			●								●
Rust	Try lemon juice or use a commercial rust remover										
Sauce – bottled		●		●							
Scorch marks				●		●	Sponge when fresh with cold water				
Tar				●						●	
Tea	●		●	●	●						
Urine/vomit	●		●								
Varnish – shellac							●				
Wine	●		●	●	●		Sprinkle immediately with salt				

• For other stains, sponge or rinse through with cold or lukewarm water – never hot water, which could fix the stain.

• Blot carpets or upholstery frequently,. while you work on getting out the worst of the stain, to avoid overwetting them.

• What you should do next to complete the job depends upon what caused the stain, and what will dissolve it (see chart).

• Not all stains can be removed. If in doubt, and for delicate and valuable articles, just blot the stain and do not attempt any further treatment at home. Instead, seek advice from a professional cleaning firm.

• In general, stains on suede and leather, waterproof fabrics or rich materials such as velvets, satins and silks should be left to a professional cleaner.

• With other fabrics and surfaces, start with the mildest treatment and test first on a hidden area. Some solvents can damage certain materials, such as rayon.

• Use a white absorbent pad for applying solvents. Where possible, work from the underside of the stain, holding another pad on the topside to absorb it.

• Dab at the stain. Rubbing can spread the mark and damage the surface. Work inward from the edge to avoid spreading the stain.

• If a stain has become dried, try to soften it. Rub in some glycerin solution (equal amounts of glycerin and warm water) and leave it for an hour. Then sponge with cold water.

• Once the substance has been loosened, treat it as a freshly made stain.

Emergency alternatives

If you find in an emergency that you do not have the substances mentioned in the chart, there are other ways, using more common household items, to get rid of some stains.

• If somebody spills wine, for example, on your carpet, flush it out immediately with bottled soda water or by sponging with warm water.

• If you get wine on a washable fabric – a tablecloth, say – immediately sprinkle it with salt to stop the stain spreading. Then, as soon as possible afterward, stretch the stained area over a bowl and pour hot water through the fabric. If it is red wine, you can also pour white wine over the stain; this will make it easier to remove.

• If a pet or a baby urinates on your carpet, immediately sponge the area with bottled soda water. Blot up the soda water. Then sponge with warm water with a few drops of antiseptic added.

• Use lemon juice for tea and coffee stains on washable fabrics. Rub the juice into the stain and wash the fabric in warm soapy water.

• If you get chewing gum on your clothes, put the article of clothing in a plastic bag and leave it in the freezer section of the refrigerator until the gum has hardened. You will then be able to pick it off easily.

Elevator emergency

When an elevator breaks down with people trapped inside, the greatest danger is from panic.

• Stay calm and try to reassure anyone who shows signs of panic.

• Explain that you and they are not in danger, that help can be summoned in several ways, and that there is no possibility of the elevator falling out of control down the shaft.

• Tell the others in the elevator that automatic brakes, usually fitted underneath the elevator, prevent this happening by clamping onto the steel guide rails that run down each side of the elevator shaft. The brakes work even if there is a power cut and the lights go out.

• Use the alarm button or the telephone inside the elevator to call for help.

• If there is no alarm system, bang on the doors and shout. Use a shoe to bang with.

• Once you contact someone outside, explain what has happened and ask him to call the company that services the elevator. A company mechanic can lower the elevator manually and open the doors to let you out.

• If expert help is unavailable, elevator rescues are often handled by the fire department. Tell your contact to dial 911. The firemen will usually open the doors just above the stalled elevator and rescue you through the hatch in the elevator.

• Never try to escape from the elevator without help from an expert outside.

• Do not try to force the inner elevator doors open. Even if you managed to do so, it is unlikely that you would be able to reach and open the outer doors onto a landing, let alone climb out safely. There is also the danger that you might slip on the oil and grease that accumulates on the outside of an elevator. Having shoes with a good grip or bare feet is no guarantee that you would be able to balance steadily.

• Do not be tempted, either, to climb out of any hatch there may be in the elevator's ceiling. When an elevator hatch is opened, an electrical contact prevents the elevator from moving. But if the open hatch falls shut by accident the elevator could move without warning, throwing you off balance. In the darkness of the shaft, you could also trip over the elevator cables or slip on grease and fall off the roof of the elevator.

If you cannot raise the alarm

It is very rare for calls for help to go unanswered for long, particularly in an apartment building where there are other people within earshot. But in an office building late at night or at the start of a weekend, it may happen that nobody passes near the elevator for hours – or even days.

• The safest course in this situation is to stay put, stay calm and wait. You may get hungry, thirsty and hot – but you will survive.

• Listen for a caretaker and try to attract his attention. If that fails, wait for the building to open again, then bang on the doors and shout for help.

Intruders in your home

The vast majority of people who are likely to visit your home are law-abiding citizens. But it is worth being cautious always, just in case the visitor is a thief or a confidence trickster.

If a stranger calls at your door
• Use a peephole to check anyone who knocks at your door. Keep the chain on the door if the caller is someone you do not know.
• Never let in strangers who call unexpectedly until you have checked their credentials.
• If the person gives you a telephone number to call to check his credentials, look up the name of his organization in the directory – the number he gave you may be that of an accomplice. Ask the stranger to wait outside, door closed and chain on, while you call.
• If you are still in doubt about the caller's identity, ring the local police department and explain your suspicions. Suspect anybody who protests at your caution.
• Remember that the longer you draw out the process of identification, the better your chances of scaring off a potential wrongdoer.
• Always be fully clothed before opening the door. Close the door on a stranger before going for your purse or to make a phone call.
• If you live in an apartment, do not automatically "buzz open" the main door if a stranger calls your apartment on the intercom with a plausible excuse.

If you return to see signs of a break-in
• If you notice or suspect that somebody is inside your home just as you arrive – you see movement, perhaps, or notice an open door – avoid entering the house at all.
• If you have driven in by car, back out of the driveway again and drive off. The intruder may think you were just turning round.
• If you are on foot, walk on down the sidewalk.
• Go to a neighbor's house at once and call the police. Follow the same drill if you find strangers outside your house.

If you get indoors to find an intruder inside
• Ask the intruder what he wants.
• Do not, the police advise, give any impression that you intend to fight over money or possessions – you may get hurt. Try not to anger or provoke him.
• Memorize the intruder's appearance, and call the police as soon as he has gone.

If you hear an intruder inside house
• If you hear someone breaking into your home at night, put on all the lights and make a lot of noise by moving about. Most burglars will flee empty-handed rather than face their intended victim.
• If you wake at night to hear an intruder already in the house, lock your bedroom door. Move as quietly as possible to avoid attracting the intruder's attention. Find something that you can

use as a weapon – a heavy brush, a vase, a knitting needle or a bunch of keys – but plan to use it only if you cannot avoid a fight (see *if you are attacked on the street,* page 314).
• Look out of your window after you hear the intruder leave and try to note what he looks like, what direction he heads in and what car, if any, he gets into. Then call the police, if you have not already done so.

How to give a description to the police
Anyone who contacts the police to report a crime suspect – an intruder, say, or someone behaving suspiciously near his or a neighbor's home – may need to give a description of the person he has seen, or of the person's vehicle. This is a checklist of details useful to police:
• Male/female
• Color of skin
• Complexion
• Height
• Hair (color, length, straight/curly, receding)
• Build
• Age
• Eye color
• Glasses
• Face (long, thin, round, clean-shaven, mustache, beard)
• Marks (scars, tattoos)
• Mouth (narrow/wide)
• Dress (description of clothing)
• Any other distinguishing features (mannerisms, say, such as a limp or a stutter).

If you see a suspicious vehicle, try to note these details:
• Car/van/truck/motorcycle
• Color
• License plate
• Other details (damage marks, any company name on it and so on)
• Make/model
• Body type (sedan, convertible, number of doors)
• Direction it was traveling.

Securing doors and windows
Your best defense against burglary is secure points of entry. If a burglar finds your windows and doors hold fast, he will likely go elsewhere.
• Replace any hollow wooden doors – particularly if they lead to the outside or to the garage – with solid-core or metal doors and firm frames.
• Equip exterior doors with a 1 in. (2.5 cm) deadbolt lock. Make sure that you also have strong locks on the doors to the garage and porch.
• Add a metal grille to any glass door that might give access to an intruder.
• To prevent a sliding glass door from being lifted, install a metal bar to prevent it from moving on its tracks. You can also put a length of pipe or broomstick along the bottom track.
• Windows are as vulnerable to forced entry as doors. So consider fitting window locks to all windows that are on the ground floor or can be

reached by an easy climb. If you live in an apartment, fit locks to all windows or doors opening to balconies, fire escapes, or roofs.

• Consider using strong screws to make improvised locks. On a sash window, drive a screw about 1 in. (2.5 cm) into the wood beside the lock. This will prevent the lock from being moved by an intruder who has broken or cut through the glass to reach it.

• Secure a sash window with a nail that slips into a hole where the top and bottom sashes meet. With the window closed firmly, drill a hole through the top of the bottom sash and part of the way into the bottom of the upper sash. Insert a nail that is long enough to penetrate the entire thickness. The nail should protrude slightly so

it can be removed easily. Alternatively, use a clipped-off nail and draw it out with a magnet.

Installing home security systems
If your area suffers many break-ins, or if you are away from home a lot, install a security system (see chart, below). There are two basic types – the perimeter and the motion-detector systems. The perimeter system sounds an alarm when an intruder opens windows and outside doors; the motion detector, when an intruder moves around inside. Both systems are set off by infrared, magnetic, microwave or ultrasonic sensors. You can select a local or central alarm, or a police hookup. To select the best for your home, consult a security firm or the police.

In the home and at work

HOME SECURITY SYSTEMS AND ALARMS

Type	How it works	Advantages/Disadvantages
System		
Perimeter detectors (exterior protection)	Alarm is set off when an intruder attempts to open doors or accessible windows that have magnetic sensors, which are connected to an electric circuit	Perimeter sensors are visible deterrents, which detect intrusion immediately. But they require elaborate wiring and are easily penetrated by an expert burglar
Motion detectors (interior protection)	Alarm is set off when infrared, microwave or ultrasonic sensors detect an intruder who is moving through given areas or "trap zones" inside a house	Motion detectors are difficult to spot and elude, but they are easily set off by pets, children, or air conditioners
Alarm		
Local	Alarm and flashing lights are set off on the premises	Local alarm sets off sudden and conspicuous noise and light, which is intended to frighten the intruder and to alert the occupants of the house. It is ineffective if no one is nearby, and it often goes off when no intruder is present
Central	Switchboard operator is alerted to call home, office, or police	Central alarm makes no sound in the house, only at a central point such as a security firm. It reduces false alarms. But any delay in answering the alarm could provide time for an intruder to act and escape
Police hookup	Police switchboard operator is alerted to dispatch unit	Police hookup provides fast assistance, but frequent false alarms may incur fines

PROTECTING YOUR HOME

If you are going away or leaving the house for a period, the central rule is: do not advertise your absence.

• Cancel deliveries of milk and newspapers.

• Consider hiring a telephone answering service, so that your telephone gives no clue that you are absent. If you have a telephone answering machine, word your announcement as though you were merely away for an hour or two.

• With timing devices, you can have lights burning at certain hours, even when you are away. A photoelectric cell will turn on exterior lights when darkness falls.

• Ask a neighbor to keep an eye on the house – to collect mail and other material left in the mailbox, to mow the lawn, sweep up leaves, leave footprints in the snow and generally make the house look lived in. Offer to do the same for the neighbor.

• Do not put your name on the mailbox. Burglars will phone to find out if you are at home. If they reach your answering service, they may learn too much about your whereabouts.

• If you are going away for only a short period, consider leaving your car locked outside. It may fool a prowling thief into thinking that the house is occupied. But if you will be away for a long holiday, remember that a dusty car may itself become an indication that the house is empty.

• Tell the local police department that you will be away. Many police departments like to know your home is vacant, particularly if it has an alarm.

How to deter burglars

Each year, around 3.5 million burglaries are reported to the police in North America – an average of about 9,500 every day. However, these figures do not really tell how many are committed because only 50 percent of burglaries in the United States are reported.

A skilled professional burglar will always find a way into a house if he wants to – and has the time. But many burglaries are committed by unskilled and often young opportunists who are looking for easy pickings. You may deter both kinds of burglar by offering stiff resistance in the form of security devices. If a burglar has to make a lot of noise or spend a lot of time breaking in, he is likely to give up and look elsewhere.

• Never leave a door unlocked and do not leave keys under doormats.

• Make sure that all your windows and doors have strong locks (see *Securing doors and windows*, page 178).

• Consider installing lighting at all outside entrances and in the yard to discourage intruders. If you suspect that there is a prowler outside, turn the lights on.

• Trim any shrubbery that hides any possible entry points to your house – for example, the basement windows.

• Do not put your name on your key ring. That way if you lose your house keys nobody will know which house they belong to (you can use a postal code marking to identify them if they are handed in to the police).

• Keys should not be carried in a handbag. If it is stolen, letters or documents also in the bag could tell the thief your address.

Neighborhood Watch: how it works

Neighborhood Watch, Crime Watch, Business Watch, Apartment Watch and other self-help crime prevention groups now operate in many parts of North America. The first groups were organized in California in the 1970s. Their primary aim is to stem the rising tide of burglaries by encouraging people to keep an eye out for suspicious activities near their homes – by being, in other words, good neighbors.

The police say that neighborhoods which have joined crime prevention schemes – and announced the fact publicly by putting up stickers visible from the street – have considerably lower crime rates than similar areas which have not joined.

The schemes do not encourage people to take the law into their own hands if they see anyone behaving suspiciously. But the schemes do encourage householders to phone the police at once by dialing 911, or to contact their street coordinator.

As a further deterrent to thieves, police also recommend that you should mark anything valuable you own – car, bicycle, furniture, household appliances and so on – with an indelible identification. Check with your local police department or neighborhood watch group about the form of identification – for example, license plate numbers – used in your area.

The marking can be done at home by using a do-it-yourself engraving tool, or an invisible marker (available from many hardware shops) whose ink shows up only under ultraviolet light. The presence of the marks should be advertised through stickers placed in the windows of your house.

Stickers, leaflets and detailed advice about joining or setting up a local neighborhood watch group, and about making your home more secure, are usually available from your local police.

Caring for a sick or injured animal

There are almost as many pet dogs and cats in the United States and Canada as there are people in the five most populous American states. Across the continent, the estimated total for these pets is 81 million – nearly 44 million dogs and about 37 million cats – compared with about 83.8 million people in California, New York, Texas, Pennsylvania, and Illinois. In addition, there are some 5.7 million domesticated horses, including about 175,000 which are used for pleasure and sport.

If a pet animal becomes seriously ill or is seriously injured in an accident, the safest course is to take it to a vet as soon as possible. But you can do much to alleviate its distress before you get there by using the first aid advice given here.

In some circumstances, swift action can save the pet's life. When a cat or dog gives birth, on the other hand, the best course is to leave the mother alone, and to call a vet only if the birth seems to be going wrong.

The section that begins on these pages describes the commonest emergencies that arise with a pet dog, cat or horse, and explains how to cope with each. It also explains what to do if you are attacked by bees and wasps, and how you can help an injured bird or wild animal.

How to handle an injured cat or dog

Any dog or cat which has been injured is almost certain to be in pain. As a result, even the most loving, placid pet is liable to bite or scratch, or to run off, if it is given the chance. The priority, therefore, is to get the animal under control and into a safe, escape-proof place where you can examine its injuries.
• Approach the animal slowly and carefully, talking soothingly as you do.
• If it is a dog, have with you a rope, string or bandage fastened into a noose at one end.
• Drop the noose over the dog's head and draw it tight on the neck. Lead the dog to a safe place.
• If the dog is unable to stand, slide it onto an improvised stretcher – a large blanket or towel. Get someone to help you to lift the blanket by

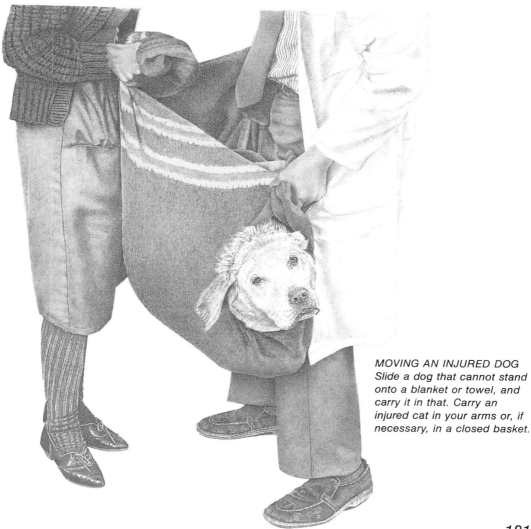

MOVING AN INJURED DOG
Slide a dog that cannot stand onto a blanket or towel, and carry it in that. Carry an injured cat in your arms or, if necessary, in a closed basket.

the corners and carry the dog to a safe place.
• In the case of a cat, grasp it by the scruff of the neck with one hand and support its bottom with the other.
• Take it – in a closed basket, if necessary – to a safe place.

Preparing for treatment

• Before you start to examine a cat's or dog's injuries, get it onto a smooth surface such as a table or, if it is a heavy dog, on a slippery floor such as lino.
• Get someone else to help you to hold the animal – the slippery surface will stop it getting a grip and lessen its ability to escape.
• Put a collar on the animal to give yourself an easy handhold.
• Grip the animal firmly. Better still, get a helper to hold the animal so that you have both hands free to tend the injury.
• With a dog, tie a handkerchief or bandage firmly around its muzzle as well, so that it cannot open its mouth to bite.

Treating the injury

The principles of giving first aid to animals are much the same as they are for humans. Do what you can to stop the injury getting any worse, and then take the animal to a vet as soon as possible. The commonest serious injuries are bleeding or a broken leg.

How to stop bleeding

• If an animal is bleeding badly, cover the wound with a clean pad – a handkerchief or gauze – and bind it on with a bandage. If you cannot bandage the wound, hold the pad in place by hand.
• If the wound is on a leg, and pressure does not stop the bleeding, apply a tourniquet above the wound. A bandage tightened by twisting a stick is effective. Tighten the tourniquet only

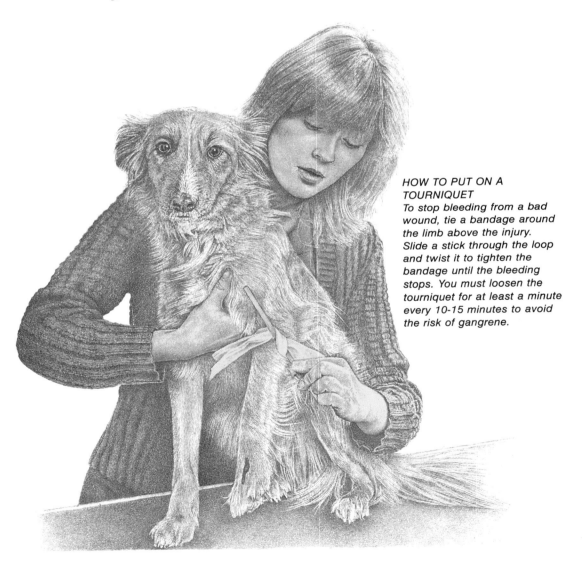

HOW TO PUT ON A TOURNIQUET
To stop bleeding from a bad wound, tie a bandage around the limb above the injury. Slide a stick through the loop and twist it to tighten the bandage until the bleeding stops. You must loosen the tourniquet for at least a minute every 10-15 minutes to avoid the risk of gangrene.

until the bleeding stops, and relax it every 10-15 minutes to avoid the risk of gangrene.
• Get the animal to a vet at once. If possible, have someone phone the vet's office to alert the staff that an emergency case is on the way.

How to treat a broken leg

If a leg is lying at an awkward angle, it may mean that a bone is broken.
• Stop any bleeding. Ease the leg into as comfortable a position as possible. Warn whoever is holding the animal before you move the leg. The pain may make the animal bite or scratch.
• Straighten the leg gently into a more normal position. Then splint it by bandaging it gently but firmly to a piece of wood or hardboard of roughly the same shape as the leg.
• Take the animal to a vet.

Giving medicine to a cat or dog

When you give medicine to a pet, prepare in the same way as you would when you examine an injured pet. Put a cat or small dog on a smooth-topped table. Put a large dog on a smooth floor with its back to a wall. Ask someone else to help you to hold the animal still.

Giving pills

• With a cat, grasp its head from behind with one hand. Place your thumb and forefinger at the corners of its mouth. Tilt its head back and push down on the lower jaw with your other hand. Use your thumb and forefinger to keep the cat's mouth open. Push the pill to the back of the tongue and close the mouth.
• With a dog, use one hand to hold it across the top of its muzzle just in front of the eyes, and push your thumb into the side of its mouth. Push up on the roof of its mouth. Use the middle

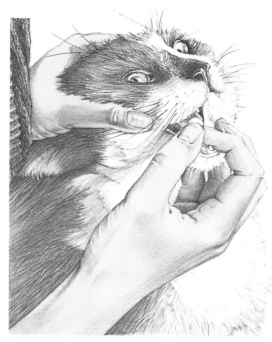

HOW TO GIVE A CAT A PILL
Tilt the cat's head up with one hand, and with the other press down on its lower jaw to open its mouth. Push the pill to the back of the tongue, then close the mouth. Hold it shut until the cat swallows.

finger of the other hand to hold down the front of the lower jaw while you push the pill to the back of the tongue. Close the mouth and hold the jaws shut until the pill is swallowed. Rub the throat if necessary to encourage this.

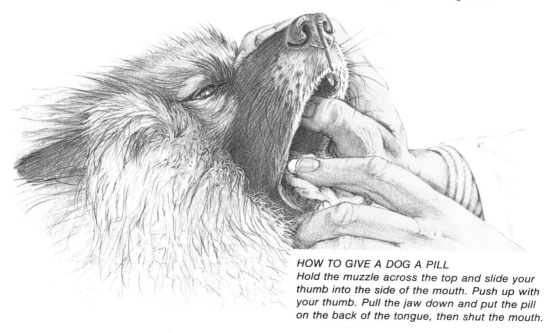

HOW TO GIVE A DOG A PILL
Hold the muzzle across the top and slide your thumb into the side of the mouth. Push up with your thumb. Pull the jaw down and put the pill on the back of the tongue, then shut the mouth.

183

Giving liquid medicine

• Buy a disposable plastic syringe without a needle. They are available from vets and most druggists.
• Load the medicine into the syringe.
• Hold the animal firmly and calm it by talking gently to it.
• With a cat, push the nozzle into the side of the mouth behind the large canine teeth and trickle the liquid in slowly. Hold the mouth up while you do this so that the medicine does not dribble out.
• With a dog, push the nozzle in where the lips meet at the side of the mouth. Pull the cheek back with one finger and hold the mouth up while you trickle the liquid in slowly.

Giving eye drops or eye ointment

• With both a cat and a dog, ask someone to hold the animal's head steady, or – if you are confident you will not be clawed or bitten – hold it steady against your body.
• Use two fingers above and below the eye to open the lids, and apply the drop or ointment directly onto the eyeball.

Giving ear drops or ear ointment

• With either pet, hold the ear flap with one hand to expose the ear canal and administer the medicine directly into the ear.
• Once the medicine is in, massage the base of the ear gently to ensure that the medicine gets well down into the ear.

• Never try to clean out the inner part of the ear canal of a cat or dog. You will damage the ear no matter how gentle you are, and the animal will resent the pain you cause.

When an animal has a fit

Fits are not uncommon in dogs; they are rarer in cats. They can have any of a number of causes, including brain tumors and epilepsy. With either animal, the basic principle of treatment is not to interfere more than necessary.
• Make sure the pet is not in danger – from knocking things over, for example.
• Try to keep it quiet and cool. Draw the curtains in the room to reduce the light.
• Get it to a vet as soon as you can, but do not try to move it while it is still convulsing.
• Take care when you do move it. An animal that is ill is more likely to bite or scratch unexpectedly.

If your cat or dog is poisoned

Ordinary vomiting and bad diarrhea in pets are only rarely signs of poisoning. The usual symptoms of genuine poisoning are persistent vomiting and diarrhea, often combined with shivering tremors or convulsions, leading later to coma.
• If your pet is already in a coma, get veterinary help at once.
• If your pet is still conscious and you know that it has swallowed a corrosive poison, such as acid or caustic soda, wash the mouth out rapidly

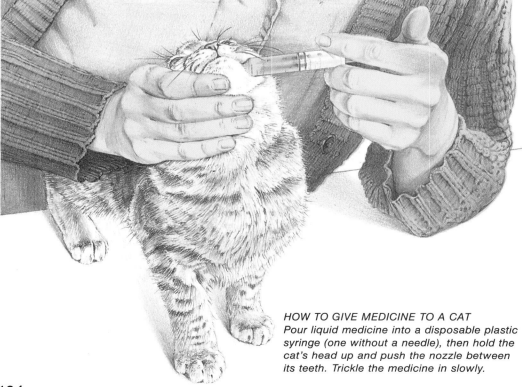

HOW TO GIVE MEDICINE TO A CAT
Pour liquid medicine into a disposable plastic syringe (one without a needle), then hold the cat's head up and push the nozzle between its teeth. Trickle the medicine in slowly.

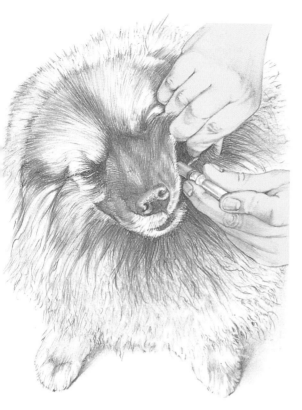

HOW TO GIVE MEDICINE TO A DOG
Use a syringe for a dog, in much the same way
as for a cat. But instead of pushing the nozzle
between its teeth, slide it alongside the teeth,
so that the medicine trickles into its cheek.

with milk or water. If you have a syringe handy, use that to wash the mouth out. Otherwise hold the animal's mouth open and pour in the liquid from a jug or cup.

• After washing the mouth out, give the animal plenty of milk or water to drink. The aim is to dilute the poison without causing vomiting – because vomiting up a corrosive poison will burn the mouth and throat for a second time.

• Follow up the drink with a meal of bread and water or porridge.

• If you are certain that the animal has swallowed a noncorrosive poison, make it vomit as soon as possible.

• To make a pet vomit give it hydrogen peroxide. Repeat the dose every 10 to 15 minutes until the pet vomits. Use a syringe to administer hydrogen peroxide – 1 teaspoon for cats, and 1 to 2 teaspoons for dogs. Most pets usually vomit after the first or second dose.

• With either type of poisoning, take the animal to a vet and take with you labels or samples of the poison.

• If you are not sure what type of poison is involved, treat the animal as if it had swallowed a corrosive poison.

Dealing with a choking animal

The priority in treating a choking animal is the same as for a choking human: speed.

• If there is something tight around the neck, remove it at once.

• If something is lodged in the mouth or throat – a bone, say – hold the animal's mouth open and pull the obstruction out. Use a bar such as a spoon handle to stop the jaws closing while you work. Push the bar to the back of the animal's mouth and between the teeth like a gag.

• If a ball gets stuck in a dog's throat, the obstruction tends to make the dog salivate profusely, which makes the ball slippery and difficult to get hold of.

• Open the mouth wide and try to get a finger behind the ball. Alternatively, put the fingers of both hands on the outside of the dog's cheeks as far back as you can and press forward from behind the ball.

• If the dog is choking on a sharp stick which has pierced its mouth or the back of its throat, pull the stick free.

• Keep the dog warm, do not let it eat or drink and get it to a vet as fast as possible.

• If the animal is likely to bite or cannot be controlled when you try to remove an object from its throat, take it to the vet immediately.

Treating a limp

If a cat or dog develops a limp for no obvious cause, examine the injured leg gently (see *How to handle an injured cat or dog*, page 181).

• Feel the limb from the paw upward, looking for swelling, heat and pain.

• Look for cuts too, especially in the pads of

CHOKING – AVOIDING RISKS

• Check regularly that the collar on a young, growing animal does not become too tight.

• Never leave a choke chain on an unattended dog.

• If your dog enjoys chasing a ball, use one that is far too big for it to swallow. Never use a small, solid, hard rubber ball.

• If you throw sticks for a dog, use one with blunt ends. A sharp one can land end-on in the ground and a running dog can impale itself.

• Never give any animal cooked bones to chew. They can splinter and cause the animal to choke or to cut itself severely. Pork and chicken bones are particularly dangerous – even if they have not been cooked. The only safe bones for an animal are raw beef bones.

the feet, and for splinters, grit and thorns. Clean any cuts in cold water.
• Remove any foreign bodies you find, if you can do so easily. If you cannot remove them easily, get veterinary help.
• Bending and straightening the leg may reveal painful areas and help you to find the cause of the problem. But again, if you cannot find the cause easily, take the animal to a vet.
• If a cat or dog develops a limp, particularly if part of the affected leg is swollen, the chances are that it has been bitten in a fight. This is much more likely to happen to a cat than a dog.
• Shave the hair around the wound. Clean the swollen area with hot water containing a little salt or with hydrogen peroxide.
• After bathing the affected area, contact a vet immediately.
• If a septic wound is obvious, apply a warm pad to reduce the risk of inflammation, especially if there is any delay in getting to the vet.
• To prepare the warm pad, use a clean cloth that has been squeezed out in water as hot as you can stand and then bandage the pad over the wound.

Removing a barb from a paw
Barbed objects such as fishhooks that become embedded in the skin of a cat or dog need special treatment, to avoid making the injury worse when the barb is removed.
• Get the animal to a safe, escape-proof place before you start trying to treat it (see *How to handle an injured cat or dog*, page 181).
• Cut the hook free from any fishing line it is attached to.
• If the hook will not pull out easily, push it through until the barb is exposed.
• Cut off the barb with the wire-cutting section of a pair of pliers.
• Remove the rest of the hook by pulling the shank back out through the original incision.
• Clean the wound, cover it with a clean dressing and consult a vet.
• Do not try to remove a hook that has pierced a particularly sensitive part of the body such as the lips or eyes. Treatment of these areas may require an anesthetic and is best left to a vet.

If a dog gets heatstroke
Never leave a dog in a car on a hot day. It can quite rapidly become seriously overheated, to the point of collapse.
• If a dog is obviously in distress, get it at once into a cool place and soak it in cold water, using towels or sponges. Wrap cold, wet towels round its head and body as well.
• If possible, put it in a bath or paddling pool – but do not do this if the dog is unconscious.
• If you have small lumps of ice handy, push them up the dog's bottom.
• Get the dog to a vet as soon as possible. Keep it cool on the journey by wrapping it in more wet towels. Use more ice if you have any.

If your cat or dog is bitten
A pet that has been bitten or scratched in a fight may have several small wounds which are not easily visible through the fur.
• Use your fingers to find the site of the injury.
• Clip away the fur around the wound, but do not pull the hair away if it seems to be part of a scab or clot. You may start the wound bleeding again.
• Clean the wound with warm water containing a little salt or with hydrogen peroxide.
• Cover and bandage the wound if it looks serious.
• Have the injuries checked by a vet. Bites and scratches suffered in a fight may go septic without treatment.
• With cats particularly, the first evidence of a bite may be an abscess, which often develops behind a tiny wound. You may notice the swelling, or the cat may become listless and off its food. The cat will need antibiotics – get it to a vet for treatment as soon as possible. If there is any delay, bathe the swelling with warm water to reduce the inflammation.

How to stop a dogfight
• Intervene in a dogfight only if the dog is your own or is well known to you. Most dogs usually stop fighting of their own accord fairly quickly.
• If you do decide to intervene, take care not to get bitten yourself.
• Make a loud noise, such as a shrill whistle. Alternatively, throw a bucket of water over both contestants or turn a hose on them.
• If the owner of the other dog is available to help, ask him to move in behind one of the dogs at the same time as you move in behind the other.
• Grab the dog by the collar, if it is wearing one, or the scruff of the neck.
• Do not pull the dogs apart because this will worsen any wounds – if one has its teeth in the other, say. Instead, hit the dog in the side of the chest to make it let go, then pull it away.
• Once the dogs have been parted, keep a firm grip on them to make sure that they do not start fighting again.

If cats fight
• Stop a cat fight by chasing the combatants and shouting and shooing at them. Cat fights rarely last long.
• Do not try to get hold of a fighting cat – you are very likely to be scratched or bitten.

If a pet is stung
Cats and dogs often chase wasps and bees. So when they are stung, it is often on or around the face.
• If the sting is on the skin, rub on an antihistamine cream. It is as effective on animals as on humans. Do not use a cream of this kind near the eyes or mouth, however.
• If the sting is inside the mouth, get the animal

HOW TO GET A HOOK OUT OF A PAW

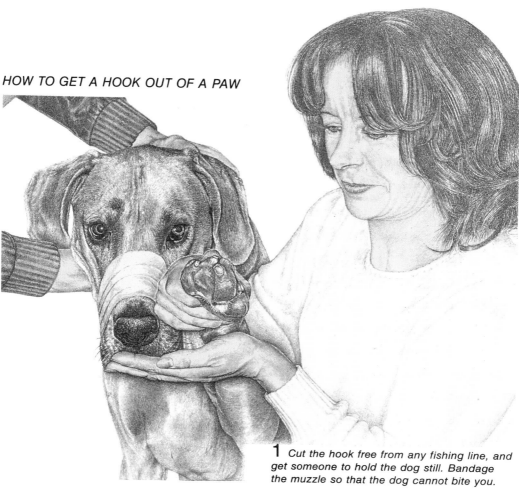

1 Cut the hook free from any fishing line, and get someone to hold the dog still. Bandage the muzzle so that the dog cannot bite you.

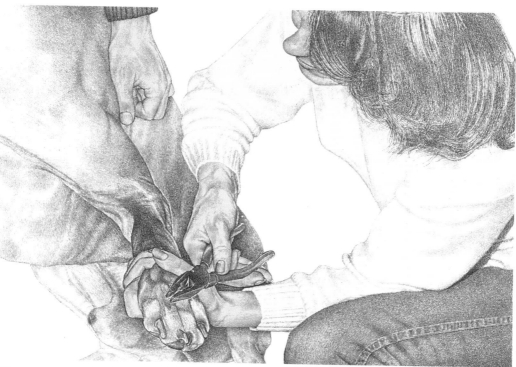

2 If the hook will not pull free easily, push it through until the barb is exposed. Cut the barb off with a pair of pliers, then pull the shank back and out. Dress the wound and see a vet.

187

to a vet at once. A sting in the mouth is much more serious because the swelling could block the animal's airway and choke it.

Coping with wasps or bees

• If you are attacked by bees or wasps – and this is likely to happen only if a nearby colony has been disturbed for some reason – the safest course depends on where you are.

• If you are indoors, open a window and leave the room quickly, closing the door. The bees and wasps will probably fly out after a few minutes. Never swat a bee or wasp – just move away slowly and calmly. Striking out in alarm may simply excite its attack.

• If you are in a garden, retreat indoors quickly but calmly, closing doors and windows behind you. Stay inside until the insects disperse, which they will do within a few minutes.

• If you are in open country away from any building, plunge into the nearest patch of dense undergrowth or bushes. Keep going until you leave the insects behind. This will usually happen within 50 yd. (45 m) because the insects will be disorientated by the moving branches. When you are clear, wait until the insects disperse.

• A swarm of bees on its way to found a new colony will not normally attack a person. If you are in the path of a swarm, move out of its way, or lie flat and cover yourself with a coat in case any bees settle on you.

• If wasps have built a nest in or near your house – for example, in an attic or porch ceiling, or in a tree in your yard – spray the nest with carbaryl or malathion, or with a commercially available wasp-and-hornet formula. Spray at night when the insects are sluggish. Wear protective clothing.

• Alternatively, get a local exterminator to destroy the wasp nest. You will find exterminators listed in the *Yellow Pages* of your telephone book.

• If a swarm of bees settles near your house, contact the police or your municipal office. They will put you in touch with a local beekeeper who will remove the swarm.

Caring for an injured bird or wild animal

If you come across an injured bird or wild animal such as a rabbit, stop and analyze the cause of its distress and then get expert help.

• Never approach a fully grown wild mammal or a bird of prey, such as an owl. It may attack you or harm itself further by trying to escape.

• Avoid a wild animal such as a raccoon that behaves abnormally or that seems tame but is not wary of your presence. It may have rabies.

• If the creature is young and helpless but apparently abandoned, do not handle it. If the mother is about she will help and feed it, but if you handle it she may be frightened away.

• Even if an injured animal appears harmless, report its condition and location to the local wildlife officer, who will provide appropriate help – or advise you what to do. You may also get help from a veterinarian or a branch of the Society for the Prevention of Cruelty to Animals.

Handling a sick or injured horse

Like any animal in pain, a horse is likely to become vicious and turn on even a person who knows it well. So get it under control first.

• Approach the horse quietly with a halter, talking to it steadily and looking at it all the time. Let it see you coming. Slip the halter on and hold the rope firmly. But do not wind the rope around your hand. If the horse jerks back, it could give you a painful rope burn.

• If further restraint is necessary, use one hand to hold it around the soft tip of its muzzle.

• If someone else is with you, ask him to hold the horse by an uninjured foreleg and bend it to lift it off the ground. This will help to immobilize the animal. Once the horse is under control, examine it for injuries.

• If the horse is standing on three legs, it may mean that it has gone lame, or the leg may be broken if it is at an awkward angle or badly swollen. Do not move the horse unless it is in danger of further injury (on a road, for example). Get veterinary help at once.

• If the horse is lying down and cannot get up, leave it alone and get veterinary help.

• If the horse is lying down and thrashing about, try to restrain it from causing itself further injury. Get hold of its head and lie on it to hold it still. But stay well away from the forefeet. Get veterinary help at once.

Dealing with a horse that has gone lame

Lameness in a horse usually happens when the lower leg or the foot is damaged and the tissues inside the hoof swell up. The rigid hoof constricts the swollen tissues, causing much pain.

• If you are riding a horse that goes lame (you can tell because the animal's gait becomes awkward and lopsided as it tries to guard the painful foot), dismount at once.

• Pick up the foot of the affected leg and examine it for injuries. A nail may have penetrated the sole, or a stone may have caught in the hoof.

• Remove any foreign body you find, then lead the horse home.

• Once you get there, apply a hot pad to the foot and call a vet. Use a cloth pad that has been squeezed out in hot water and bandage it around the horse's foot.

• If you find nothing in the foot, feel the rest of the leg for areas that feel hot or swollen or that seem to cause the horse pain. Whether or not you can find the source of the trouble, call a vet. Rest the horse until the vet arrives.

If a horse is caught on barbed wire

• Restrain the horse and hold it firmly to stop it tearing itself away from the wire and making its injuries worse.

• Restrict its movement by lifting its foreleg as well, if you can.

• Ease the barbed wire free, making all your movements slow so as not to startle or hurt the horse. Once the horse is free, clean any cuts with warm water containing a mild antiseptic (the same antiseptics that work on people work on horses, too).

• Ask a vet to come and look the horse over. Horses are highly susceptible to tetanus, and even minor cuts can easily become infected.

Treating a horse for colic

When a horse suffers from colic or acute abdominal pain, the animal has usually eaten or been fed something other than its natural diet of grass and vegetation.

The symptoms of internal pain are: restlessness; pawing and scraping at the ground; looking around at the flanks; getting up and down frequently; rolling; sweating; and rapid breathing. In addition, a horse suffering from colic may strain as it tries, unsuccessfully, to defecate.

• Once you have the horse under control, get it walking gently and try to keep it on the move.

• If possible, stop the horse rolling on the ground. This could worsen its condition.

• Call a vet. Keep the horse on its feet and moving until the vet arrives.

If fire breaks out in a stable

• Dial 911 and ask for the fire department, or get someone else to make the call.

• Open the stable door and chase the horse out, but only if you can do so without endangering yourself. Do not wait for it to bolt out – it will probably be too terrified to move and may need a prod with a pitchfork.

• Shut the door once the horse is out. A horse panic-stricken by the flames may well try to get back into its stall unless you prevent it by shutting the door.

• Let the horse or horses run free if necessary.

• Once all the animals are safe, fight the blaze as best you can until firemen arrive. But do so from the outside. Do not enter the burning stable.

In the home and at work

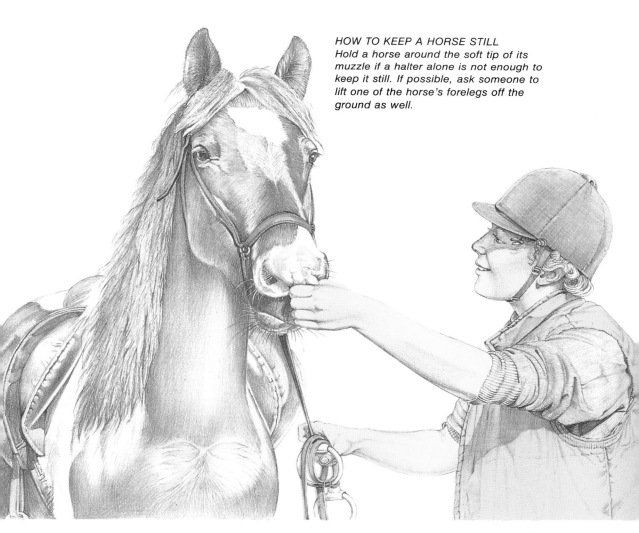

HOW TO KEEP A HORSE STILL
Hold a horse around the soft tip of its muzzle if a halter alone is not enough to keep it still. If possible, ask someone to lift one of the horse's forelegs off the ground as well.

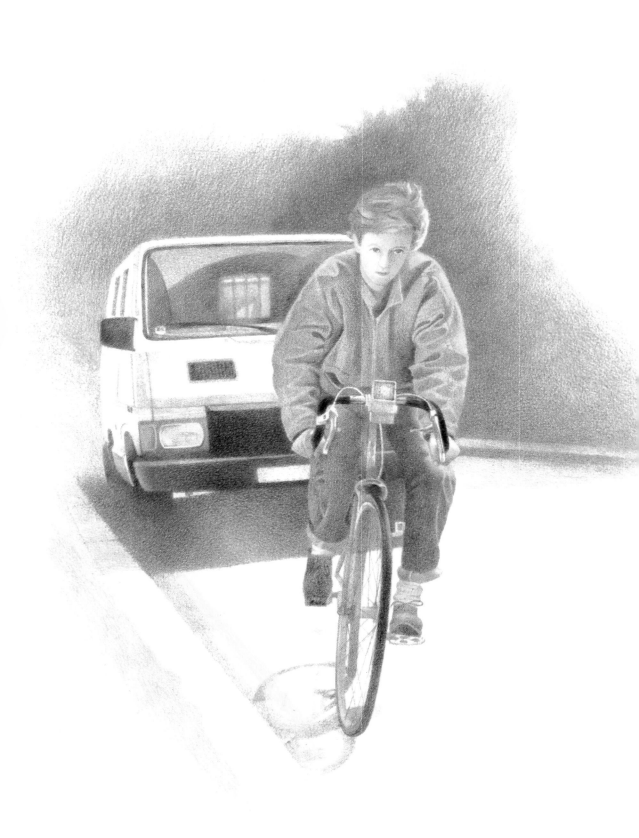

Emergencies on the road

192   At the scene of an accident
194   If you are involved in an accident
196   Defensive driving
198   What to do if you hit an animal
199   What to do if someone collapses
200   Controlling a skid
202   Brake failure at speed
203   If you have a blowout
203   Driving through fog
204   If you feel drowsy at the wheel
205   Fire in your car
205   Stuck on a rail crossing
206   Stuck in snow
208   Escaping from a car underwater
210   Driving through floodwater
211   Emergency repairs
216   Menaced by a hitchhiker
216   Safety on two wheels
217   If police stop you

At the scene of an accident

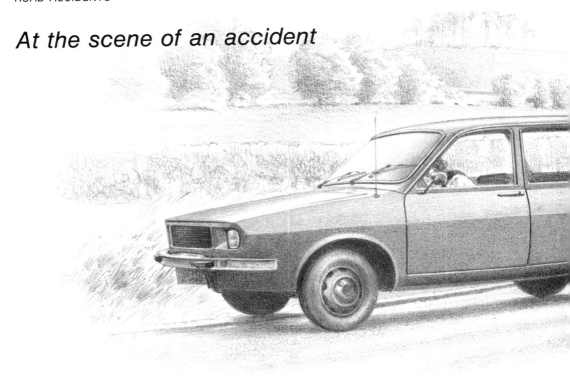

If you are the first on the scene of a crash, do not dash headlong from your car to the aid of an injured person – you or your car may be struck by another vehicle and add to the disaster.

For this reason, the first thing to do at the scene of any accident is to protect the area from approaching traffic. Once you have warned other motorists, send for the police and an ambulance, turn off the ignition in the crashed vehicles, and help the injured.

Warn other traffic
• If you arrive first at an accident, park your car on the shoulder, wheels toward the ditch, well away from the crash. Put on your brakes and your emergency flashers and take charge of the accident scene.
• If one of the crashed vehicles is on fire, keep clear in case its gas tank explodes.
• Keeping well to the side of the road, warn traffic approaching from behind, redirecting it into another lane. At night use a flashlight.
• On a two-lane highway, ask someone to warn traffic coming the other way.
• Put out as many flares or reflectors as possible. Position them according to the situation. On a two-lane or undivided highway, for example, you might place them from 10 ft. (3 m) to 200 ft. (60 m) behind the wrecked vehicles, and the same distance in the opposite direction. On a divided highway, where vehicles may be approaching from behind at high speeds, position all flares or reflectors up to 300 ft. (90 m) or more behind the cars.

Send for the police
• Check the number of vehicles involved, and the number of victims, noting whether anyone is trapped. Then ask a passing driver or anyone living nearby to call for assistance or do so yourself. In some places you will be able to use one of the highway phones, which are connected to a central emergency headquarters. In others you will use the 911 emergency number or ask the operator to assist you.
• If you make the call yourself, describe the accident location as exactly as you can. Say how many vehicles are involved, whether any vehicle is on fire, how many people are injured and whether anyone is trapped.

Immobilize the crashed vehicles
• Switch off each vehicle, but leave the key in the ignition.
• Check that the parking brake of each car is on. If it is not, put it on.
• Do not smoke, and warn others not to – even away from the cars. Gas may be leaking from a ruptured fuel tank.

Help the injured
• Do not move anyone unless he is in immediate danger – from a burning car or excessive bleeding, for example.
• Do not attempt to pick out glass from face or body wounds. The glass may be plugging the wound against bleeding.
• Check that each victim can breathe freely. Loosen clothing that is tight around the neck.
• Do not give anyone anything to eat or drink.

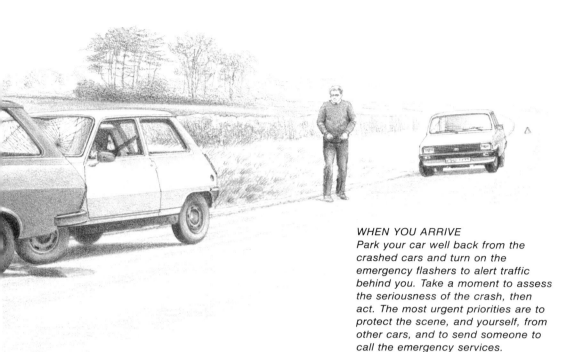

WHEN YOU ARRIVE
Park your car well back from the
crashed cars and turn on the
emergency flashers to alert traffic
behind you. Take a moment to assess
the seriousness of the crash, then
act. The most urgent priorities are to
protect the scene, and yourself, from
other cars, and to send someone to
call the emergency services.

WHY ACCIDENTS HAPPEN

Thousands of North Americans die each year in highway accidents. In 1986 alone, 18 million were injured and 50,000 died in this way. One in three of those killed was between 15 and 24 years of age.

In Canada, the commonest time for an accident is 5 p.m., and the safest time is 6 a.m. In the United States, however, most accidents take place at 3 p.m., the fewest at 3 a.m. The accident toll in both countries is highest on weekends.

The accident black spots
Most accidents need not happen. If improper practices such as the following could be corrected, many lives might be saved.
SPEEDING This is a factor in some 18 percent of all accidents and about 26 percent of all fatal accidents.

IGNORING RIGHT-OF-WAY This is the cause of about 21 percent of all accidents on the highway.

TAILGATING This is responsible for about 6 percent of all accidents.

PASSING Improper passing and driving to the left of center accounts for about 4 percent of all accidents.

MAKING IMPROPER TURNS This is to blame for about 3 percent of accidents.

It might cause problems if the victim has to have an anesthetic soon afterward.

Treatment priorities
• Treat victims in the following order:
1. Unconscious and not breathing (see *Artificial respiration*, page 50).
2. Bleeding severely (see page 60).
3. Unconscious but breathing (see page 136).
• Persuade anyone wandering around in a state of shock to lie down.
• Cover each injured person lightly with a blanket or coat.
• Reassure them that help is on the way. Keep each victim as safe and as calm as possible until the ambulance arrives.
• If possible, do not leave the victims alone after you have treated them. Get someone to stay with each victim until help arrives.

At the scene of a highway crash
Because of the volume of traffic on North American highways, traffic can back up quickly if motorists stop at the scene of a crash. The resulting traffic jam can delay the arrival of police and ambulance services.

For this reason, and because of the risks for rescuers from speeding traffic, safety experts recommend that you should stop at the scene of a highway accident only if you believe it is absolutely necessary – if, for example, someone is lying injured in the path of traffic, or struggling to get out of a car on fire.
• Find a telephone at the nearest rest area, toll booth or exit ramp and call 911.

193

If you are involved in an accident

A traffic accident may involve only your vehicle and damage to property, such as a lamppost. Or it may involve other vehicles and perhaps injury to people or animals. Whatever the involvement, there are certain steps the law requires you to take and others that are advisable for insurance purposes.

Try to keep cool and note down essential information, even though you will probably be feeling shocked and flustered by the incident.

At the scene

• Stop as soon as you safely can. You must stop even if you have been only indirectly involved and your vehicle is undamaged – if, for example, one car collided with another after swerving to avoid you.

• Whatever the circumstances, do not become involved in arguments with other drivers or onlookers about what happened. Particularly, do not make any statement admitting liability. If you think you may have been at fault, it is wisest to say as little as possible.

• Dial 911, or call the police directly, and report the accident. Ask them to alert any other emergency services, such as an ambulance, that may be required.

• Before any vehicles are moved, make a sketch, noting the cars' positions on the road and their relation to the other vehicles involved. Note, for example, if any car has crossed the central dividing line. If any car has skidded, make an estimate of the length of skid marks.

• Examine your vehicle and the others involved and make a note of the damage each has sustained. Look, too, at the condition of the other cars. Were all their lights working at the time, for instance, and were their tires in good condition?

• The police will want to see your driver's license, registration and, if anyone is injured, your automobile insurance card.

These should be carried with you at all times.

• Give your name and address and the name of your insurance company to other motorists involved and to anyone else who has reasonable grounds for asking, such as the owners of any damaged property. If you are not the owner of the car you are driving, give the owner's name and address as well.

• Collect the same information from other motorists involved. If anyone refuses, write down his car's license plate number: the owner can be traced through the number.

• Try to find an independent witness (not someone traveling in your car) who is willing to make a statement about the incident to your insurance company. Take his name and address.

After the accident

• If you hit and damage an unoccupied car – in a parking lot, say – report it to the police. If you fail to do so and are eventually traced, you could face not only a claim for repair of the damage you caused, but also criminal charges as a hit-and-run driver.

• Notify your insurance company of the accident as soon as possible, preferably within 24 hours, whether or not you or anyone else will be making a claim on your policy.

• Ask the company to send you an accident report form on which you can fill in the details.

• Ask a garage to give you a written estimate of the cost of repairs to your car, but do not get any repairs done at once if you plan to claim the cost from an insurance company. The insurers will probably want the damage inspected first by a professional insurance adjuster.

• Send any bills or letters you get from other motorists involved to your insurance company. Do not write to or contact the other motorists or their insurers.

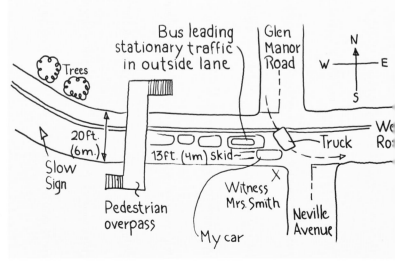

MAKING A SKETCH OF THE ACCIDENT
A sketch of the accident scene, made on the spot, will be useful in any later court case and for making an insurance claim. Show the road layout and the cars' positions. Mark where any witness was standing. Add the compass points, too (get them from a map if necessary); official reports often refer to them.

• Let your insurance company know if you receive a summons to appear in court. This would likely arrive within 30 days of the accident. It is possible, too, that accidents involving injury or property damage might give rise to civil suits at a later date.

If you have an accident abroad
The legal requirements about what to do if you are involved in an accident vary in detail from country to country. Nevertheless, if you follow these general guidelines, you will be doing at least as much as the law requires in any country.

• Stop at the scene of the accident.

• Warn approaching traffic of the obstruction by setting up flares, or warning reflectors, about 200 ft. (60 m) from the crash site. Place one in each direction on a two-lane highway, but place them behind the accident on a divided highway, where your main concern is traffic approaching at speed from the rear.

• Call the police, or ask a passing motorist to call them. Even if this is not obligatory under local laws, it is always advisable.

• Help anyone who has been injured (see *At the scene of an accident*, page 192). Call an ambulance if necessary.

• Generally, do not move the car or cars from the positions in which they have come to rest. But if they are seriously obstructing other traffic, mark the positions on the road and get the details confirmed by independent witnesses before moving them.

• Do not leave the scene of the accident until the police arrive, unless there is an overriding reason for doing so. If you think there is such a reason, discuss it with the police by telephone, and get their permission before leaving.

• Give your name and address, and any other details requested, to others involved in the accident. Collect the same details from them.

• Cooperate with the police when they arrive. Answer their questions as fully as you can, but avoid saying anything which could be construed as an admission of liability.

• Make notes or a sketch of the accident to help you fill in your insurance company's accident form later. If you have a camera, back up your notes with photographs of the cars and the scene. Try particularly to show any factors which might have helped to cause the accident – a concealed road sign, for instance. Take close-up pictures of the damage, too; they may be useful evidence if you want to claim compensation from the other driver or from your insurance company.

• Report the accident to your insurance agent by telephone. The agent's number should be on the motor vehicle liability insurance card issued by the insuring company. Give your insurance policy number and some preliminary details of the accident. Make the report as soon as possible after the accident, preferably within 24 hours.

• If you have additional insurance coverage, through a travel agent or automobile association, for example, report the accident to that insurer as well. The policy will tell you how soon after the accident you should let the firm know. If the time limit is short, make the first report by phone, then follow up with a letter.

• Some insurance companies provide extended insurance policies. These may cover repairs to your car, medical expenses and a variety of other accident-related costs and services such as roadside emergency help and delivery of replacement parts. The extent of your coverage may vary from country to country. Check with your agent about this and about how and where you should get your car repaired, and how medical bills will be settled. (See also *Seeing a doctor overseas*, page 273.)

HOW TO AVOID A HEAD-ON COLLISION

If you see another vehicle coming toward you on the wrong side of the road, whose driver seems to be either unwilling or unable to get out of your way, you must act quickly and coolly to avoid a head-on collision. Head-on collisions are the most dangerous of all road accidents.

• As soon as you see the danger, sound your horn or flash your headlights to warn of your presence.

• Brake firmly but not violently. Unless your car has an antiskid brake system, it may start to skid if you slam your brakes on, and you could lose steering control.

• As you reduce speed, scan the road ahead to see if there is anywhere to get out of the way safely – a shoulder, say, or a side road.

• Start to pull right, but do not commit yourself until you see which way the other car is going. There is a danger that both of you could pull onto the shoulder and collide there.

• As soon as you see which way the other vehicle is swerving, turn away from it – even if this means sideswiping another car. Sideswiping is far less likely to kill you and your passengers than a head-on smash.

• If a collision is unavoidable, try to scrape the side of the other vehicle rather than meet it head-on.

Defensive driving

The best way to avoid an accident is to be alert to what might cause one – to develop your powers of observation so that you can see danger coming and react to it in time. The principle of the technique known as defensive driving is to be prepared for the unexpected by observation and anticipation. These pages show how to apply the principle in practice.

Other motorists – watch for:
- Taxi ahead – it may slow down and move to the right with little warning. Keep an eye open for someone hailing it from the sidewalk.
- Learner stopped on a hill – do not get too close. He may roll back when starting off.
- Bus ahead – beware of people running to catch it or jumping off just as the bus pulls away from the stop.
- Motorcyclists at an intersection ahead – if you see two ready to come out and one emerges safely, watch for the other. Will he follow?
- Bicyclist ahead – if he glances over his shoulder he is probably preparing to pull out to the left, and may hesitate and wobble. Watch his movements.
- Turn signal on a car ahead – never rely on the driver doing as he has signaled. He may have forgotten to cancel a previous signal, or may change his mind.
- Turn signal on a car to your left – if you are waiting to emerge from a side road onto a main road, never assume that it is safe to pull out just because an oncoming driver is signaling right. Wait until he slows down and is obviously going to turn.
- Brake lights coming on ahead – touch your own to warn traffic behind. There may be an accident or obstruction ahead.
- Headlight flashed as signal – never assume another driver means: "You go ahead, I will wait." He may mean: "I'm going ahead. You

wait." Such a signal is easily misinterpreted and could lead to an accident. Headlight flashing should be used only to let another driver know you are there.
- Siren sounding on police car, ambulance or fire truck – if you do not know where the sound is coming from, slow down and keep to the side of the road. Do not move across an intersection until you are certain you will not be in the path of the emergency vehicle.
- Headlight dazzle – if a car approaches with headlights on high beam, do not look at them directly. Look slightly to the right. Do not retaliate by switching your own headlights to high beam. Flashing them will usually bring an appropriate response.
- Slow vehicle ahead very close behind another – the rear vehicle is probably being towed, even if the emergency flashers are not operating. Be careful about passing.
- Moving out from a side road onto a main road – watch for bicycles and motorcycles near the shoulder as well as for cars. A cyclist or motorcyclist is easy to overlook if you are trying to nose out of a side road in heavy traffic.

Approaching a parked car – watch for:
- People inside – the door may be opened.
- Flashing indicator – the car may pull out into your path.
- Wisps of smoke from the exhaust – the car may be about to move off.

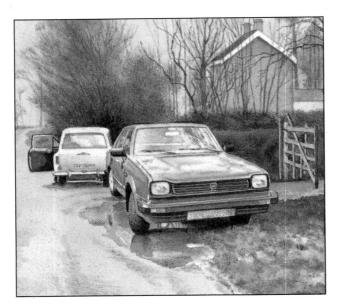

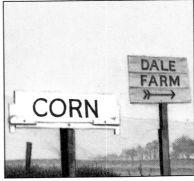

Farm produce
Slow down whenever you see a sign advertising farm produce. Cars ahead may be backed up at a farm lane, or they may be carelessly, even illegally, parked at roadside stand or farmhouse entrance.

• Feet that can be seen beneath vehicles – a child may run into the road.
• Mobile ice-cream vendors – there are bound to be children around, and they may dart across the road without warning.

Roadside signs – watch for:
• Bus stops – people may run across the road from the left.
• School signs – children may run across the road, especially in the morning and afternoon, when school is opening and closing, or during the midday recess. But look out for a lone child near the school at any time of day.
• Pedestrian crossings – scan the sidewalks on both sides to see if anyone is preparing to cross.
• Garage or bar and tavern entrances – vehicles are likely to pull in and out without signaling, especially late at night.
• Red traffic light – stop. Before starting off again, watch the cross traffic and pedestrians, in case someone tries to rush through at the last second.
• Yellow traffic light – be decisive. Slow down and stop unless you are almost at the lights. In that case, continue on through; otherwise traffic behind may run into you.
• Green traffic light – do not treat it as an open door; it may change. Reduce speed as you approach, and look right and left to make sure that nothing is coming through.
• Construction sign – prepare to slow down or stop; the work may be some distance ahead around a bend, or masked by parked cars.
• Road-narrows sign – get into the through lane in good time, and watch for other drivers cutting across.

Making use of clues – watch for:
• Mud or hay on a country road – there may be a slow-moving tractor ahead.
• Droppings on a country road – there may be horses or cattle ahead.
• Telephone poles – in rural areas, the line of poles ahead of you can sometimes alert you to bends in the road that may be masked by trees or hedges. Do not rely on them, however; the lines sometimes cut across country, and so can mislead you.
• Boundary sign – the road surface is quite likely to change from one state or province to another; sometimes even from one municipality to another. At night the street lighting ahead may be different.
• Shop-window reflections – in urban areas, make full use of reflections in windows and on shiny vehicles. They can help you to see around bends and around corners at awkward intersections, and to see how close you are to the car behind when parking on the street.

Approaching animals – watch for:
• Dog not on leash – it may wander into the road or run across, especially if there is another dog (or a cat) on the other side.
• Cat crouching on footpath watching traffic – it may be planning to cross the road, and may dash in front of your car.
• Horses ahead – slow down and give them room as you pass. Do not toot your horn or accelerate hard, or they may shy into your car.
• Herd of cattle ahead – stop until they have gone around you or off the road. Do not sound your horn or rev your engine. If you startle them, they may blunder into your car and damage it.

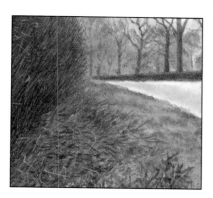

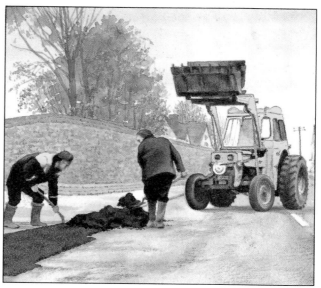

Road crews
Look out for workers and machinery blocking the road around the next corner. Slow down, too, if you see newly mowed grass or hedge clippings. There may be a work crew on the road ahead.

What to do if you hit an animal

If you suddenly find an animal in your path – a pet, a straying farm animal or a wild animal – there may be no time to avoid it. In heavy traffic or bad weather, there may be no choice but to hit it rather than to swerve and risk a serious accident.

• Pull over onto the shoulder of the road, stop as soon as you can after the impact, and switch on your emergency flashers. Find out whether the animal is dead or injured.

• If it is injured, do not approach it or try to restrain it. The animal might be rabid. Even if it is not, its pain may cause it to attack you (see *Caring for a sick or injured animal*, page 181).

• Whether the animal is dead or injured, it is best to call the police.

• If the animal is a pet or a farm animal, and you are in a rural area, you might alert the residents of the nearest house or farmhouse. Even if the animal is not theirs, they may recognize it as belonging to one of their neighbors.

• An animal that has fallen on the road is endangering itself and passing traffic. For the protection of both, you should set up flares or reflectors at the accident site while you wait for the police to reach the scene.

PET OWNERS AND THE LAW

Anyone who owns or looks after a pet is obliged to keep it from hurting anyone or damaging property. If it does – if it bites someone, for example, or if it runs in front of a car and causes an accident – the victim could sue the pet owner for compensation.

Although laws vary from jurisdiction to jurisdiction, pet owners in most areas of North America are responsible for the actions of their animals. In many circumstances, you will be responsible for any damage or injury caused by your pet, no matter who released it from your property. Keep it well fenced in or otherwise under control at all times.

• If you own or look after what the law calls a dangerous animal – a poisonous snake, or a vicious dog, for example – you might be liable if it attacks someone, even a burglar, on your property. Some communities have bylaws designed to control vicious dogs and prohibit certain exotic pets from residential areas.

• Make sure your dog and cat are vaccinated against rabies. Keep the certificates in a safe place.

• Most communities require that dogs be licensed. This serves to identify the pet if it strays. And some authorities will not issue a license until the animal has been immunized against rabies and distemper.

• In the past, owners of cats have rarely been held responsible for damage done by their pets: the law recognizes that cats are very difficult to control. This may change, however, now that more and more communities are considering legislation to control their cat populations.

• You must keep your pet reasonably quiet, particularly at night.

• In most communities you must clean up your animal's droppings.

• Keep your dog on a leash in crowded places and anywhere there is livestock. Some communities require a dog to be leashed whenever it is off its owner's property.

• Train your dog properly. Your vet will probably know about nearby obedience classes. Check also with your local kennel club or humane society: many sponsor reasonably priced obedience classes.

• Avoid an obedience school that promises to take your dog and return it trained: the owner and the dog must learn the commands together.

• Consider taking out insurance against your pet doing harm. Some household insurance policies include such cover as a matter of course.

Motorists and the law on animals

Although you are not always obliged to call the police if you hit an animal on the road, you would be wise to do so. They can help trace the owner, and will arrange for the removal and treatment of the injured creature. Besides, you may need a copy of their report if you ask your insurance company to compensate you for injuries or damages arising from the accident.

• A police report will be useful, too, if you collide with an animal such as a horse, cow, steer, sheep, pig or goat. Damage to your car could be extensive from such a collision and the animal owner might be liable since it was his responsibility to keep the animals under control.

• Calling the police is equally wise when wildlife is involved. The accident may have to be reported to certain government agencies, especially if an animal or bird of a protected species is wounded or killed. The police will see that such obligations are fulfilled.

• If it is apparent that a wild animal is too badly hurt to recover, the local humane society will kill it in the quickest way possible.

What to do if someone collapses

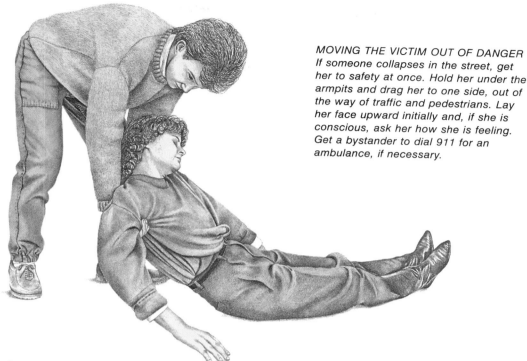

MOVING THE VICTIM OUT OF DANGER
If someone collapses in the street, get her to safety at once. Hold her under the armpits and drag her to one side, out of the way of traffic and pedestrians. Lay her face upward initially and, if she is conscious, ask her how she is feeling. Get a bystander to dial 911 for an ambulance, if necessary.

Emergencies on the road

A person may collapse in the street for any of a number of reasons. The most common cause is fainting (see page 96). Less often the cause may be an epileptic seizure (see page 94). More rarely still, it could be a heart attack (see page 105) or a stroke (see page 134). Whatever the cause, the priority is always the same: move the victim to a safe place out of the way of traffic.
• Lift or drag the victim to the side of the road, unless you suspect a head or neck injury. Persons with such injuries should not be moved at all. Once the victim is out of immediate danger, lay her down on her back.
• If the victim is conscious, ask her to describe her symptoms. If necessary, call an ambulance, or get a passerby to do so.
• If she is unconscious, tilt her head well back by putting one hand on her forehead while you lift her chin with the other. This will open her airway.
• Listen for breathing. See if the chest rises and falls.
• Put your ear near her mouth so that you can hear and feel her breath.

If the victim is breathing
• Someone who is unconscious but breathing should be placed in the recovery position (see page 136). Do not make a fainting victim sit up unless she wants to.
• Ask a bystander to dial 911 for an ambulance. Ask him to return afterward to confirm that he has done so. Anyone who has been unconscious, even for a short time, should have immediate medical treatment.

If the victim is not breathing
• If the victim's breathing stops, perform mouth-to-mouth respiration (see page 50).
• Give two full breaths, then check for breathing.
• If there is no response, reposition the head and reattempt ventilation.
• If there is still no chest movement, suspect an obstruction (see *Choking*, page 15) and perform a finger sweep of the mouth.
• If there is chest movement, check the pulse at the carotid (neck) artery.
• If you cannot detect a pulse, give chest compressions as well (see page 52).
• Once the victim is breathing, loosen her clothing at the neck, chest and waist.
• Turn her into the recovery position.
• Stay with her until an ambulance comes. Do not give her anything to eat or drink – you could make hospital treatment more difficult.

Helping the victim of an epileptic seizure
• If the victim is having an epileptic seizure, do not try to push anything into her mouth.
• Do not try to restrain her either. Muscle spasms – twitching or convulsing limbs – and the breath-holding often associated with seizures rarely last more than a minute.
• Once the seizure passes, the victim may fall into a deep sleep. Use a finger to clear any blood, mucus or vomit from her mouth.
• If she is breathing normally, turn her into the recovery position.
• Get someone to call an ambulance. Stay with the victim until help arrives.

Controlling a skid

A car skids because the tires lose their grip and begin to slide over the road surface instead of rolling along it. What you do to control a skid depends on which tires are skidding and whether or not the car has front-wheel drive. The "natural" reaction – jamming the brakes on hard – may be the worst thing you can do.

How to stop a rear-wheel skid
In a rear-wheel skid the back of the car slides sideways and the vehicle begins to swing around back to front. This usually happens when you drive too fast around a bend or corner, but can occur if you brake harshly on an uneven surface or a road with a steep gradient. It is most likely to happen in vehicles such as empty pickup trucks and small front-wheel-drive vehicles, which have little weight on the rear wheels.

Whether the car has front-wheel or rear-wheel drive, you take the same action.
• Suppress the instinct to brake and take your foot off the accelerator.
• Turn the steering wheel in the direction the back of the car is sliding (turn right if it is sliding to the right, for example). Do not turn it too far or you may start a second skid in the opposite direction. When all four wheels are back in line, accelerate gently.

How to stop a front-wheel skid
In a front-wheel skid, the front of the car keeps straight on, even though you have turned the steering wheel to right or left.

Front-wheel skids usually happen when the driver accelerates too harshly around a bend. What you do depends on whether the car has rear-wheel or front-wheel drive.

IN A CAR WITH REAR-WHEEL DRIVE Take your foot off the accelerator. Do not apply the brake.
• Turn the steering wheel so that the front wheels are straightened – pointing again in the direction the car is moving. Do not turn it too far or you could cause the rear wheels to skid.
• Once the front wheels are gripping again, accelerate gently and steer in the direction you wish to go.

IN A CAR WITH FRONT-WHEEL DRIVE Ease off the accelerator smoothly. Do not downshift or brake. Instead, steer smoothly in the direction you were headed. As the car slows down and you feel the steering respond, accelerate very gently.
• Continue steering smoothly in the direction you want to turn, but do not turn the wheel violently or too far.
• As the car moves back on course, straighten the wheels and accelerate gently.

How to stop a four-wheel skid
In a four-wheel skid – which usually happens during hard braking – the wheels lock and the car slides forward not seeming to lose speed. It may skid in a more or less straight line, or off to the side if the road is crowned and slopes steeply from the center to the edges.
• To control a four-wheel skid, ease off on the brake pedal until the wheels start to roll again.

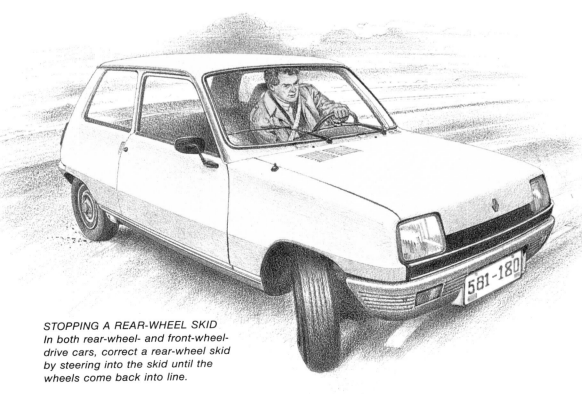

STOPPING A REAR-WHEEL SKID
In both rear-wheel- and front-wheel-drive cars, correct a rear-wheel skid by steering into the skid until the wheels come back into line.

• Once steering control is restored, straighten the wheels.
• Reapply the brakes until the wheels begin to lock, then ease up just enough to let the car keep rolling. Increase brake pressure as the car slows down. This technique of threshold braking prevents the wheels from locking.

Use of *Neutral*

Putting your car into *Neutral* can also be an effective reaction when your car begins to skid. In many cars nowadays, electronic antipollution controls continue to govern the engine even after you have removed your foot from the accelerator. This is particularly the case when the engine is warming up.

There are times then when you might be better to shift an automatic transmission to *Neutral,* or to declutch a manual transmission. It might be appropriate, for example, if all four wheels begin skidding on ice just as you approach a stop sign.

Note, however, that not all automatic transmissions can be shifted to *Neutral* without the risk of engaging *Reverse*.

How to avoid skidding

• Make sure your car has good all-round vision before you drive. Misty glass can prevent you from seeing a hazard in good time.
• Drive smoothly and steadily.
• Read the road ahead and adjust speed in good time to avoid hazards.
• Make allowances for road conditions. Braking distances are greater in wet weather, and longer still on snow-covered or icy surfaces.

HOW LONG IT TAKES TO STOP

This chart shows how road conditions and tires affect the distance a car takes to stop. Keep in mind that damp roads – such as occur in misty conditions – can be even more dangerous than wet roads, largely because light moisture combines with the rubber residue and oil on the road to create a slippery film. Heavy rain washes the film away.

Note that on ice, snow tires have slightly less traction than summer tires.

On dry and wet roads – see the first six entries – distances are for an emergency stop made from 60 mph (100 km/h). The figures include reaction time that eats up 60 ft. (18 m) – the minimum distance traveled from the time you recognize a hazard until you brake.

The snow and ice section of the chart shows how tires and chains perform in an emergency stop made from 20 mph (32 km/h) on two common winter surfaces: loosely packed snow and glare ice.

Road condition	Tires	Stopping distance
Dry concrete or asphalt	Summer tires with good treads	190 ft. (58 m)
Wet road	Summer tires with good treads	310 ft. (94 m)
Wet road	Summer tires: treads caked with dirt and oil	760 ft. (232 m)
Very wet road	Summer tires with good treads	360 ft. (110 m)
Very wet road	All-season tires with good treads	490 ft. (149 m)
Very wet road	Nearly bald tires	1,360 ft. (414 m)
Snow	Summer tires	60 ft. (18 m)
Snow	Snow tires	52 ft. (16 m)
Snow	Chains	38 ft. (12 m)
Ice	Summer tires	145 ft. (44 m)
Ice	Snow tires	151 ft. (46 m)
Ice	Chains	75 ft. (23 m)

Brake failure at speed

If you have an automatic transmission and your brakes fail when you try to stop the car at speed, your options are to use the parking brake, the engine, and possibly the terrain – a steep upward slope, for example – to slow down.

Do not switch off the engine. If you have power steering and power-assisted brakes, neither will work properly once the engine is switched off.

• First pump the brakes hard: often this will build up enough pressure to get back at least partial braking. Apply the parking brake smoothly. If you have a hand model, pump it hard. You can prevent it from locking by keeping the release mechanism in position.

• Keep a firm grip on the steering wheel while you do this: using the parking brake at speed may lock the rear wheels and cause a skid (see page 200).

If your car still has not stopped, shift momentarily into *Reverse*. Do *not* slip into *Park*, since this could damage your transmission.

• Switch off the ignition as soon as the car stops. Look for a safe place to park the car and, as you steer it there, use your horn, flashers and lights to warn other drivers and pedestrians that you have lost your brakes.

• If these procedures fail, try sideswiping something – curb, guardrails, even parked cars in an emergency – to help you bring the car to a stop.

• With manual transmission, you also pump the brakes and apply the parking brake to slow the car. If this does not work, ease in the clutch and downshift. As engine drag slows the car, continue shifting down until you are in first gear. To engage lower gears at speed, try double-clutching (see box, this page).

• Finally, pull off the road and switch off the ignition.

• If you cannot slow down or stop fast enough to avoid a collision, try to run the car up a slope.

If the parking brake fails on a steep hill
If the parking brake fails when you stop on your way up a steep hill, starting off again is difficult in a car with manual transmission. If you know how to find the friction point on the clutch pedal, all is well. This friction point holds the car and prevents it from rolling backward.

• Otherwise, swivel your right foot so that your toe remains on the brake pedal while you place your heel on the accelerator.

• As you release the clutch pedal, ease your right toe off the brake and press your heel down on the accelerator. This should allow you to hold the car until you move forward and can release the brake completely.

WHY BRAKES FAIL

Complete brake failure is rare because modern cars have two separate circuits of hydraulic fluid operating the brakes. If one circuit is damaged, the other can operate the brakes on its own, although less effectively. Nevertheless, water, driving habits or inadequate maintenance can all cause brakes to become dangerously unreliable.

Brakes may become temporarily ineffective after driving through floods (see page 210) because the disks or shoes get wet.

They may also fail temporarily on a steep descent or after prolonged use because the fluid gets hot and may partially vaporize; if this happens, the pedal feels spongy when it is depressed.

Repeated pumping of the brakes usually restores pressure in these circumstances. Use a low gear on a long or steep descent and brake gently to lessen the chances of the brakes overheating.

Sometimes hard braking causes the brake pads to get so hot that they temporarily lose their friction quality. When this happens, the pedal does not feel spongy, and the brakes will work again after a short stop to let them cool off.

How to double-clutch
Shifting to a lower gear enables you to use the engine as a brake, but downshifting at high speed puts considerable extra strain on the transmission.

On a manual transmission, it is possible to minimize this strain and to make downshifting at speed easier by using the technique known as double-clutching. Its purpose is to match the speed of the road wheels with the speed of the engine in the new gear and so make it easier for the gear teeth to engage. To double-clutch down through the gears:

• Take your foot off the accelerator.
• Press in the clutch pedal.
• Move the gear lever to *Neutral*.
• Release the clutch pedal.
• Give the accelerator a quick burst, then remove your foot.
• Press in the clutch pedal.
• Move the gear lever into the lower gear.
• Gently release the clutch.

With an automatic transmission, double-clutching is impossible. The only option is to move the gear lever into a lower gear and risk some mechanical damage.

If you have a blowout

A blowout may be caused by a fault in the tire structure, by underinflated tires, or by a sharp object piercing the tire. It occurs suddenly, often accompanied by a loud bang. The tire instantly loses its cushion of air, the wheel rim drops to the pavement, and the car is thrown out of balance.

If it is a front-tire blowout, the car pulls strongly to one side (the side on which the tire has burst). In a rear-tire blowout, the car may skid, or the back end may slide to one side.

• With a front blowout, avoid braking if possible. Lift your foot off the accelerator, and keep a firm grip on the steering wheel, which will wobble fiercely.

• The car will veer toward the side of the blowout, putting you at risk of swinging into another traffic lane. Steer in the opposite direction to maintain a straight course.

• Once you have the vehicle under control, apply the brakes gently, all the time keeping a firm grip on the steering wheel to keep the car on course.

• Finally, pull off the road, turn on your emergency flashers, and park the car on solid, level ground.

• In the event of a rear blowout, brake gently – not suddenly or fiercely – and keep a firm grip on the steering wheel to keep the car on course.

• Then steer the car onto the shoulder, switch on your emergency flashers, and park someplace where you will be able to install your spare wheel, without endangering yourself or other motorists.

A pierced tire does not always burst; it may deflate gradually, giving the driver the impression he is traveling over a bumpy surface. The steering, however, is affected the same way as in a blowout. Therefore you should follow the above steps to get off the road safely.

Avoiding tire trouble

A tire goes flat when a nail or screw or some other sharp object lying in the road punctures the tire. Flats tend to occur more in wet weather, probably because the water lubricates the screw or nail and helps it to penetrate.

• Check tires regularly for embedded stones, nails or other objects that might result in a flat, and remove them.

• If anything has pierced the casing, change the wheel and get the tire repaired.

• Check also for cuts, cracks or bulges in the sidewalls that might cause tire failure, and get damaged or worn tires repaired or replaced. A tire that develops a bulge affects the car much the same way as a flat tire: there is a repeated slapping sound against the road.

• Have wheels and tires balanced by a tire dealer or garage and maintain tires at the pressure recommended by the manufacturer. Get the pressure checked for prolonged highway driving, and when the temperature drops below $-4°F$ ($-20°C$).

Driving through fog

Fog occurs in many parts of North America, especially in densely populated and industrial areas and along the coasts. In these regions, you can check if there are foggy conditions ahead by listening to the weather and highway reports on your radio.

The main hazards of fog are limited vision and distortion of objects, great variation in fog density, and disorientation.

In foggy conditions, being seen – particularly by drivers behind you – is as important as seeing. When fog is forecast, make sure all your car lights, front and rear, are clean and bright. Dust and dirt from road spray can form a film capable of cutting the light intensity of your headlight beam by half.

• By day or night, drive through fog with dipped headlights. High beams will reflect from fog particles and may dazzle you.

• Use fog lights if they are installed. A single fog lamp must be used in conjunction with headlights, otherwise your car may be mistaken for a motorcycle.

• Occasional use of the windshield wipers will keep the windshield clear. Operate the windshield washers as necessary, and use the fan and defroster, too.

• Keep your speed low. You should be able to stop within your range of vision, which could limit you to 5 mph (8 km/h).

• Drive with your window open. You may hear something coming, or hear a warning toot from a horn, even if you cannot see another vehicle. You need to glean every scrap of information in order to avoid obstacles and other traffic.

• Do not hunch over the wheel and peer forward. You will see better if you sit relaxed in your normal driving position.

• Try to drive in line with the curb or shoulder; if you have a passenger, ask him to keep you informed of your distance from the roadside.

• Avoid getting too close to the vehicle in front. With vision restricted, you will not be able to anticipate it making an emergency stop. You therefore need more reaction time before braking than in normal conditions.

• Remember that fog makes road surfaces even more slippery than rain. So braking distances will be greater, too (see *How long it takes to stop*, page 201).

• Beware of blindly following red lights in front; if the driver ahead gets into trouble, you could follow him into it. Plot your own course. Do not pass unless you are sure it is safe to do so.

• Turn left with extreme care. Signal in plenty of time, and put your head out of the window to look and listen for oncoming traffic first.

• If a large truck is going in your direction, follow behind it at a safe distance. In a high cab the driver has a better view of the road and may be able to see above the worst of low-lying fog.

• When you have to stop in fog, try to park off the road. If you are forced to stop on the highway shoulder, switch on the car's hazard lights.

Emergencies on the road

If you feel drowsy at the wheel

If you find yourself beginning to nod off while driving, you must make an urgent effort to revive yourself until you can stop the car safely and wake yourself up. Fatigue can seriously affect a driver's judgment and is a leading cause of accidents.

Danger signs

Cruising for long periods in a warm car – particularly on a wide, straight highway – can be more hazardous than negotiating busy urban streets. With little to do, you can be tempted to daydream and let your attention wander dangerously. And the road sliding unvaryingly past the windshield can exert a hypnotic effect powerful enough to put you into a mental state not unlike a trance.

Since fatigue builds up only gradually, judging when it has reached a dangerous level – in yourself or someone else – can be very difficult. These are the symptoms to watch for. If you notice any of them, take action at once.

- Continual yawning.
- Eyes feel heavy and are difficult to keep open.
- Difficulty in concentrating, especially on a monotonous stretch of road.
- Suddenly realizing that you have no recollection of the last few miles you have traveled.
- A spasmodic jerk of the body, recalling you from the brink of sleep.

- The car begins to wander off course and you have to correct the steering hurriedly.
- You have to take rapid action to avoid a hazard you had not noticed.
- You start at a shadow, reacting to an imagined hazard.

Reviving yourself at the wheel

- If you do find yourself becoming drowsy, pull off the road to a safe parking place as soon as possible. Do not stop on the shoulder of the highway, however – it is only for emergencies such as breakdowns.
- In the meantime, slow down.
- Direct the dashboard air vents onto your face. The blast of cold air will help to wake you up.
- Lick your finger and dampen your forehead and your eyelids – particularly at the inner corner of each eye.
- Take a deep breath, purse your lips, and then breathe out again very slowly.
- Encourage passengers to chat with you.
- Wind down the window if the road is quiet and the weather dry. On a highway or a busy road, however, let in blasts of fresh air only for short spells, because the extra noise increases fatigue.
- Play the radio or taped music only if it is something you will respond to positively. Some sounds can send you to sleep.

HOW TO STAY WIDE AWAKE ON A JOURNEY

- Before starting out, do not drink alcohol or take medication that makes you sleepy or otherwise affects your judgment.
- Do not eat a heavy meal immediately before a journey; the process of digestion encourages sleep.
- Before a long journey, eat a light meal and take a rest. Do not set off on an empty stomach. You need to be comfortable to concentrate well.
- If you intend to drive through the night, make sure you have at least three hours of sleep first.
- At the outset, adjust the seat to ensure a comfortable driving position for the journey.
- Avoid wearing tight clothes. When you sit for long periods, the stomach and ankles tend to swell up.
- If you are driving in bright sunshine, wear sunglasses that do not distort images or colors. Glare puts extra strain on the eyes and adds to fatigue. But do not wear dark glasses of any kind after dark; although they may reduce the dazzle of oncoming headlights, they restrict your ability to see dimly lit objects.

- Make sure the car is well ventilated.
- In heavy traffic, take advantage of slowdowns by exercising your limbs gently. For example, curl your toes, rotate your wrists and stretch your shoulders and neck. This helps the blood circulation and relieves boredom and frustration.
- On a long journey, alternate the driving with someone else, if possible.
- Suck hard candies occasionally for refreshment while you are driving.
- Make regular stops on a long run – never drive for more than three hours without a break.
- If you are driving abroad, take breaks more frequently than normal. Interpreting unfamiliar signs demands extra concentration and so will tire you more quickly.
- When you stop for a break, take a short nap if you feel you need it. But always get out of the car and go for a stroll to exercise cramped limbs and pep up circulation. A hot drink is also beneficial.
- On a brief stop, try taking your shoes and socks off for a while. Relaxing and cooling the feet helps to clear the head.

Fire in your car

A car fire must be put out very quickly because of the danger of the gas tank exploding if the gasoline vapor should ignite. As with any fire, the way to extinguish it quickly is to cut off its air and fuel supply.

• As soon as you notice smoke or flames, switch off the ignition but leave the key in position to avoid locking the steering.
• If the car is moving, coast to the side of the road if possible and stop.
• Get everyone out and away from the car.
• Disconnect the battery if you can, by pulling the wires off the terminals. But do not open the hood wide if the fire is underneath, as air will increase the flames.
• If you do not have a fire extinguisher, try to smother the flames with a car blanket or any thick material.
• If this is not successful, dial 911 and ask that firemen be sent to the scene.

Using a fire extinguisher
• If the fire is in the engine compartment, lift the hood just enough to aim the extinguisher under it.
• Direct the extinguisher at the base of the flames and work methodically from side to side and from the edge inward.
• Do not leave a patch uncovered, otherwise the flames may spring up again.

FITTING A FIRE EXTINGUISHER IN YOUR CAR

Every year, about one half-million cars are damaged or destroyed by fire in North America. Most automobile fires are caused by a short circuit in the electrical system, or by leakage in the fuel system. Others result mainly from collisions or are started by cigarettes.

Fire extinguishers for cars may contain either dry powder or a gas, such as halon. You will need a powder extinguisher of about 3 lb. (1.4 kg) for most car fires. In the gas models, a 2-lb. (1-kg) container should suffice.

Both the dry powder and gas models are nontoxic and can be used safely on electrical equipment. The halon model leaves no residue.

A car fire extinguisher needs to be mounted in an easily accessible place, such as on the dashboard or in the driver's footwell – not in the trunk.

Powder extinguishers must be checked once a year by the manufacturer to ensure that the filling is kept up to capacity. Halon models do not need an annual inspection.

Stuck on a rail crossing

Your chances of surviving a crash with a train are minimal. If your car stalls or breaks down on a rail crossing, therefore, the priority is to protect yourself and your passengers – not the car. Even if the engineer can see you, he is unlikely to be able to stop in time. A 150-car freight train traveling at 60 mph (100 km/h) takes up to 1½ miles (2.5 km) to stop.

• Get everyone out of the car and off the crossing as quickly as possible.
• If visibility is good, and there is no sight or sound of a train in either direction, get your passengers or passersby to help you push the car to safety.
• If you cannot move the car, send someone to the nearest telephone to call 911. Give the location of the crossing and ask that the train company be notified. They may be able to alert approaching trains.
• If you see a train coming, run alongside the tracks toward it. This way you will not be hit by flying metal when the train hits the car. Wave your arms and point to the crossing to warn the engineer.
• If the train does crash into the car, go to the nearest telephone and call 911.

If the barriers come down
• If the alarms start to sound, the lights flash or the barriers come down while the car is still on the crossing, get everyone right away from the tracks. A derailed train or the wreckage from a crash can travel incredible distances from the point of impact.
• Abandon the car and everything in it. The train might be at the crossing within a matter of seconds. Usually only about 10 seconds elapse between the bells' and flashers' start-up and the barriers' descent. The train may arrive in another 12 seconds.

Safety on crossings
There are about 385,000 rail crossings in North America, and each year they are the scene of about 6,000 accidents. These cost the lives of about 600 persons and seriously injure some 2,500 more. Most of the victims are local people. Motoring experts recommend five rules for crossing the tracks safely.
• Approach at a moderate speed.
• At an open rail crossing – one with no barriers or warning lights – treat the crossing as if it were a major intersection. Stop, look both ways and listen carefully before you cross.
• Do not drive nose to tail over a crossing. Start to cross only when you can see that the road on the other side is clear.
• Do not stop on a rail crossing for any reason. If you are already on the crossing when the lights start to flash or the alarms sound, carry on over at once.
• Do not assume that the way is clear once a train passes. Another one may be coming in the opposite direction.

Emergencies on the road

205

Stuck in snow

If you are forced to stop in snow or on ice, it is often difficult to start off again because the tires cannot grip the surface. It is particularly easy to get stuck if you stop while driving up a hill.

The techniques described here for getting out of snow also apply to getting out of mud or sand.

If you get stuck on hard snow or ice
• Do not accelerate hard in an attempt to pull away. The spinning of the wheels will compact the snow and make gripping even more difficult; snow may also become packed into the tire treads, lowering their gripping ability.

• Ensure that the wheels are straight so that the treads are in the best position for gripping the surface.

• Find something to pack under the driving wheels to improve their grip, such as sand, grit, sacking or twigs.

• Press the accelerator gently, just enough to

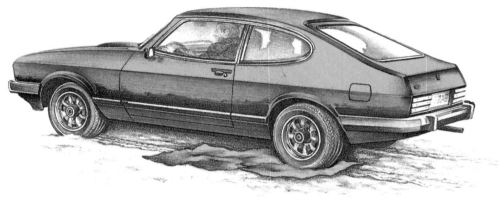

GETTING UNSTUCK
Give a stuck car's driving wheels something to grip by packing gunny sacks, say, in front of them.

DRIVING ON SNOW AND ICE

• Make sure that tires are inflated to the recommended pressures. Underinflated tires do not give as good a grip. Winter radial tires, which have wide grooves, may grip snow better if they are inflated to a slightly higher pressure than normal.

• Accelerate slowly, avoiding sudden turns which may trigger a skid. Inexperienced drivers often take off too quickly on slippery surfaces. With automatic transmission, put it in drive to reduce wheelspin. With manual transmission, accelerating in second gear instead of first will give you better traction on icy surfaces.

• Keep your speed low because it takes much longer to pull up than on a normal surface. On ice, the braking distance can be ten times longer than normal.

• Stay well behind the vehicle in front to give yourself plenty of room for braking.

• Do not brake and steer at the same time.

• Use the brakes gently.

• Try to avoid stopping on an icy hill. If necessary, wait at the bottom until you can climb without interruption.

• Descend a steep hill very slowly in low gear, and use the brakes very gently and cautiously.

• Gently tap your brakes occasionally to test for traction on snow and ice.

• Where permitted, snow chains or snow traction clamps can greatly improve tire grip.

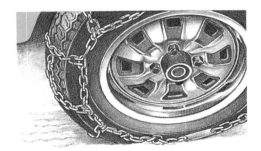

GETTING A GRIP ON ICE OR SNOW
Where permitted, snow chains fitted around a car's tires help to improve traction on icy or snowbound roads.

move the car forward slowly. On manual transmissions, slip the clutch as necessary to keep the engine revving.

• If there are any passengers in the car, they may be able to help by pushing the car forward as you drive off. Tell them to stand at the sides – so that the car does not roll or slide into them – but well away from the driving wheels or they will be sprayed with dirt, snow and packing material.

• Once the car gets moving, do not stop to pick up passengers or luggage until you have reached a firmer, level surface.

Getting out of deep snow

• It is sometimes possible to drive out of snow about 12 in. (30 cm) or so deep by moving the car backward and forward to build up a track – a technique known as rocking.

• Try to move forward a little bit by shifting to low gear and then revving gently.

• While the car is as far forward as it will go, quickly shift to *Reverse* and move slowly a little bit backward.

• Repeat the backward and forward movements until you can mount the piled up snow and drive out of the trough.

• If this method fails, the alternative is to dig the snow away from all four wheels, and use the techniques recommended above for moving off on hard snow or ice.

If you are trapped in a snowbound car

Driving is usually impossible in a blizzard, or if snow becomes deeper than about 12 in. (30 cm). In a snowbound car, the main things to concentrate on are keeping warm and keeping awake.

• Stay in the car; it will give you shelter. Do not try to walk for help – you risk falling into a snowdrift or getting lost in a blizzard, and could die of exposure only a short distance from a building.

• Before the snow gets too deep, try to clear the snow from around the exhaust pipe. Otherwise poisonous fumes are likely to enter the car when you run the engine to use the heater.

• Bring anything you need from the trunk into the seating area. Look for an implement that you can use to make an air channel should the car become completely buried – a snow shovel or a jack handle, for example.

• Keep warm by wrapping yourself up in clothing, blankets, or coats. Wrap your head up as well. More heat is lost from the head than from any other part of the body.

• Newspaper wrapped around limbs or stuffed into clothing helps to conserve body heat; it can also be used to improvise a hat.

• To help you warm up, run the engine and heater for only about ten minutes every hour. Do not run them constantly; not only will the warmth make you drowsy, but you need to conserve fuel in case you are trapped for a long time. There is also a higher risk of exhaust fumes entering the car.

• Keep awake. If you doze off, you are more likely to succumb to frostbite or hypothermia (excessive loss of body heat). Or you could suffocate if the car became buried by snow.

• Open a window occasionally to let in air. Use a window on the side away from drifting snow.

• Avoid drinking alcohol in the hope that it will warm you up. It dilates the blood vessels and so encourages the loss of body heat. It may also make you sleepy.

• Exercising gently from time to time will help you to keep awake and keep your blood circulating. For example, stretch or wriggle your toes, fingers, knees, shoulders and neck.

• Do not attempt strenuous exercise, as this will increase your need for oxygen, use up your body heat and make you tired.

• Do not keep the radio or car lights on constantly, or you may drain the battery.

• If the car gets completely buried by snow, open a window and poke an air channel through the snow. Use an implement such as an umbrella or jack handle if necessary. Keep the channel clear.

• If a number of cars are snowbound together, join forces with the other occupants. Sitting together in one vehicle generates warmth, boosts morale and helps you to keep awake.

SURVIVAL PACK

When motoring in snowy weather, make sure the car is well equipped to keep you moving on a slippery surface and to keep you warm and occupied if you break down or become snowbound in cold, icy conditions. This is a list of useful equipment to keep in the car.

• Shovel.
• Sacking or bag of sand.
• Snow chains or traction clamps.
• Snow boots.
• Extra clothing.
• Flashlight and spare batteries.
• Survival or space blanket.

If you are going on a long journey – especially at night – and conditions are such that you might experience delays along the way, consider taking some additional items:

• A hot drink in a thermos bottle.
• Emergency high-energy rations such as chocolate, cookies or hard candies.
• Something to pass the time – for example, a novel, a battery-powered tape player or radio, a quiz book, a book of crosswords or pencil and paper.

Escaping from a car underwater

IF IT SINKS BEFORE YOU CAN GET OUT

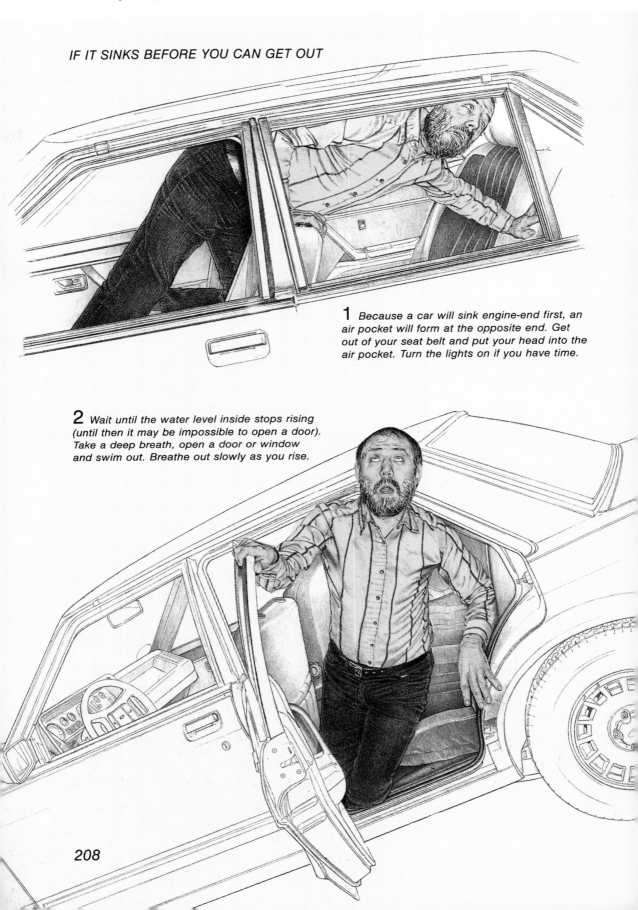

1 *Because a car will sink engine-end first, an air pocket will form at the opposite end. Get out of your seat belt and put your head into the air pocket. Turn the lights on if you have time.*

2 *Wait until the water level inside stops rising (until then it may be impossible to open a door). Take a deep breath, open a door or window and swim out. Breathe out slowly as you rise.*

If your car plunges into deep water, you may be able to escape through a door or window before it sinks – usually within a minute or so. But even if the car sinks with you inside, you can still escape because it may take a few minutes to fill up with water. Precisely how long it takes depends on whether the windows are open, how well sealed the car is and how deep the water is. The deeper the car sinks, the higher is the pressure of the surrounding water and the faster it will force its way in.

How to get out of a sunken car

• A car will sink engine-end first, and a pocket of air will form inside at the opposite end near the roof. Use this pocket of air to escape.

• Release your seat belt and any child safety restraints. If there is time, turn on the headlights, the interior lights and the emergency flashers. They will enable you to see better and will help rescuers to find the vehicle.

• Place yourself so that you can put your head into the air pocket and breathe. In a front-engined car, climb into the back seat.

• Close any open windows and ventilation ducts, if there is time, to retain air in the car.

• As the car settles, water will find its way in through cracks and holes until the pressure inside and outside the car equalizes. Keep calm and wait until the pressures equalize – when the water level inside stops rising. Until then it will be extremely difficult to open a door – and failure to do so might lead to panic.

• When the level stops rising, take a deep breath, open a window or door and swim out.

• As you swim to the surface, allow air to bubble slowly out of your mouth. Because the air pocket in the car was under pressure, the air in your lungs will be as well – and will expand as you rise. If the excess is not allowed to escape, it could damage your lungs.

LIFESAVING BUBBLE
When Kenneth Hope's car plunged into the river at Mark in Somerset, England, in November 1982, it turned over, trapping him inside. He crawled into the trunk of the car where there was a large enough air pocket to keep him alive until he was rescued by emergency services several hours later.

He was suffering from exposure because of the chilly water, but was otherwise unharmed.

Emergencies on the road

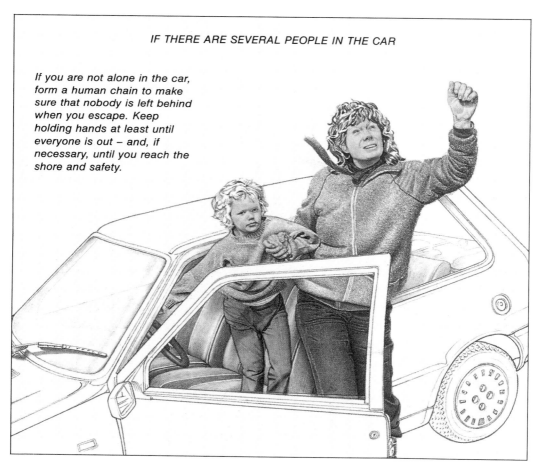

IF THERE ARE SEVERAL PEOPLE IN THE CAR

If you are not alone in the car, form a human chain to make sure that nobody is left behind when you escape. Keep holding hands at least until everyone is out – and, if necessary, until you reach the shore and safety.

Driving through floodwater

Flooding is likely on many low-lying roads after heavy rain and sudden thaws. The pools of water on some roads can be quite deep.

• Should you see a sheet of water ahead, slow down. If you hit still water at high speed, the impact could jerk the car into a skid. Reducing your speed will also keep the water from splashing under the hood and possibly stalling the engine.

• If the water is obviously not very deep – other traffic may be going through, for example – there is no need to stop and check the depth. Wait until the car in front is clear of the water, then drive through slowly.

• Stop if you are uncertain of the depth. It is not advisable to drive on if the water level is higher than the bottom edge of the cooling-fan blades, because they will send a fine spray of water over the engine and could short-circuit the spark plug leads or crack the hot engine block. In some cars, the blades are only 10-12 in. (25-30 cm) above the ground – about as high as the midpoint of the wheels.

• Enter the water on the crown of a road so that you keep to the shallowest part.

• Drive slowly in L (*Low*) or 1 (first gear) in a car with automatic transmission – in first or second gear with a manual transmission – so that as little water as possible is splashed on the engine. But do not let the engine stall.

• Maintain a steady speed until you are clear of the water.

• As soon as you drive out of the water, test the brakes. They are likely to be soaked and useless. To dry them out, drive slowly with your left foot pressing lightly on the brake pedal. Do not pick up speed until you have tested the brakes several times and are sure they are pulling evenly on all wheels.

HOW FLOODWATER CAN DAMAGE YOUR CAR

If you drive through even quite shallow water at speed, the car will throw up a considerable wave. The wave can be heavy enough to obscure your vision, and the water may wrench the front wheels to one side so that you risk losing steering control.

The surge of water may also swamp the engine compartment, damaging the electric system and causing the engine to stall. If this happens, you will either have to push the car out or wait for a tow.

If the engine stalls, water may enter the exhaust system and do extensive damage.

Driving slowly through a flood does not guarantee a trouble-free passage either. Your brake drums are quite likely to become flooded, leaving you without braking power when you emerge.

Where the risk is greatest
Flooding is most likely: on roads beside rivers and lakes; in dips on undulating roads; on roads liable to subsidence (this is sometimes signposted); under bridges, where the road often dips.

After heavy rain, keep an eye out for flood warning signs. Look out, too, wherever roadside fences and buildings ahead seem unnaturally low. These are occasionally found near reservoirs and places where flooding happens regularly.

SAFELY THROUGH THE FLOOD
Drive slowly but at a steady speed. Remember to dry out your brake linings as soon as you get out of the water. Simply brake gently as you drive slowly away.

Emergency repairs

When a car breaks down miles from help, there may be little or nothing you can do about it unless you happen to be carrying the necessary spare parts.

But some common causes of breakdown can be repaired temporarily on the spot with little more than ingenuity, and others can be dealt with merely by know-how.

All the methods described here have been used successfully by motorists in an emergency to get them home or to a garage.

If the fan belt breaks

If the ignition light comes on while you are driving, indicating that the alternator is not charging the battery, the reason may be a broken drive belt or fan belt.
• This should not happen if the belt is regularly checked during the car's normal servicing. Check it at least once a year, and replace it as a matter of course every five years – even if it is showing no signs of wear. And carry a spare fan belt in the car.
• Do not be tempted, if the fan belt breaks, to improvise one from string, nylon tights or cord. These substitutes are often recommended, but they do not work properly and may simply add to your troubles.
• Modern fan belts work under much greater tension than the belts on older cars. This means that the substitutes are likely to break within a minute or two. And the broken pieces can cause expensive damage – by getting tangled around the pulleys, for instance.
• If you do not have a proper replacement fan belt – or if you do not have the tools necessary to install it – get to a telephone and call an automobile association or a garage for help.
• If getting to a telephone is impossible, you can, in an emergency, drive on without the belt.
• If you decide to do this, wait first of all for the engine to cool off – a process which usually takes about half an hour. Remove any loose pieces of belt from the engine compartment while you are waiting.
• After that period, drive on – keeping the motor at a low, steady speed – for no more than 3 miles (5 km). If you drive farther than this, you risk overheating the engine and causing expensive damage.
• Then stop and let the engine cool off again for half an hour. Repeat the process until you reach a garage.
• One good way to extend the driving range of the engine between stops is by turning the car heater to maximum. The heater will draw more heat from the engine, preventing the engine from overheating so quickly even if you get uncomfortably warm, and allowing you to drive a few extra miles before stopping.
• During the journey, the battery will not be charging. So keep lights, air conditioning, radio – all the car's electrical systems – turned off as much as possible. Otherwise you will in time drain the battery and, without electrical power for the spark, the engine will not work.
• Many cars today have more than one drive belt, and have electric fans, not belt-driven ones. In a modern car, if your ignition light comes on and stays on, it probably means that the belt driving the alternator is broken. If this is the case, the engine will not overheat if you drive on without the belt. But you will, in time, drain the battery.
• Stop and remove any loose pieces of belt from the engine. Turn off all unnecessary electrical systems – including the heater fan and any radio – so as to preserve the battery's charge for as long as possible.
• Drive on to the nearest telephone or garage and get the belt replaced.
• At night, a fully charged battery will usually keep the engine going, with the headlights on, for at least an hour – although the lights will become progressively dimmer. During the day, if no lights or other electrical systems are being used, a fully charged battery will keep the engine going for several hours.
• If the ignition light comes on only intermittently or dimly, the reason is not a broken drive belt. Usually, it means that the engine is turning over too slowly. Rev up the engine a little and the light should go out.

If the gas gets low

If the gas gauge reads very low, you may, by careful driving, be able to conserve fuel long enough to reach a service station.
• Drive smoothly, but not fast – about 25-30 mph (40-50 km/h). In a manual shift car, use top gear but not, however, an overdrive or a fifth gear.
• Avoid stopping and starting if you can. Anticipate conditions ahead so that you can slow down as much as possible simply by taking your foot off the accelerator. The more the accelerator is pressed, the more gas is consumed.
• Try to approach traffic lights at such a speed that you can cruise through without stopping. If you have to stop and start again, get into top gear smoothly and as early as practicable.
• When approaching a hill, gently build up speed beforehand, then allow your car to slow down rather than pressing the gas pedal further. With a manual shift, do not stay in top gear too long as you go up the slope so that you lose speed and have to increase acceleration. Instead, downshift so that you can keep going in a lower gear without having to press hard on the accelerator.
• Coasting down hills with the motor switched off is not recommended. On automatic cars, it can lead to the transmission overheating. On cars with power brakes and power steering, the effort required to operate the brakes and steering will be alarmingly increased. On a car with a steering lock, you could lock the steering as well.

For manual shift cars, coasting in neutral with

the engine off limits your control of the car and, without power braking help provided by the engine vacuum, you may need to press twice as hard on the brake pedal to achieve the same braking effect.

• Try to avoid driving until the gas runs out completely, because dirt and moisture from the tank bottom will be dragged through the fuel system and probably cause a blockage.

• If the gas does run out, the engine is likely to splutter and falter a little before it finally stops. Pull off the road if this happens.

• If you are stranded on a highway, pull onto the emergency lane or shoulder and wait for a police patrol or use the nearest emergency telephone to call for assistance.

• On other roads, you may find somewhere to buy a can of gas as quickly as you can find a telephone. This will save you waiting around for a garage or automobile association to come to your aid.

• It may be difficult to pour gas into your tank from the can. If necessary, improvise a funnel from a rolled-up newspaper or magazine.

If the windshield wipers fail

If the windshield wipers break down in rain and you cannot get them to work, you may be able – on older cars – to improvise a way of operating them manually. The problem may be that the drive cable from the wiper motor has broken. If it has not, disconnect the cable anyway – it is usually under the dashboard or hood near the base of the wipers. Otherwise the arms will be too stiff to pull.

• Tie a piece of string or cord to the wiper arm on the driver's side and stretch it through the open driver's window. An alternative could be a scarf or belt.

• Tie another string from the driver's wiper to the passenger-side arm and run it through the passenger window into the car.

• Ask the front passenger to pull the wipers back and forth across the windscreen by hand as needed to clear it. A driver alone should not attempt this, because it would limit his control of the steering.

• Alternatively, improvise a return spring such as linked elastic bands or a pair of suspenders from one of the wiper arms. Retain it against the jamb of the closed door on the same side. This may make the arms easier to operate manually by a driver alone, because he only has to pull one string. Again, though, it is safer for a passenger to operate the arms so that the driver has both hands free for steering.

• On a late-model car, it may be impossible to disconnect the wiper arms from the motor without an array of tools and considerable time. Either wait for the rain to stop or, if you have to continue your journey for some overriding reason, drive on very slowly without the wipers. Have them repaired or replaced as soon as possible. Driving a car with faulty wipers is against the law.

If you lose the wheel nuts

• If you lose the nuts on a wheel, perhaps while changing a wheel at night, remove one nut from each of the other three wheels, and use them

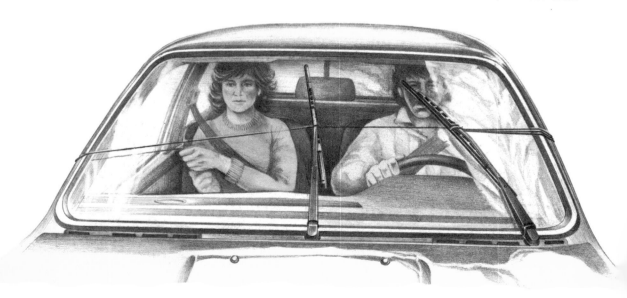

HOW TO WORK BROKEN WIPERS BY HAND
On older cars, disconnect the cable that drives the wipers, and tie something elastic such as a pair of suspenders to the driver's wiper. Clamp the other end in the door. Tie string between the *arms and run it through the passenger's window. If the wipers are stiff, though this is unlikely on an older car, do not force them. Wait until the rain stops.*

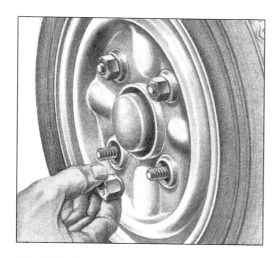

SHARING OUT WHEEL NUTS
If you lose wheel nuts while changing a wheel,
share out the remainder, putting any extra on
the front wheels. You can do this even with
small imports that have only four nuts per
wheel.

as replacements. This works even with small European cars that have only four nuts per wheel. North American-made cars, however, have at least five nuts per wheel.
• If the wheel has only three nuts (or bolts) to start with – as on a small Renault, for example – it is still possible to borrow from the other wheels. But it is not advisable unless you have no alternative, because the strain on the remaining two nuts is very great.
• If you lose only some of the wheel nuts so that you have a total of, say, 18 nuts between the four wheels, put the extra nuts on the front wheels rather than the back, because the front wheels have to take the additional strain of the steering. Also, in many late-model cars, the drive is through the front wheels.
• Drive on smoothly – braking gradually and using only gentle acceleration – at no more than 30 mph (50 km/h), to lessen the strain on the remaining nuts.
• Get a full set of nuts on each wheel as soon as possible.

If the engine is flooded with gasoline
If you pump the accelerator too much when trying to start a car with carburetors, the tips of the spark plugs can become soaked with gas, and they will not fire.

Similarly, if the car stalls when you stop at an intersection shortly after setting off, and will not start again, pumping the accelerator has probably fouled the spark plugs.
• Slowly press the accelerator to the floor and hold it there. This also increases the airflow.
• With the accelerator held down, turn the starter for a few seconds. This should blast the

plug ends dry and clear any overrich mixture from the combustion cylinders. The engine should then fire.
• If it does not fire, wait for about ten minutes and then repeat the operation.
• Before pressing the accelerator on cars with a manual choke, push the choke right in to increase the flow of air to the cylinders.

If the engine fades out because of vapor lock
When it is very hot, gas sometimes vaporizes in a car's fuel lines or pump, sending bubbles of vapor instead of liquid fuel to the carburetor. This restricted fuel supply will cause the engine to misfire or cut out altogether.

Such a vapor lock might occur on an older car after a long drive at high speed, or in a lengthy traffic jam, or in unusually hot weather.
• Cooling is the only answer, so park safely in the shade and wait for the engine to cool and the fuel to condense. This will probably take at least half an hour. Then start up again.
• There is no need to cool the intake manifold and carburetor by wrapping a wet cloth around them. Waiting will do the job almost as quickly, and with much less effort.
• If the trouble recurs, get the car checked. The solution may be as simple as adding coolant to your cooling system.

If the engine does not turn over
If your car won't start and has an automatic transmission, make sure that you have not forgotten to put the gearshift lever in *Park*. If you still have a problem, one of the following steps may provide the solution.
• Jiggle the lever in each gear, beginning with *Neutral*. A safety switch may have become misaligned.
• Test the battery. Turn on the headlights and try to start the car. If the lights burn brightly, your battery is most likely all right and the trouble is probably in some other part of the starting system. If the headlights dim or flicker when you try to start the motor, however, your battery is most likely almost dead.
• Check the heavy cable running from the battery's positive terminal to the starter and make sure that the connection is tight. Make a similar check of the cable from the negative side of the battery. Tighten its connection to the engine if necessary.
• Is there a clicking sound when you turn the key? This could mean a problem within the starter itself. Try tapping the starter casing. Sometimes this may be all that is needed to realign a loose connection.

If the accelerator jams
If the accelerator stays down when you ease off it while driving, the return spring near the pedal or the carburetor may be broken. This means the engine will continue at high revs – it will not slow down automatically.

Emergencies on the road

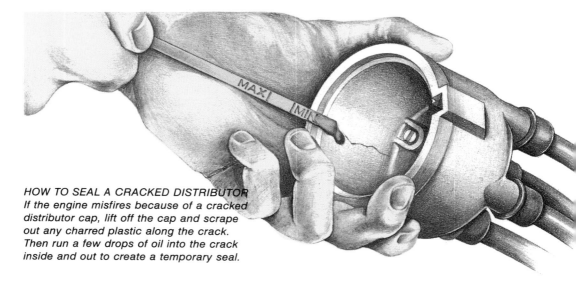

HOW TO SEAL A CRACKED DISTRIBUTOR
If the engine misfires because of a cracked
distributor cap, lift off the cap and scrape
out any charred plastic along the crack.
Then run a few drops of oil into the crack
inside and out to create a temporary seal.

• Try to hook your toe under the accelerator pedal and raise it. Better still, have a passenger pull the pedal up. You should not take your eyes off the road, nor should you reach down with your hand to free the pedal.

• Raising the pedal will slow down the revs and stop the engine racing. Signal right, check your rearview mirror and pull off the road when it is safe to do so.

• Switch off the ignition as soon as possible to prevent engine damage. But until you have pulled over and braked to a stop, be careful not to turn the key so far that it engages any steering lock on the car: switch it to the *Off* rather than the *Lock* position.

• If you cannot pull over and switch off immediately – if you are on the left lane of a highway, for example – keep going until you can, braking if necessary.

• Remember, though, that the car's braking power will be below normal because of the counter-effect of the high engine speed.

• If you, or your passenger, are unable to get the pedal unstuck, shift into *Neutral* and hit the accelerator pedal a few times with your foot. If it still remains stuck, turn the ignition to the *Off* position (not *Lock,* which will freeze the steering). Be prepared for stiff braking and steering if these are power-assisted. Coast to a spot where you can stop to investigate.

• You cannot risk turning off your engine in heavy traffic, where you will need your power-assisted brakes and steering for maneuvering. Shift into *Neutral* – in a manual transmission, depress the clutch – then apply the brakes.

• Once you have stopped and switched off your ignition, switch on your emergency flashers. If necessary, set up flares or reflectors to warn other motorists.

• Find out what is holding down the pedal linkage, and free it if possible. If you cannot find and fix the problem, call a garage.

If the distributor cap is cracked
A hairline crack may develop in the distributor cap because of damage or old age. This gives the high-tension current to the spark plugs an easy alternative path, so the engine misfires or becomes difficult to start.

• Lift off the cap and look inside for a telltale blackened track burned into the plastic along the line of the crack by the escaping current.

• Scrape away as much of the burned plastic as possible with something sharp, such as a small screwdriver or a nail file.

• Seal the crack with nail varnish, if you have any at hand, or run a small amount of oil from the end of the dipstick into it.

• If it is a bad crack, put the sealant on both sides – inside and outside the cap.

• Have a new distributor cap installed as soon as possible.

If a fuse blows and you have no spare
If one part of the car's electrical system fails but others do not – if, for example, the lights go out but the brake lights and indicators work – the reason is most likely a blown fuse.

• Open the fuse box. Your car's manual will tell you where it is – usually inside the car under the dashboard or under the hood near the firewall. Sometimes there is a spare fuse supplied in the box. The blown fuse will probably be obvious because it will show signs of burning. If not, take out each fuse and inspect it to see which has its wire strip burned out.

• If possible, use a fuse of the same rating from a circuit you can temporarily manage without – for example, the fuse covering the rear window heater. In most fuse boxes there are labels or a chart indicating which fuse covers which circuit. If the fuse you have transferred blows as well, there is a short circuit in the system – perhaps a chafed wire or a faulty switch. Try to find it and rectify it.

• If you cannot discover the problem, either drive on if possible – without using the faulty circuit – or call a garage or an automobile association to which you belong. Do not try to replace the blown fuse with a temporary fuse that is too strong for the circuit. It will not blow, but cables will probably overheat and you risk starting a fire.

• Neither should you try wrapping a layer of metal foil from a cigarette package or chocolate bar around the fuse holder – a method someone may suggest. This may damage a major component or set the car on fire.

Thawing a frozen door lock

If you cannot get the door key in the lock on a frosty or snowy morning – or if it will not turn when it is inserted – the lock is probably frozen. To free it, use one of the following methods:

• Thaw the frozen lock with an aerosol that squirts a mixture of alcohol and lubricant into the keyhole.

• Heat the end of the key with a match or cigarette lighter, then put the key into the frozen lock. To avoid burned fingers, wear gloves or hold the key with pliers. Repeat the process several times until the frozen car lock turns freely. Do not force it.

• Squirt a few drops of lighter fuel or antifreeze into the lock, but take care not to get it on the paintwork. Using a deicer spray is not recommended because you cannot avoid spraying it on the surrounding paintwork, and it may damage the surface.

SPARE PARTS FOR EVERYDAY MOTORING

Carrying a few spares of the parts most likely to fail, as well as some tools and a few repair aids, can save any motorist hours of trouble. Whether you use it or not, a well-stocked emergency kit will bring peace of mind on car trips.

• Drive belt (or fan belt) – a replacement of the type used for your make of car. Emergency fan belts are also available, but are not recommended. They do not last long and may be awkward to fit.

• Fuses – one or two of each type of fuse used in your make of car.

• Light bulbs – packaged sets are available for different makes.

• Spark plug – one of the type suitable for your car. You do not need to carry a complete set, because it is rare for all to fail at once.

• High-tension wire – a length of heavily insulated wire of the type used between the coil, distributor cap and spark plugs. Carry a length equal to the longest high-tension wire in your car, and any tools you will need to install it.

• Duplicate ignition key – keep it in a magnetic box, which can be fixed to the outside of the car in a concealed spot.

• Can of fuel. Carry this only in remote areas where you may be cut off from a gas station. The can must conform to approved specifications – CSA B376-M1980 in Canada; ASTM-F852 in the United States. Replace the gasoline every three months or so. Gas quality deteriorates in time.

• Tools – a straight-bladed and a Phillips screwdriver; a circuit tester; wrenches of the sizes most common on your car; and a wrench for removing spark plugs.

Useful extras

• Heavy-duty flashlight and spare batteries.
• Worklight that plugs into the cigarette lighter.
• Radiator sealant.
• Water-repellent lubricant.
• Exhaust bandage and sealing cement.
• Strong adhesive tape.
• Insulating tape.
• Tire inflators. These commercially sold cans of compressed air and sealant are useful if you get a flat tire and have difficulty changing a wheel. But if there is any damage to the tire structure, their use may make the tire difficult to repair later, and garages may be reluctant to handle the job.
• Magnet – for retrieving small metal parts dropped into inaccessible areas.
• Coil of baling wire – soft, galvanized iron or steel wire suitable for innumerable small repairs such as fashioning a temporary exhaust hanger.
• Jumper cables – useful for getting a start from another car if your battery is dead. But before you buy a set, check your owner's manual, because it may not be safe to use jumper cables on some modern cars equipped with fully electronic ignition and fuel injection. When you use jumper cables, always follow the procedure spelled out in your owner's manual.
• Tow rope.
• Length of cord.
• Pocket knife.
• Packet of strong elastic bands.
• Spare container of coolant.
• Spare windshield washer fluid.
• Six flares, or three reflectors.
• Car-type fire extinguisher.

Menaced by a hitchhiker

More often than not, someone hitching a ride is quite harmless and intent only on being helped on his way. But there is always a risk that he is planning to rob you, and even if not, there have been cases of hitchhikers slashing the back seat or doing other damage.

Hitchhiking is also illegal on many roads and highways. Even where this is not so, crime prevention experts advise motorists never to give a lift to a stranger.

• If a hitchhiker you have picked up threatens you with a weapon, do as you are told and drive on. Do not attempt to struggle with him.

• Look for the first opportunity to get out of the situation. The police suggest that, if possible, you stop the car at a place where there are a lot of people about – a bus station, say – and attract attention by yelling and screaming.

• Another way is to stall the car deliberately at busy traffic lights and pretend it will not restart. With the buildup of other traffic and irate drivers, the attacker may run off, or you may manage to get away from the car.

• If you cannot shake off the attacker, hand over money, car keys or other possessions if ordered to do so.

• As soon as the hitchhiker leaves or you escape, write down all you can remember about the incident – where and when it happened, what the hitchhiker looked like, and what was said. Sign and date what you have written, and take it to the police; it will be useful evidence if the hitchhiker is later caught and prosecuted.

If a girl tries to blackmail you
If a man gives a ride to a girl and she threatens to rip her blouse and scream "rape" unless he gives her money, he should remain calm and neither touch her nor argue with her.

• Drive straight to the nearest police station or flag down a passing police car.

• Alternatively, stop where there is a large crowd and ask someone to call the police.

If you are flagged down at night
There is a possibility that what appears to be an accident or someone in need of help is a ruse to stop a car and rob the driver. This is most likely to happen to a motorist who is known to be carrying money and who regularly uses a particular route.

• Lock all doors as you approach the person flagging you down.

• Slow down, or change to a low gear, so that you can accelerate away if necessary.

• Turn your headlights to full beam to light up the scene so that you can assess the situation.

• If you stop, do not turn off the engine or get out of the car until you are satisfied that the situation is genuine. Be ready to drive off quickly.

• If you are not sure whether the situation is genuine, drive on and call the police from the nearest telephone.

Safety on two wheels

Motorcyclists are far more likely to be injured or killed in a crash than are motorists. The death rate per 100,000,000 miles (161,000,000 km) traveled is ten times greater for motorcyclists than it is for drivers of other motor vehicles. And there are about 500,000 motorcycle accidents in North America every year.

The commonest motorcycle accident is a collision with a motorist turning onto a major road, and it happens because the car driver simply fails to see the motorcyclist in time – even in daylight on an urban road. The same circumstances account for numerous bicycle accidents. Many occur at or near an intersection.

For this reason the most important safety rule for motorcyclists and cyclists is: be visible.

On a motorcycle
• Make sure you can be seen. Wear brighty colored clothing, or a fluorescent sash or vest.

• Although your headlight should be on constantly while riding, do not assume that it alone will make you conspicuous. On smaller machines – particularly 250 cc and under – the light is not very powerful.

• Before overtaking, flash your headlight to make sure the driver has seen you. If you have been riding behind the left edge of the car, his view of you may have been masked.

• Do not overtake on the right. The driver may not see you and could pull over toward the curb or turn right in front of you.

• If the car in front of you turns right, beware of another vehicle pulling out across your path from the same side road. The driver may not have seen you behind the turning car.

• When motorcyclists ride in a group, the one in front should take up the best position on the road. Those behind should be staggered to right and left so that they have as much vision and braking space as possible.

• For a safe braking distance in dry weather, road safety experts recommend keeping as far behind the vehicle in front as you can travel in two seconds, which means allowing about 1 yd. for each 1 mph (2 m for every 3 km/h). You can measure the distance using a roadside landmark – a mailbox, say – as a marker. You should be able to say: "Only a fool forgets the two-second rule," which takes about two seconds to repeat, in the time between the vehicle in front passing the marker, and passing it yourself.

• In wet weather, braking distances may be doubled, so you need a four-second gap between your machine and a vehicle ahead.

• If you want to brake when riding upright on a firm, dry surface, the safest and most effective way is to pull more firmly on the front brake than on the rear brake. On a firm but wet surface, put even pressure on both front and rear brakes.

• When riding with the machine leaning to one side, when turning, or when riding on a poor surface such as loose gravel, avoid using the front brake at all.

On a bicycle

• Wear brightly colored clothing, and a fluorescent sash and arm or leg bands.

• At night, make sure your lights are on. Local laws may require that you have some or all of the following: working front and back lights, and reflectors on both wheels and the front and back of the pedals. You must, by law, have working front and back lights and a rear reflector.

• Slow down when you approach a turn and look out for vehicles coming unexpectedly across your path. Be ready to brake suddenly.

• Keep at least 1 yd. (1 m) from the curb – to give yourself space to swerve into if a passing car comes too close. A red flag on a light rod that extends 30 in. (75 cm) laterally or 2 yd. (2 m) vertically alerts motorists.

• Remember that a bicycle is a road vehicle like any other. It is just as illegal for a cyclist to cross against a red light or to go the wrong way up a one-way street as it would be for a driver.

PROTECTIVE CLOTHING: WHAT TO WEAR ON A MOTORCYCLE

• Your safety helmet, which is required by law in many states – at least for certain age groups – and in all provinces, should conform to certain standards. Depending on where you live, this will be Canadian Standards Asssociation specification D230, or U.S. motor vehicle safety standard 218.

• Wear goggles or a visor, whether part of the helmet or not. Even though the law does not require you to wear them, it is highly desirable that you do.

• A well-fitting, two-piece windproof suit (jacket and leggings) is convenient for normal use on a motorcycle. Leather gives the best protection from abrasions if you fall from the machine and slide on the road, but it will not keep out the cold and wet for long. For riding long distances or in very wet weather, wear vinyl coveralls over your normal riding gear.

• Protect your hands with gloves whatever the weather. In summer wear thin, unlined leather. In cold weather, wear leather lined with silk or lamb's wool. Alternatively, you can buy handlebars with attached mitts that can be heated with power from your motorcycle battery.

• It is also possible to buy heated motorcycle suits, which are also powered by your motorcyle battery.

• Wear strong, waterproof boots. When you buy them, make sure there is room for extra socks in cold weather.

If police stop you

The police can stop any motorist and question him – whether or not they suspect him of an offense. But they are not entitled to delay him for longer than he reasonably consents to stay, unless they make an arrest or have some other authority, such as a search warrant.

• You are not obliged to stop if you are flagged down by a civilian, even if he is a plainclothes police officer, because you have no way of knowing whether he is a policeman or a thief.

• If a uniformed policeman stops you, give your name and address when asked. If you are genuinely in a hurry – rushing to see someone seriously ill in hospital, say – explain your haste and ask to give the details later.

• If the policeman does not agree to this, though, he can insist on taking your name and address on the spot anyway.

• Motorists and motorcyclists are obliged to carry driving licenses, and insurance and registration certificates. They must produce them when police request that they do so. Bicyclists are not usually obliged to carry documents, although many local authorities require that bicycles be fitted with registration plates.

• You must obey a policeman if he asks you to move your vehicle. Otherwise you can be prosecuted for obstructing the police – regardless of whether or not you were blocking the road and regardless of whether or not you were legally parked.

• If the police are looking for a stolen car, they may ask questions about your car, such as the registration number or the make of the tires. Answer the questions as best you can – you will be helping to confirm that the car is yours.

• Be polite and cooperative, but do not answer any questions that you think might incriminate you. You are under no legal obligation to do so.

• If the police arrest you, they must give you the reason for the arrest, and they must read you your rights. Do not resist, even if you are innocent, otherwise you could be charged with resisting arrest or obstructing the police. And you could be convicted of that even if the courts find you not guilty of the charge for which you were arrested.

• Make a note of the reason you are given for the arrest – it could help your defense later – and when you reach the police station, ask to see a lawyer.

If you are asked to take a breathalyzer test

• Only a police officer can ask you to take a breathalyzer test.

• If you refuse to take the test, you can be arrested and are liable to be fined, jailed or to lose your license – regardless of whether or not you were over the limit.

• If the breath test proves positive, you will be taken to a police station for further tests, but you will not be officially arrested unless you are uncooperative.

Emergencies on the road

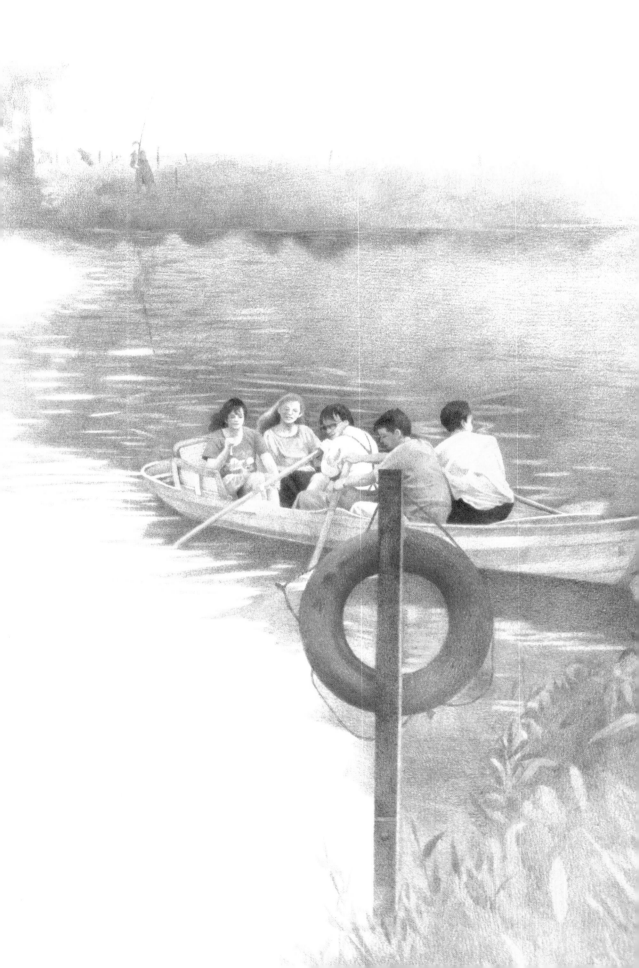

Emergencies in the water

220   If you fall into a river or lake
221   Rescuing someone from a river or lake
222   If you get into difficulties while swimming
224   Getting out of trouble in surf
226   Skin diving: what to do if things go wrong
227   Menaced by a shark
228   How to deal with a panicking swimmer
232   If you fall through thin ice
234   If someone falls through the ice
236   If you fall overboard
238   Man overboard
240   Safety for windsurfers
240   Righting a capsized dinghy
242   Avoiding collisions on the water
244   Running aground
248   Dealing with a hole or leak
250   Fire on board
252   Deciding what to do in heavy weather
254   Wind and weather
258   Caught in a storm
260   Abandoning ship
263   Safe canoeing
264   Kayak emergencies

If you fall into a river or lake

Shock and cold are the biggest hazards in North American waters. Lakes and rivers are often very cold well into summer, and cold quickly saps the strength of even a good swimmer. Concentrate your efforts on getting out as fast as possible. Deep, steady breathing will help to calm you. Keep your strokes slow and steady as you swim or tread water. Apart from these unavoidable movements, move as little as possible to slow up heat loss.

• After you fall in a river or lake, try to stand up; the water may not be very deep.

• If the water is too deep for standing and you cannot reach the bank at once, keep afloat by treading water. See if there is any floating debris at hand to cling to. If there is, use it.

• Do not remove any clothing; you need it to keep warm. Air trapped between clothing layers may also aid buoyancy. But do discard heavy shoes and anything heavy in your pockets.

• Remove rubber boots if you are wearing them – they will fill with water and weigh you down. But do not discard them. If you cannot swim, you may be able to use the boots as air cushions to help keep you afloat; turn them upside down, empty them of water and hold them under your arms.

• If you can swim, make for the nearest suitable bank. If there is a current, do not waste strength fighting it. Go with the flow and swim diagonally across it to work your way to a bank. If the river curves, head for the inside of the curve where the water is likely to be shallower and the current less powerful.

• If you cannot swim, call for help but don't tire yourself by screaming frantically. Stay calm and cooperate with anyone who is trying to rescue you. If he has swum to your aid, relax and leave him to take charge. Do not cling to a rescuer, or you may both drown.

• If the side is steep and you find it difficult to get out, look for a handhold while you choose the most likely escape point. Work toward it by edging from one handhold to another. If necessary, remain clinging to a good handhold and breathe deeply in between calls for help.

How to tread water

To keep your head above water without swimming, kick your legs as if you were cycling and continually paddle with your arms to add support and balance.

Alternatively, bring both legs up, knees outward, then push down while bringing legs together (like the breaststroke kick when swimming); or keep your legs straight and use a fast, beating movement of each leg alternately below the knee, as in the crawl stroke.

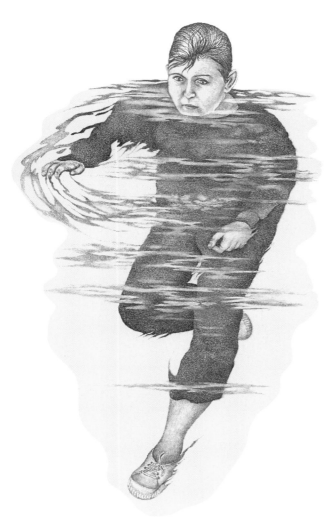

TREADING WATER
One way to stay afloat is to tread water. Pedal with your legs as if you were cycling, and scull your hands back and forth in the water. Leave your clothes on; they help to keep you warm.

AVOIDING AN ACCIDENT

Every year about 6,000 North Americans drown, mostly in rivers and lakes. Many victims did not intend going into the water – they fell in while fishing, walking, playing, boating or cycling. The Red Cross believes that nearly 75 percent of North Americans cannot swim well enough to save themselves or others.

• Be cautious when alongside water. Banks are often wet and slippery, or may crumble underfoot.

• Never disregard danger notices. Do not be overconfident because you can swim. Swimming in cold water is very different from swimming in a pool.

• Do not go fishing on your own.

Rescuing someone from a river or lake

Water-safety experts use a four-word rhyme to summarize the safest ways of getting to someone who has fallen in the water. It is: reach, throw, wade, row.

Never get into the water yourself unless there is no alternative and you are a strong swimmer. The shock of the cold water, the possibility of injury from submerged obstacles, and the risk of being pulled under by a panicking victim could put you in danger as well.

Reach
• If the person is not far from reach, give him encouragement while you find something to stretch out to him, such as a strong stick, an oar, a pole, a rope, or a piece of clothing.
• Lie on your front at the water's edge and anchor yourself in some way if possible. Hook your ankle round a post, or get someone to hold you. Tell the person in the water to grasp the stick or rope. Then haul him in steadily.

Throw
• If the person is out of reach, throw something, such as a life preserver or a child's rubber ring, to keep him afloat while you get help.

Wade
• If you decide to wade out to get nearer to the person in trouble, first test the temperature of the water and note any currents.
• Test the bottom with a stick before each step forward. There could be submerged obstacles or sudden changes of depth.

Row
• If a boat is available and you have the skill to manage it, use it to get near to the person, but take care not to get too close. Otherwise the weight of the boat may push him under, knock him out or injure him. To lessen the risk of capsizing the boat as you haul him aboard, bring him in over the stern.
• If no other method is possible and you are a good swimmer, swim out with something buoyant such as a life preserver, preferably with a line attached to the shore (see also *How to deal with a panicking swimmer*, page 228).
• Keep your clothing on to combat the cold, but discard heavy shoes and anything heavy in your pockets before you enter the water.
• Tell the person to hold on to the life preserver ring and then tow it back. But let go if he attempts to climb on it or to grab hold of you.

Getting the victim ashore
• If there is a strong current, it may be difficult to haul the person straight to the bank. Instead, move downstream and haul him diagonally across the current. If there is a bend, aim for the inside bank where the current is less powerful.
• If the side is steep, try to tow the person to something he can grasp – a chain, for example.
• Lifting a person out where the side is steep is very difficult on your own. Keep him from submerging by tying a line round him under the armpits. Explain why you are doing this; the cold and shock may have made him confused.
• Climb out of the water, holding the other end of the line; then tow him to a better landing point, or secure him while you get help.

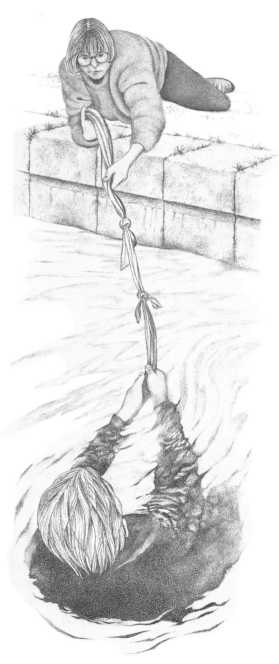

USING AN IMPROVISED ROPE
Reach from the bank using anything at hand. Tie pairs of pants, jackets, scarves or towels together to make an improvised rope.

If you get into difficulties while swimming

Cramp, exhaustion and strong currents are the commonest problems facing swimmers. Cramp and exhaustion can both be caused by cold.

If you get cramp
• Stop swimming. Turn on your back and float.
• Stretch the cramped muscle. If the cramp is at the front of your leg, point your toes and straighten the leg. If the cramp is in your calf or the back of your thigh, turn your toes upward and straighten the leg. Use your hands if necessary to pull your foot upward.
• When the cramp goes, swim to shore using a different stroke. If you must use the same stroke, keep alert in case the cramp returns.
• If the cramp in your leg continues, swim to shore slowly, using only your arms.
• If a stomach cramp occurs, stay calm – just swim slowly to shore on your back.

If you become exhausted
• Swim ashore as soon as you begin to feel cold or tired. If you are too far out, or are too exhausted to reach the shore at once, turn on your back and float to conserve your strength.
• Raise one arm, keep it straight, and move it from side to side as a distress signal.
• When someone comes to help you, relax and let him take control. Do not try to cling to him.
• If nobody comes, float until you feel better, then make for the shore.

Caught in a current
• Do not try to swim against a current.
• If you are swimming in a river, swim diagonally across it to land farther downstream. If the river bends, aim for the bank on the inside edge. The current will be at its weakest there.
• On the coast, waves piling into the beach can trap water behind offshore sandbanks. The sandbanks may be submerged at some or all stages of the tide. Gaps in the sandbanks then become outlets for the water, generating riptides which may be invisible from the beach. Riptides can flow out to sea at 4-5 mph (6-8 km/h) – impossible to swim against. But they usually dissipate within a short distance of the gap. If you are caught in a riptide, let the current take you, then strike vigorously across it parallel to the beach. Once you are free of the current, turn back toward the beach.

If you get caught in waterweeds
• Unless you are carrying a knife with which to hack away weeds, try to kick yourself free.
• If kicking fails, try to roll the weeds from your limbs as if rolling down a sock. Duck your head under the water when you do this so that you can see what you are doing.
• Once free of the weeds, swim with a shallow kick until you are clear of them.

How cold water affects a swimmer
When you plunge into cold water, the first few seconds are taken up by huge, involuntary gasps (doctors call this hyperventilation), followed by anything up to several minutes of increased blood pressure and faster heartbeats as your body responds to the shock. At this time, there is a high risk of breathing water into

---

DO'S AND DON'TS OF SAFE SWIMMING

The highest proportion of drownings in North America – more than one-third – occurs among adults aged between 15 and 35, who are often the strongest swimmers. They die usually because they have ignored the safety rules recommended by experts.
• Test the water temperature before you get in. Do not swim if it is too cold.
• Always swim in a group, not by yourself.
• Look out for warning flags or markers indicating areas that are unsafe for swimming. Be sure to check what flags and markers of different colors signify. In some areas, they denote patrolled areas, surfing areas and so on.
• Do not swim in water-filled gravel or sand pits, or in flooded quarries. They are cold and often deep with steeply shelving sides that may be impossible to climb out of. There may also be submerged obstacles.
• Never dive into water unless you are sure that the water is deep enough – at least 10 ft. (3 m) – and free from underwater hazards such as weeds, rocks or other obstacles. Climb down or wade in if you can, but if you have to jump, do so feet first.
• Swim parallel to the shore and keep within easy reach of standing depth. Unless you are a strong swimmer, do not go out of your depth at sea at all. Wade out, then swim back.
• Watch for underwater hazards. Their presence is sometimes, but not always, indicated by visible breaks in the usual pattern of waves or currents.
• Keep an eye on a shore mark so that you can see if you are being carried out to sea or along the beach. Do not swim out with a current. You may not be able to swim back.
• Do not swim in the ocean using inflatable swimming aids. You may be carried out of your depth without realizing it – and be unable to get back.

your lungs and drowning. Hyperventilation also reduces the amount of carbon dioxide in the blood, and this can lead to cramp.

Loss of body heat is very fast in water. Even with a water temperature of around 68°F (20°C), the loss can outpace the body's capacity to produce heat. The body reacts to cold-water immersion by forming a cold outer shell to insulate the inner core, and the consequent cooling of muscles and nerves in the arms, legs and outer trunk weakens movement and reduces coordination. Even a good swimmer may drown quickly under these circumstances, and in water below 50°F (10°C), swimming ability commonly fails in less than 15 minutes.

The length of time you can hold your breath underwater is also severely affected by the temperature. In cold water it is likely to be only one-third as long as in a heated swimming pool; in water below 60°F (15°C) the average time is about 15-25 seconds.

In an indoor swimming pool the water temperature is generally between 80 and 84°F (27 and 29°C). The waters off the seacoasts of the United States and the milder regions of Canada, as well as the lakes and rivers in both countries, vary greatly in temperature. But many lakes and rivers never warm up to 50°F (10°C) during the year. And even the oceans, except in semitropical regions, remain cool.

If you have to swim in cold water, it is best to get in gradually, keeping your head well above water until the initial shock is over, and to try to control your breathing consciously. Wear a wetsuit as well, if possible. It will lessen the effects of the cold on your body.

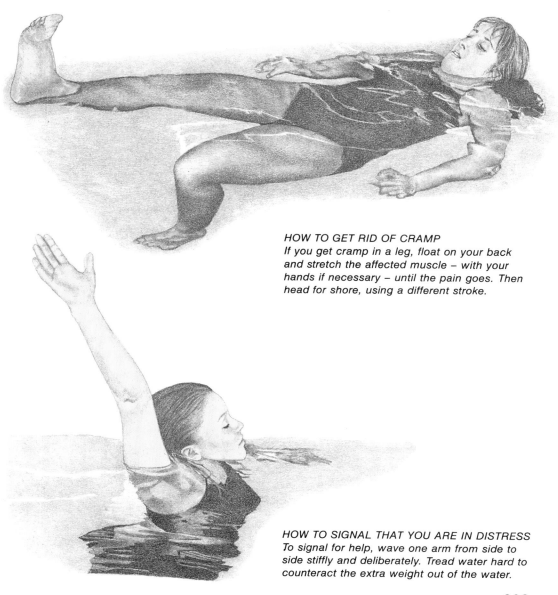

HOW TO GET RID OF CRAMP
If you get cramp in a leg, float on your back and stretch the affected muscle – with your hands if necessary – until the pain goes. Then head for shore, using a different stroke.

HOW TO SIGNAL THAT YOU ARE IN DISTRESS
To signal for help, wave one arm from side to side stiffly and deliberately. Tread water hard to counteract the extra weight out of the water.

223

Getting out of trouble in surf

The continuous pounding of heavy breakers soon saps the energy of an inexperienced swimmer, and can be hazardous even for a strong and proficient swimmer. Do not be tempted to swim in heavy surf if your swimming ability and experience do not go beyond swimming in a pool or in sheltered water.

How to swim ashore through surf
• Use the waves to get ashore. Between waves rest and wait, then swim vigorously shoreward as each wave crest approaches and keep kicking to get the maximum ride forward.
• To increase the forward motion, use a technique known as bodysurfing. Just as the wave catches you, stiffen your body. Hold your head up with chin thrust forward. Either hold your arms straight in front of your head, or back beneath your body, to make your body into a living surfboard.
• When the wave has gone past, tread water, and watch over your shoulder for the next wave.
• Once you are able to stand up, brace yourself against the strong pull of the water as it flows backward between the waves. If necessary, crouch and hold onto the bottom.

How to get out onto rocks
• Time your landing so that you go ashore just behind the crest of a wave, to avoid being hurled against the rocks.
• Quickly get a good handhold on a rock so that you are not pulled back into the water as the wave falls back.

BODYSURFING TO GET ASHORE

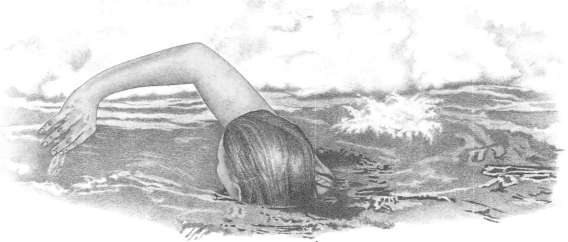

1 *To bodysurf on a wave, swim hard toward the shore as the wave crest approaches. Watch it over your shoulder as you go.*

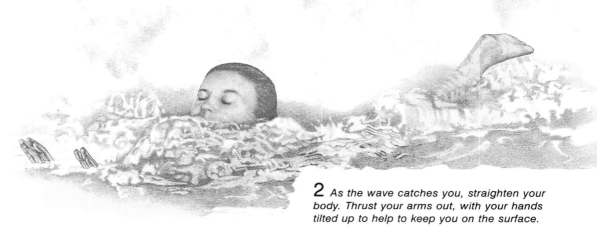

2 *As the wave catches you, straighten your body. Thrust your arms out, with your hands tilted up to help to keep you on the surface.*

- Hold on while the wave recedes.
- Scramble up the rocks as quickly as you can before the next wave reaches you.

How to cope with turbulent breakers
Waves become turbulent and thus difficult to swim through only after they get close to the shore and break. Before then, the easiest way to swim seaward past a wave – or to hold your position while the wave passes you – is to jump, float or swim over its crest.

Once the wave has broken, however, the water forms a turbulent tube, rolling over and over as it foams toward the beach.

Any swimmer caught in this turbulence can be tumbled helplessly, losing his sense of up and down, being unable to breathe, and risking – in shallow water – being hurled against the bottom and stunned.

A wave's turbulence usually affects only the upper layers of the water. So a swimmer who wants to get past the wave without being caught in the turbulence needs to get below it.

- As the wave approaches, dive well below the surface. The heavier the surf, the deeper you will need to dive.
- If necessary, dive right to the seabed and hold on by digging your hands into the sand while the wave passes overhead. It is often possible to feel the turbulent water skim your back as it passes.
- When the wave has gone by, gather your legs beneath you and push back to the surface. Watch for the next wave as soon as you emerge.

SWIMMING OUT THROUGH LARGE WAVES

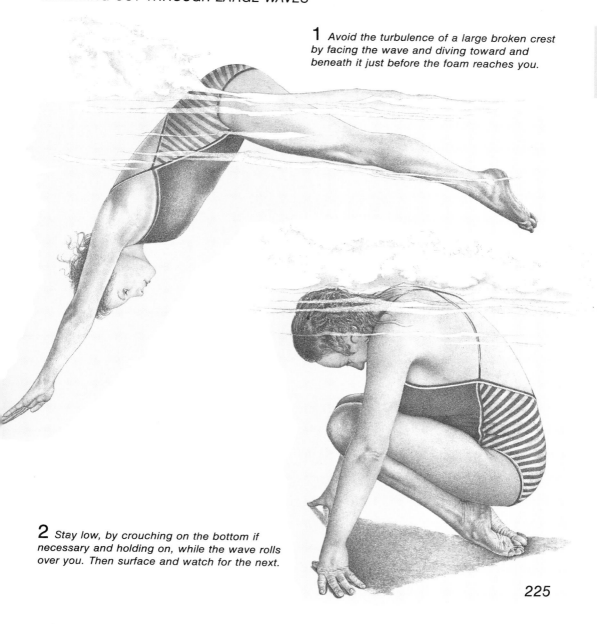

1 *Avoid the turbulence of a large broken crest by facing the wave and diving toward and beneath it just before the foam reaches you.*

2 *Stay low, by crouching on the bottom if necessary and holding on, while the wave rolls over you. Then surface and watch for the next.*

225

Skin diving: what to do if things go wrong

With a face mask, a snorkel (breathing tube) and a pair of fins, a swimmer can breathe just below the surface of the water and so watch the underwater world without interruption. But difficulties can arise, particularly in open water. All need prompt, calm action.

If water fills the snorkel

An unexpected wave or a careless dip of the head can send water down the snorkel without warning.

• If this happens, do not breathe in. Make sure that the end of the snorkel is above water.

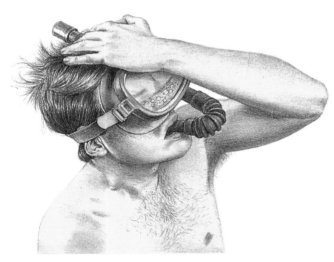

HOW TO CLEAR THE MASK UNDERWATER
Tilt your head back, hold the top of the mask and breathe out slowly through your nose. The air will force the water out of the bottom.

• Tilt your head up so that water can flow more easily from the snorkel.
• Blow out forcefully to expel the water.

If water leaks into the mask

• On the surface, one easy way to clear water from a mask is to lift your head above the water and pull the mask away from your face with your hands to drain it. Tread water with your legs while you do this.
• To clear the mask while you are still below the surface – during a dive, say – tilt your head well back until you are looking upward toward the surface.
• Press the top of the mask firmly against your forehead.
• Breathe out slowly through your nose. This will fill the mask with air and force water out of the bottom. Stop breathing out as soon as the mask is clear, to retain the maximum amount of air in your lungs.

How good a swimmer you need to be

Because of the extra swimming ability needed to go snorkeling in safety, experts recommend that no one should take up the sport until he or she can:

• Swim 220 yd. (200 m) freestyle (except backstroke) without a stop.
• Swim 110 yd. (100 m) backstroke.
• Swim 55 yd. (50 m) freestyle wearing a 10 lb. (4.5 kg) weight belt.
• Float on his back for five minutes, using hands and legs if desired.
• Tread water with his hands above water and using legs alone for one minute.
• Recover six objects in succession from the deep end of a swimming pool with only one dive for each object.

CHOOSING THE RIGHT EQUIPMENT

• Before buying masks and fins, borrow or rent several models for testing. Masks and fins that are comfortable on land may not be so underwater.
• The best snorkel is a simple J shape. It should be less than 18 in. (45 cm) in length; otherwise it will be hard to breathe through.
• The snorkel should be separate from the mask. A built-in snorkel is dangerous because it can let water into the mask. It is also difficult to clear.
• Make sure that the snorkel's mouthpiece fits comfortably under your lips and between your teeth.
• Do not buy a snorkel with air valves – these often look like ping-pong balls. If a valve jams, it can cut off the air supply.

• The mask should be fitted with shatterproof safety glass – not plastic, which can scratch and mist up easily.
• The mask should cover nose and eyes only and should have a shaped nosepiece. It allows you to hold your nose through the mask, if necessary.
• Test that the mask fits by holding it against your face without putting on the straps. Breathe in through your nose. A well-fitting mask will stick to your face.
• Buy well-fitting fins, whether they have full foot pockets or open-heel straps.
• If you plan to snorkel in places where there could be weeds underwater, buy a diver's knife with a serrated edge (see *If you get into difficulties while swimming,* page 222).

Menaced by a shark

Each year there are about 30 shark attacks on humans around the world. Most of the attacks take place in tropical waters. But most victims survive; only three or four die.

Two of the largest species of shark – the basking shark, which grows as long as 45 ft. (14 m), and the gigantic whale shark, reputed to reach up to 60 ft. (18 m) – are harmless plankton-feeders. All other shark species, however – and there are some 250 of them around the world – should be treated as dangerous.

If you see a shark near someone else
• Call a warning to anyone in the water if you spot a shark nearby.
• Make a noise – it may frighten the shark away. If you are in a boat, start the engine or bang on the hull.
• Help those in the water to get ashore or aboard a boat as quickly as possible.

If you are in the water
• Do not try to swim away fast if a shark approaches you. You cannot outswim a shark, and the frantic movement may simply add to the danger by attracting its attention.
• If you are spearfishing, release at once any fish you have speared. Blood in the water tends to attract sharks.
• Make a noise in an attempt to frighten the shark away. Shout into the water, for example, or beat on diving tanks if you have them.
• Swim slowly back to the boat or to the shore. Swim backward if necessary. Keep facing the shark all the time as you go, preferably underwater, to reduce the chances of being attacked from beneath or behind.
• A shark attack is often preceded by a nudge. If this happens, strike the shark as hard as you can with your fists, feet or any object at hand in order to startle it and drive it off.

LESSENING THE CHANCES OF AN ATTACK

Along most of North America's coasts there is little danger of swimmers or skin divers being attacked by sharks. Most attacks occur in the warm coastal waters of California and Florida. Sharks are unpredictable, and there is no way of telling when they will, or will not, attack. Nevertheless, shark experts do recommend some ways of reducing the risk of an attack.
• In areas where there may be sharks, avoid murky water; sharks seem adept at detecting prey in such conditions.
• Do not swim too far from shore or near deep channels. Sharks rarely swim into water that is shallow enough for a man to wade in.
• Do not swim at dusk or at night, when sharks are more likely to be looking for food.
• Do not swim or skin-dive alone. Having another person close by helps you to keep an all-round lookout, and may deter a shark.
• Do not go into the water if you have a cut or scratch. Blood may attract a shark.
• Do not carry captured fish if you are spearfishing. Put them in a boat.
• Where there are known to be sharks, make and carry what the French oceanographer Jacques-Yves Cousteau calls a shark billy – a stout stick about as thick as a broom handle and 3 ft. (1 m) long, with a loop for the wrist at one end and a circle of small nails, points outward, at the other end.
• Jab the billy firmly into the snout of any shark that comes within reach. The nail points prevent the stick sliding off the shark's skin and help to keep it away from your body without wounding or angering it. A shark

billy rarely drives a shark off completely, however; it only keeps it at bay.
• If you see sharks in the area where you are swimming or diving and you are close to shore or a boat, leave the water quickly.
• But remember that you are in most danger as you leave the water. For this reason, try to time your exit so that any shark is well out of striking range when you climb out.
• Clothing or a diver's wet suit appears to give some protection from sharks. A naked person seems to be more liable to attack than a clothed one.
• Be careful if you have a partial suntan, with white areas exposed while swimming. Areas of light and shade also seem to attract sharks and make an attack more likely.

Other dangerous marine animals
Barracuda make direct attacks on swimmers, and their bite is deep and serious. They bask in the waters off the West Indies, Florida and Hawaii. If one appears, do not try to scare it off. Leave the water quickly.

The moray eel – "the rattlesnake of the deep" – has a poisonous bite. It inhabits tropical and semi-tropical waters, but some are found as far north as New Jersey. It is best not to poke about the underwater holes and crevices that it inhabits.

Jellyfish can inflict painful stings with their long threadlike tentacles. If you are stung, remove as much of the tentacle as possible. Wash the stung area with sea water, or rub it gently with sand. Rinse with fresh water. See a doctor at once.

How to deal with a panicking swimmer

A person in difficulties in the water is often panic-stricken and will cling with the strength of desperation to anything that offers a safe hold – including someone trying to help him. Never swim to the aid of a swimmer in distress if there is any other way of reaching him – from the shore, say, or from a boat (see *Rescuing someone from a river or lake*, page 221).

Even trained lifesavers are taught to go into the water only as a last resort. An untrained rescuer runs a still greater risk of losing his own life in the attempt to save another's.

• If you decide that you have to swim to the rescue, try to stay out of the swimmer's reach. If, however, you need to get close to him – because he does not respond to your instructions, say – and he suddenly tries to grab you,

avoid his grasp by reversing immediately into backstroke and swimming vigorously out of his reach.

• Once at a safe distance, offer him one end of a piece of clothing, a towel or one side of a life preserver ring and tell him to hold on to that. Tow him to the shore by holding the other end.

• If he tries to pull himself toward you, let go of your end and swim out of his reach.

• If you have no choice but to make contact with the swimmer, approach him from behind.

• Grasp him firmly and support him in the water. Calm him down by talking, and tow him to shore using one of the techniques shown on the pages overleaf.

• Keep an eye on him as you swim and keep talking, if you can, to calm him.

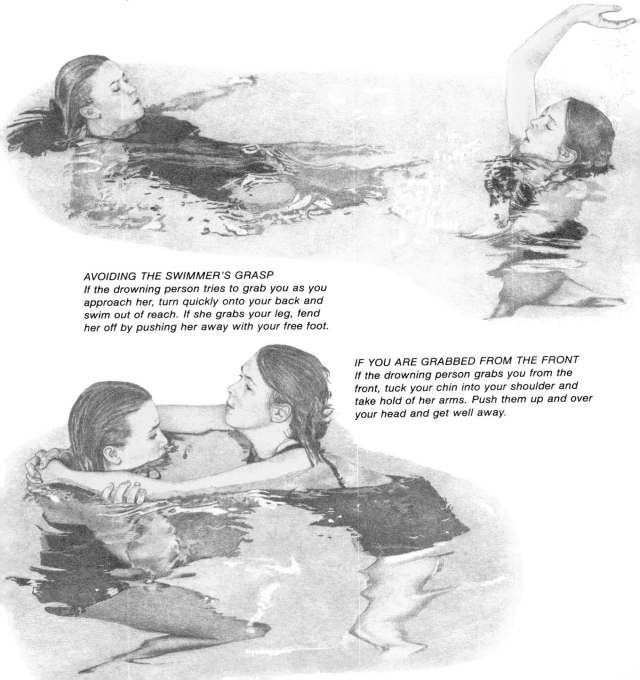

AVOIDING THE SWIMMER'S GRASP
If the drowning person tries to grab you as you approach her, turn quickly onto your back and swim out of reach. If she grabs your leg, fend her off by pushing her away with your free foot.

IF YOU ARE GRABBED FROM THE FRONT
If the drowning person grabs you from the front, tuck your chin into your shoulder and take hold of her arms. Push them up and over your head and get well away.

Breaking a hold

- If a panicking swimmer grabs you, break free at once. If he grasps your leg, push it down into the water and thrust against his shoulder with your free foot.
- If he clutches you from the front round your head and shoulders, tuck your chin down into your shoulder, grasp him under the arms and push him up and away.
- If he grasps you from behind round your head and shoulders, lower your chin to protect your throat. Then grasp him by the wrist of his uppermost arm and pull down, at the same time pushing up his elbow with your other hand. In this way you both break his clutch and keep hold of him.
- As a last resort, take a deep breath and allow yourself to be pushed underwater. The aim of most panicking swimmers is to stay on the surface. Swim downward until he lets go, then return to the surface out of his reach and grab him from behind.

Helping an unconscious or panicky person

- Tow an unconscious person by the chin from behind. Use a sidestroke and keep your towing arm straight so that your legs are clear of the victim and you can look forward regularly to see where you are going. Make sure you keep his face out of the water.
- If he is conscious but panic-stricken and needs firm control, grasp him under the chin, draw him close (ear to ear) and clamp his shoulder firmly with your elbow. If necessary,

IF YOU ARE GRABBED FROM BEHIND

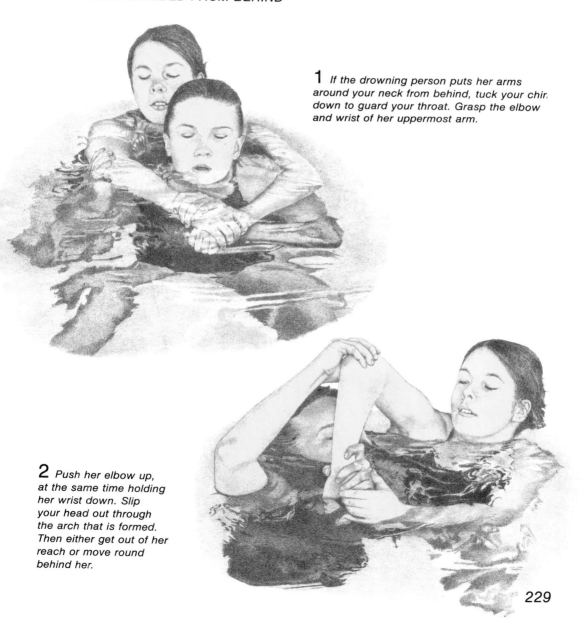

1 *If the drowning person puts her arms around your neck from behind, tuck your chin down to guard your throat. Grasp the elbow and wrist of her uppermost arm.*

2 *Push her elbow up, at the same time holding her wrist down. Slip your head out through the arch that is formed. Then either get out of her reach or move round behind her.*

restrain him with your other arm as well. Tell him to stop struggling. Keep talking to him to try to keep him calm while you swim.

• In rough water, it is better to tow the person by holding him across the chest. This enables you to swim on your side, breathe more easily, and see where you are going.

Helping a swimmer with cramp

• Support him in the water while he tries to relieve the cramp by stretching the muscles.
• If the cramp does not go, tell him to lie on his back and tow him ashore using one of the life-saving techniques shown here.
• Once ashore, wrap him in a coat, towel or blanket. Stretch the affected muscle gently and massage it to relieve the cramp.

SAFETY FIRST

The central rules for a rescuer – recommended by the Red Cross Society – are to stay out of the water if you can, and to avoid making direct physical contact with the victim if you can.

Only senior-level swimmers and people trained in lifesaving should attempt a rescue. Specialized training is available from local swimming clubs and community centers, the YMCA and YWCA, and the Red Cross Society.

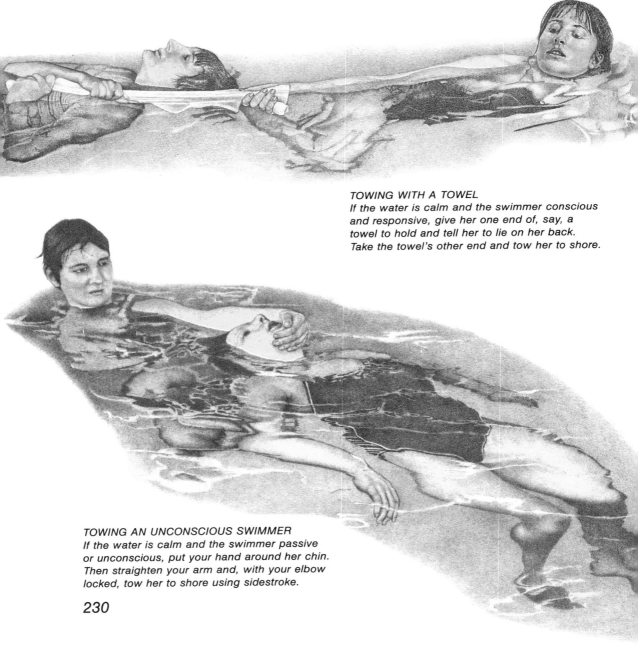

TOWING WITH A TOWEL
If the water is calm and the swimmer conscious and responsive, give her one end of, say, a towel to hold and tell her to lie on her back. Take the towel's other end and tow her to shore.

TOWING AN UNCONSCIOUS SWIMMER
If the water is calm and the swimmer passive or unconscious, put your hand around her chin. Then straighten your arm and, with your elbow locked, tow her to shore using sidestroke.

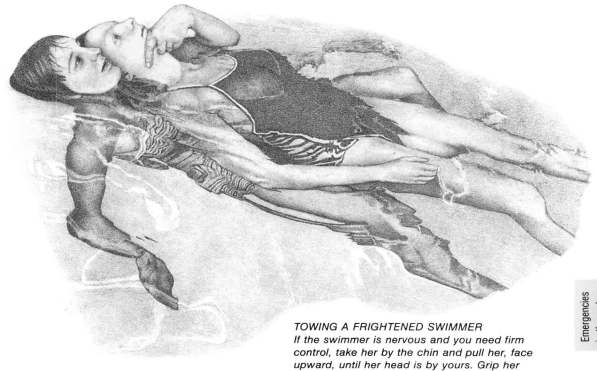

TOWING A FRIGHTENED SWIMMER
*If the swimmer is nervous and you need firm
control, take her by the chin and pull her, face
upward, until her head is by yours. Grip her
shoulder with your elbow and make for shore.*

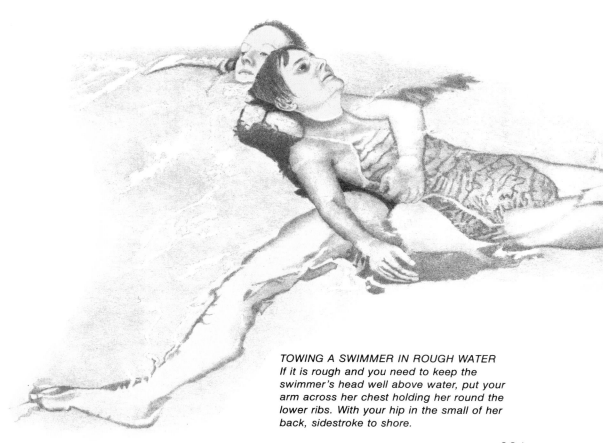

TOWING A SWIMMER IN ROUGH WATER
*If it is rough and you need to keep the
swimmer's head well above water, put your
arm across her chest holding her round the
lower ribs. With your hip in the small of her
back, sidestroke to shore.*

231

If you fall through thin ice

Every winter, rivers and lakes in Canada and the northern parts of the United States freeze solidly enough to be used safely as skating rinks. But year after year, tragedies occur because people venture onto ice while it is too thin – either at freeze-up or during spring thaw.

The biggest danger for anyone who goes onto a frozen patch of water is not an inability to swim; clothes contain enough air, initially at least, to help to keep afloat anyone who falls in. The biggest peril is the shock of the cold water, which can paralyze the muscles and render even the strongest of swimmers helpless in a matter of a few minutes.

• Do not wait to be rescued. Get yourself out of the icy water if you can. Cold will quickly sap your strength.

• Keep afloat by treading water – kick your legs as if you were cycling and continually paddle with your arms. Breathe deeply and slowly. It helps to prevent panic.

• Break the ice around you – moving generally toward the bank – until you find some that seems strong enough to hold you.

• Extend your arms forward onto the stronger ice and kick your legs behind you to bring your body up so that it is almost level.

• Keep kicking to drive your body forward, and pull at the same time until you are out of the water. If the ice cracks under you, keep flat and keep edging forward.

• When you reach ice that is firm enough to take your weight, roll away from the broken area toward the bank.

• Once safely on firm ground make for shelter and warmth. Keep moving to stay warm. If dry clothes are available, put them on. Otherwise, keep your wet clothes on until you reach somewhere warm.

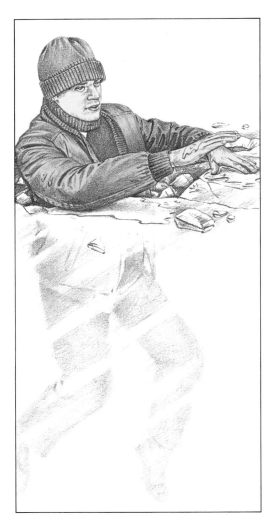

TREADING WATER TO KEEP AFLOAT
If you cannot get out at once, tread water to keep your head and neck out of the water, and to stop yourself getting trapped under the ice.

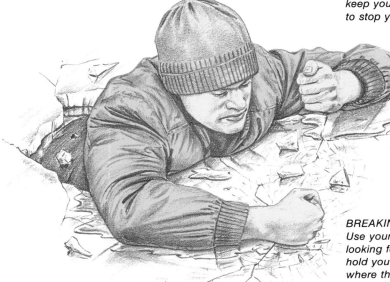

BREAKING THE ICE
Use your fists to smash the ice around you, looking for areas that are strong enough to hold you. Move generally toward the shore, where the ice is likely to be thicker.

EDGING YOUR WAY TO SAFETY

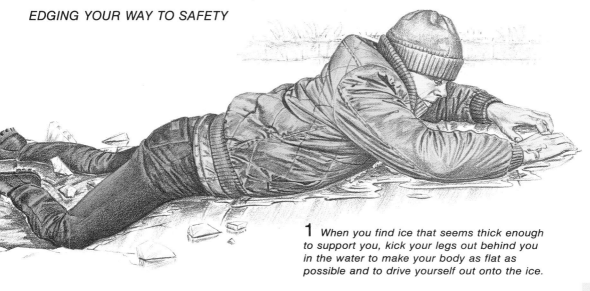

1 *When you find ice that seems thick enough to support you, kick your legs out behind you in the water to make your body as flat as possible and to drive yourself out onto the ice.*

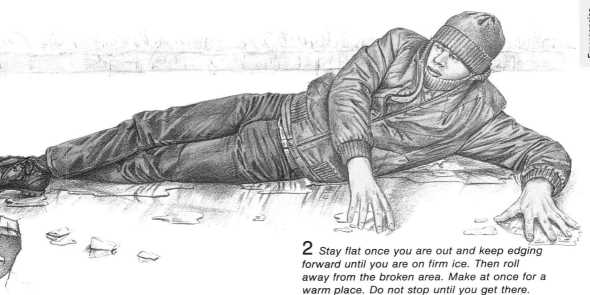

2 *Stay flat once you are out and keep edging forward until you are on firm ice. Then roll away from the broken area. Make at once for a warm place. Do not stop until you get there.*

DANGER – THIN ICE

• Never venture onto ice without first testing its strength. Find a firm handhold on the bank while you stamp with one foot at the edge in several places. Throw the largest stone you can find into the middle of the water area.

• Ice over shallow water is usually the safest. Ice over flowing water or underwater vegetation is weaker because the water is relatively warmer.

• Ice is not uniformly thick over a whole stretch of water. It gets thinner toward the center. Ice also weakens as the sun's warmth builds up during the morning and early afternoon, and if the weather gets warmer.

• Never allow children onto ice without the supervision of a responsible adult. Do not allow a child onto any ice if the water below is deeper than the height of the child's waist.

• Make sure that rescue equipment is available – a light ladder, a strong rope, or a pole with a looped line attached. Take it with you if necessary.

If someone falls through the ice

A person who falls through ice into a pond or river – even someone who is ordinarily a competent swimmer – can drown within minutes. Even if the person can keep his head above water, the shock affects breathing and the cold can paralyze the limbs (see *Drowning – the perils of the cold*, page 239). For rescuers, therefore, the priority is speed.

Helping a conscious victim

• Stay off the ice yourself unless there is no other way of reaching the victim and there is someone else to pull you back if you fall in.

• Slide a stick, with a rope attached, across the ice toward the victim. If necessary, make a rope from sweaters or scarves.

• If you cannot reach the victim from the shore, lie flat on the ice so that your weight is widely distributed.

• Slide forward cautiously, pushing the stick in front of you, until it is within the victim's reach. Do not go any farther than absolutely necessary. Ice generally gets thinner toward the center of a river or pond.

• Tell the victim to stretch her arms forward on top of the ice and kick back to keep her body as level in the water as possible. This will lessen the chance of her being pulled under the ice by any current, and make it easier for her to get out onto the ice.

• Tell her to grasp the stick or rope with one hand and break the ice in front with the other until the ice is strong enough to support her. Pull on the other end to help her haul herself out of the water.

• Tell her to kick her legs as if she were swimming and to slide forward onto the ice. Do not hold her directly or let her hold you, unless you are well anchored. Otherwise she could pull you into the water.

• Once she is on the ice, tell her to lie flat. Pull her in.

• Another way to help a conscious victim is to stretch a rope from bank to bank – of a pond, say – across the spot where he or she has fallen in. Tell her to grab hold of the rope and haul herself in, hand over hand.

Forming a human chain

• If there are several people to help and there is no other way to reach the victim, form a human chain.

• The first person should lie flat on the ice and slide toward the victim. The next should lie flat

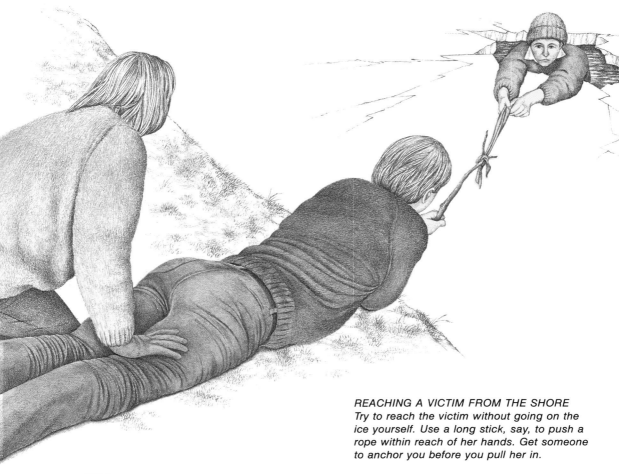

REACHING A VICTIM FROM THE SHORE
Try to reach the victim without going on the ice yourself. Use a long stick, say, to push a rope within reach of her hands. Get someone to anchor you before you pull her in.

and hold the ankles of the person in front, and so on until the chain is long enough to reach from a safe position on shore to the victim.

Using a ladder on ice
• The easiest way to rescue somebody who has fallen through ice is by using a light ladder.
• Lie on the ice with the ladder flat in front of you and push it toward the victim.
• Tell the victim to pull herself onto the ladder and lie flat. Pull the ladder back.

If the victim is too weak to hold on to a rope
• To help a weakening victim, attach a looped rope to the end of a pole or light ladder.
• Slide the pole across the ice until the loop is within reach of the person in the water. Tell her to put the loop over her head and shoulders and under her arms. Then pull her in.
• If you cannot pull her in, tie the other end of the rope to a tree or post on the bank to support her in the water while you get help.
• If you have no rope or pole, slide over the ice at full length, grab the victim's arms or clothing and try to pull her out onto the ice.
• If this is impossible, hold her so that she does not slip beneath the water. Shout for help.

Once back on shore
• As soon as the victim is out of danger, check that she is breathing. If not, begin artificial respiration at once (see page 50).
• If the victim is breathing, wrap dry clothes or blankets over her own wet clothes and move her to a warm sheltered place. If she is unconscious, put her in the recovery position (see page 136) and move her on a stretcher.
• Once in shelter, take off her wet clothes and wrap her in any dry clothes, blankets or a sleeping bag (see *Hypothermia*, page 108).

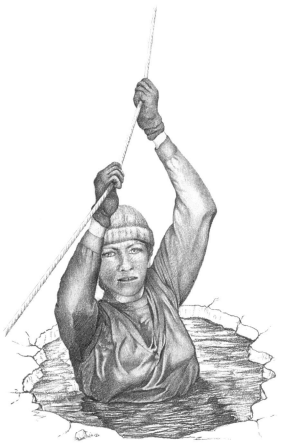

HAULING ON A ROPE OVERHEAD
On a narrow stretch of ice, hang a rope from bank to bank. Tell the victim to haul herself hand over hand to the bank, if necessary breaking the ice with her feet as she goes.

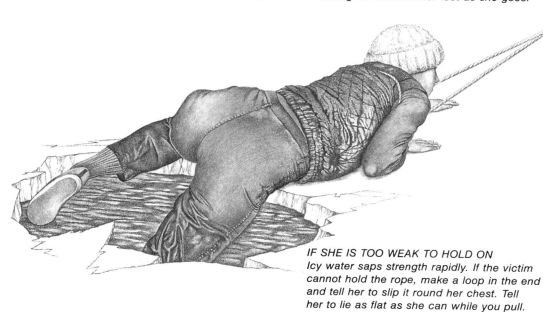

IF SHE IS TOO WEAK TO HOLD ON
Icy water saps strength rapidly. If the victim cannot hold the rope, make a loop in the end and tell her to slip it round her chest. Tell her to lie as flat as she can while you pull.

Emergencies in the water

If you fall overboard

Falling into water unexpectedly can cause shock (see page 120). Cold water also saps the strength quickly, leading to loss of coordination, confusion and exhaustion.

• Call out to alert other crew members as soon as you feel yourself start to fall.

• Once in the water, inflate your life jacket (unless it is a permanently buoyant type). It will automatically bring you back to the surface.

• If you are wearing a life jacket, keep warm by adopting a fetal position with your knees drawn up to your chest (see picture, page 262).

• Raise one arm so that you can be seen from the boat more easily. Even though you may well lose sight of the boat before it turns – particularly in rough water or at sea – other crew members will be able to pinpoint your position more easily by your arm.

• If you are not wearing a life jacket, remove heavy boots or shoes and any heavy objects from your pockets, but do not remove clothing, especially in cold water. Even soaked through, it will help to conserve vital body heat.

• Tread water if necessary to stay afloat, but otherwise conserve heat by moving as little as possible. Float on your back if you can.

• Do not try to swim after the boat whether or not you are wearing a life jacket. You will make little progress wearing clothes, and the effort will quickly exhaust you.

Ways of keeping afloat without a life jacket

• In cold water, continue to float on your back if you can, or tread water while you are waiting for the boat to return. Breathe slowly and move as little as possible; both will help to conserve energy and body heat.

• In warm water, use the drownproofing technique (see box, opposite).

• Alternatively, in warm water use a piece of clothing to construct a makeshift float. Remove pants or slacks and knot each ankle. Hold the waistband open behind your head, the legs pointing away from you, then whip the pants over your head into the water in front of you. Air will be trapped in the pant legs.

• Pull the waistband down against your chest, and float in the crotch, with the legs under your arms like a child's water wings.

• A polo-neck sweater can be used in much the same way. Remove it by bunching it up under your arms, then pulling it over your head in one movement.

• Knot the neck and both wrists, and flick it over your head to fill it with air. Hold the sweater open waist-down underwater with the sleeves under your arms and the knotted neck against your chest.

Getting into a life preserver ring

• If someone on board throws you a life preserver ring, do not duck dive and try to come up inside it. Putting your head underwater will only make you colder and tire you more quickly. Instead, stay on the surface.

• Grasp the life preserver, bend your head and lift its near edge over your head and one arm.

• Work your other arm through the life preserver so that it supports you under both armpits and across your chest.

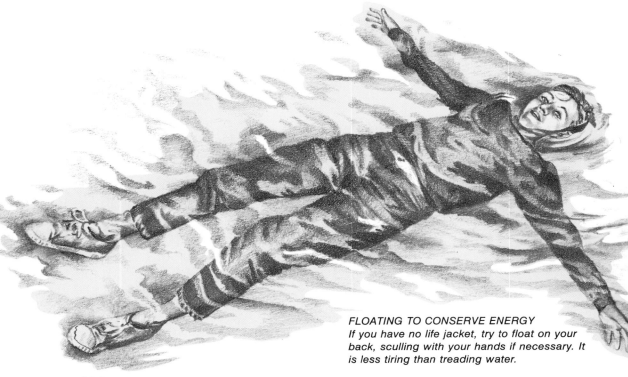

FLOATING TO CONSERVE ENERGY
If you have no life jacket, try to float on your back, sculling with your hands if necessary. It is less tiring than treading water.

HOW TO IMPROVISE A FLOAT

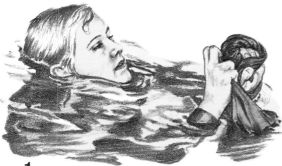

1 *Clothing can be used to make an improvised float. To make one out of a pair of pants, take them off and tie a knot in each ankle.*

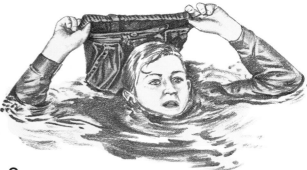

2 *Hold the pants behind your head with the waistband open, then whip them forward and down so that you trap air in the trouser legs.*

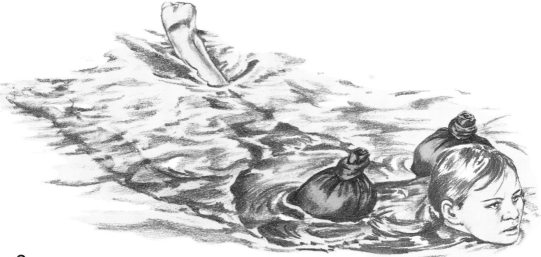

3 *Tuck the legs under your arms and float in the crotch of the pants. Air will probably leak out slowly through the fabric, so repeat the* *process as necessary. Use this technique only in warm water. In cold water, keep your clothes on to help to conserve your body heat.*

Emergencies in the water

DROWNPROOFING – A TECHNIQUE FOR SURVIVAL

In warm water – 86°F (30°C) or above – one of the easiest ways to stay afloat for an extended period without a life jacket is to use a technique known as drownproofing.
• Take a deep breath, relax, and hang in the water with your face under the surface and arms forward – as if lying over a barrel.
• To breathe again, breathe out underwater, pull down with your arms and lift your head until your mouth is just clear of the water.
• Take a deep breath, and continue alternately relaxing and breathing.

In warm water, this technique allows a swimmer to stay afloat with very little effort for hours, or even days. It works because the totally submerged human body with a lungful of air is slightly lighter than the same volume of water – and so will float naturally. Keeping part of the body constantly above the surface requires more effort and is more tiring.

Drownproofing should not be used in cold water – in northern lakes, rivers, or streams, for example – because immersing the head speeds up the rate at which the body loses heat. It is better in cold water to float on your back, using the hands if necessary, or to tread water slowly, so that your face and most of your head stays out of the water.

Man overboard

When someone falls overboard from a motor-boat or sailing dinghy, the priorities for action can be summed up in eight words: turn; shout; throw; watch; and approach to leeward.

• Start turning the boat as soon as you notice the accident.

• If there are other crew aboard, shout: "Man overboard."

• Throw a life preserver ring, or anything else that will float, to the person in the water. Make allowance for the wind when you throw.

• Keep watching the person in the water, or get someone else aboard to do so. If you lose sight of him, especially in rough water or at sea, it may be difficult to find him again.

• Steer the boat so that you approach from downwind of him. That way, there will be no danger of the boat being blown over him.

• Slacken any wire or rope guardrails around the deck so that they do not make it more difficult to get the person back on board.

• On a sailing dinghy, turn the boat into the wind as you come alongside and let the sails flap so that the boat stops. On a motorboat, stop the engine, unless the water is extremely rough.

• Before starting a rescue, put on a life jacket in case you are dragged overboard.

• Help the person in. In calm water, lift him over the stern (stop any propeller first). In rough water, though, bring him in over the side. Otherwise the drag of his body on the stern may swing the boat broadside to the wind and waves, and could cause a capsize.

• If pulling the person aboard by hand is impossible, tie a bowline in a piece of rope and put the loop over his head and under his arms.

• Get another crew member to hold the person while you tie the knot, both to keep his head above water and to stop him floating away.

• Hoist him aboard. If necessary, attach the rope to a halyard (the tackle used for hoisting the sails) to give yourself extra leverage.

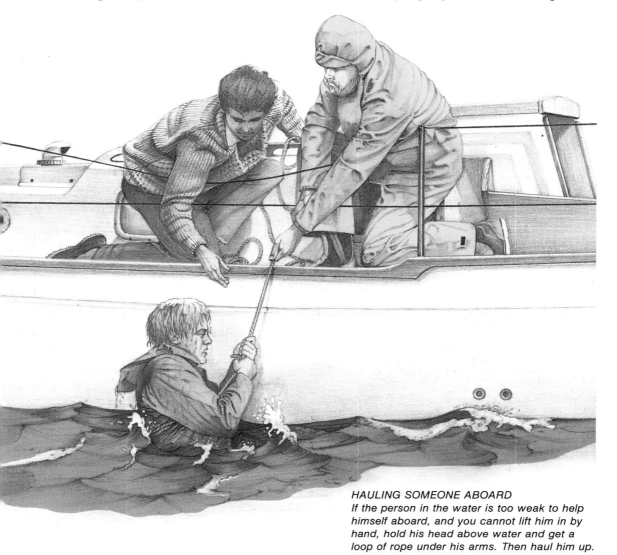

HAULING SOMEONE ABOARD
If the person in the water is too weak to help himself aboard, and you cannot lift him in by hand, hold his head above water and get a loop of rope under his arms. Then haul him up.

HOW TO MAKE A BOWLINE KNOT

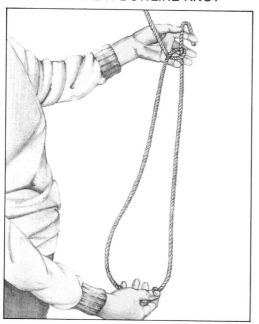

1 *To make a rope loop which will not slip, twist a small ring in the rope about 4 ft. (1.2 m) from one end, and pass the end through it.*

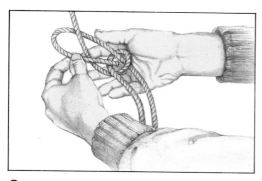

2 *Take the end round behind the rope and slip it back through the same ring.*

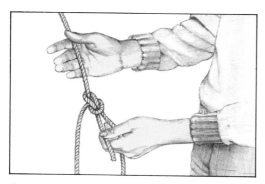

3 *Pull the rope tight to form the completed bowline knot.*

DROWNING – THE PERILS OF THE COLD

Nearly 6,000 people drown in North America each year, and many of them die not because they cannot swim, but because of the cold.

Studies by Dr. John Hayward at the University of Victoria in British Columbia show that a person submerged in cold water loses the ability to hold his breath. In a series of tests Dr. Hayward instructed volunteers to jump fully clothed into a tank of water of varying temperatures and to stay under as long as possible. Those submerged in freezing water could not hold their breath, and surfaced quickly. This result helps to explain why people in cold, deep or turbulent waters often drown before they can surface.

Dr. Hayward found that a person with his head just above the cold water breathes rapidly and may take water into his lungs. A person who is in cold water too long may lose mental and physical control. But if he tries to breathe slowly, normal breathing will return within minutes.

Dr. Hayward and others suggest that if you fall into cold water and decide that you can reach shore safely, you should not start swimming until your breathing is under control. If you are wearing a life jacket, hug your knees in a posture known as HELP while you wait for rescue (see picture, page 262).

When cold water can be a lifesaver

At swimming pool temperatures, a swimmer will die after seven minutes underwater. He will become unconscious long before that, but he can be revived with mouth-to-mouth resuscitation. At very low temperatures, however, he can survive longer, even if he appears to be dead.

Early in 1984, a four-year-old Chicago boy named Jimmy Tontlewicz was under ice for 20 minutes in Lake Michigan, before he was pulled out by divers. The rescuers thought he was dead, but doctors at a nearby hospital were able to revive him. The boy lived because the icy water had lowered his body temperature to less than 86°F (30°C) – 12.6°F (7°C) lower than normal – slowing his metabolism and reducing his brain's need for oxygen.

The message for rescuers is clear, doctors believe. Keep trying to resuscitate a drowning victim until medical help arrives. Even when all apparent signs of life have ended, the effort could save his life.

Emergencies in the water

239

Safety for windsurfers

The fast-growing sport of windsurfing – also called board sailing – has its dangers as well as its thrills. But following a few commonsense rules should keep you or get you out of trouble.
• Wear a life jacket or flotation device and, on all but the hottest days, a wet suit or dry suit.
• Do not windsurf at dusk, at night, or when visibility is poor. Never put out to sea in an offshore wind (one blowing away from the beach). The land and any buildings act as a windbreak, and by the time you feel the wind's true strength, it may be too late to get back to shore safely.
• Do not windsurf in places where there are no other people about. But do keep clear of others using the water.
• Carry a towline, in case you need to be pulled back to shore. Tie the sail rig to the board, so that you will not lose it if the foot of the mast jumps out of its housing.
• Always swim toward the board if you fall off, and stay with it if you get into trouble. If you start feeling tired, or the weather is too much for you, head for shore before you get exhausted and while you still have some energy.

What to do if you get into trouble
There are two recognized ways for a windsurfer in trouble to signal for help. Whichever you use, first lower the mast and the sail into the water.
• Kneel on the board and raise both arms above your head as if in surrender; then let your arms drop and lift them again.
• Alternatively, stand on the board. Hold on with one hand to the uphaul line (used to pull the mast up) for stability. Wave the other arm stiffly and vigorously from down by your side to above your head, and back. Some windsurfers carry a small red flag, or a red cloth, strapped to the ankle, to make the SOS message plain. Distress flares can be carried, too.
• If you are out of sight of possible rescuers and unable to sail back to shore, lower the mast and sail into the water and sit astride the board.
• Remove the foot of the mast from its housing. Hold the outer end of the wishbone – the end of the boom away from the mast – and lay the mast alongside the board in the water. Untie the sail from the wishbone and swing the wishbone up to the top of the mast.
• Roll the sail tightly toward the mast, removing the battens as you come to them and folding them into the sail.
• Lash the rolled-up sail and wishbone to the mast with the uphaul line and lay them lengthwise on the board. Tie them to the board, too.
• Lie face down on the board, with your shoulders across a narrow section near the front, and paddle back to shore.
• If the wind, tide or current is against you, aim diagonally across it, not directly into it.
• If the sail rig gets seriously in your way as you paddle, roll it overboard and abandon it; it is not worth risking your life for.

Righting a capsized dingh

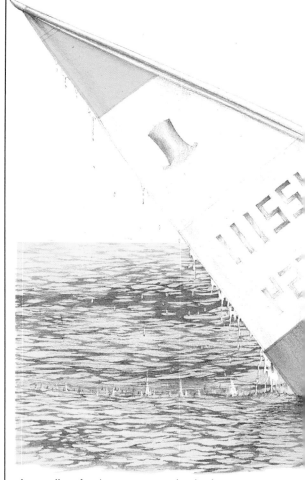

A squall, a freak wave or a mistake in maneuvering can tip a small dinghy over with little warning, throwing the crew into the water. Whatever the cause, the action to take is the same. The techniques described here are not difficult, but they do need some practice. Try them out several times by capsizing a boat deliberately in calm water close to the shore.
• Get clear of any entangling ropes or sails, and make sure that any other crew members are clear too.
• If the hull turns completely upside down, trapping you underneath, take a deep breath in the air space that will be left under the hull, then swim out underwater.
• Do not leave the boat, even if you cannot get it back upright. It will stay afloat indefinitely, and rescuers will be able to spot the hull more easily than they will see a swimmer.
• If the boat is completely upside down, a partial vacuum will be formed under the hull, sucking the boat against the water surface and making it difficult to turn onto its side. Pull down or climb onto one corner of the stern to break the vacuum, then roll the boat onto its side.
• Free the sheets – the ropes used to set the angle of the sails – so that the sails can swing

GETTING BACK ON BOARD
A practiced sailor can step straight back in
over the side of the boat as his weight on the
centerboard pulls the hull upright. For an
inexperienced sailor – especially in strong
winds – it is usually safer to drop back into the
water without letting go as the boat comes up,
then to climb aboard over the stern.

freely. Otherwise the wind will fill them as the boat comes upright, and may tip it over again.
• Check that the rudder and tiller are secure and not tangled in the ropes.
• Make sure that the centerboard is fully down, then climb onto it, keeping your feet close to the hull to avoid breaking the centerboard off.
• If it is difficult to get onto the board, ask a crew member to throw one of the jib (front sail) sheets over the hull, and use the rope to pull yourself up.
• Once on the board, hold the side of the boat – the gunwale – or the jib sheet, and lean back, pressing with your feet against the centerboard. Your weight should pull the boat back upright.
• An agile sailor can climb in over the side directly from the centerboard as the boat rolls upright, but there is a risk that he could pull the boat over again on top of him, unless there is someone else in the boat to balance it. If you have not practiced this technique, pull yourself round to the stern instead, and climb in there.
• If the weight of water on the sails prevents the boat from coming upright, lower the sails and try again.
• If there is more than one person in the boat, ask one of them to swim into the cockpit while

the boat is on its side and to lie along the inside of the hull. He or she will be scooped up into the boat when you pull it upright, and can help to stabilize it while you climb in. The crew may also need to bail out the boat partially to improve its buoyancy before you get back in.

HOW TO AVOID A CAPSIZE

If the force of the wind threatens to tip your dinghy over – in any sailing situation – let go of the sheets (the ropes from the sails) so that the sails flap freely.

At the same time, steer into the wind (if you are sitting on the windward side of the boat, this means pushing the tiller away from you) and move quickly into the center of the boat to balance it.

Whatever the situation, steering into the wind and letting the sails flap freely will end the sideways pressure on the boat and allow it to come upright again.

Avoiding collisions on the water

The "rules of the road" to prevent boat collisions appear in the *International Rules for Prevention of Collision at Sea*. Regulations for some Great Lakes and tributary rivers appear in *Rules of the Road for the Great Lakes* and Part VII of the *Canadian Small Craft Regulations*. These publications are available from the Superintendent of Documents, U.S. Government Printing Office, Washington, D.C. 20402, and the Canadian Government Publishing Center, Supply and Services Canada, Ottawa K1A 0S9. These are the main rules:

• When two sailboats are on a collision course, the one with the wind to port (coming from the left-hand side of the boat, looking forward) must keep out of the way. If two sailboats have the wind on the same side, the boat upwind must give way.

• Powerboats must give way to sailing craft if they can, but a large powerboat following a narrow channel may not be able to do so. In this case, the sailboat should keep clear.

• If a sailboat is using its engine, it is treated as a power craft, and must give way to boats under sail.

• Powerboats approaching each other end-on (or nearly end-on) should both turn to starboard (to the right). If powerboats are crossing each other's course, the one that sees the other on its starboard (right-hand) side must keep out of the way.

When there is a risk of collision, boats can also signal their intentions to other nearby boats by means of a whistle or siren. One short blast means: I am altering course to starboard. Two short blasts mean: I am altering course to port. Three short blasts mean: My engines are going astern – that is, in reverse. Five or more short blasts mean: Danger!

If a sailboat crosses your path
If you are in a sailboat with the wind coming from the left-hand (port) side of your boat, you must give way to a sailboat which is crossing your path on the opposite (starboard) tack. Steer your boat behind the other's stern to be sure of missing it.

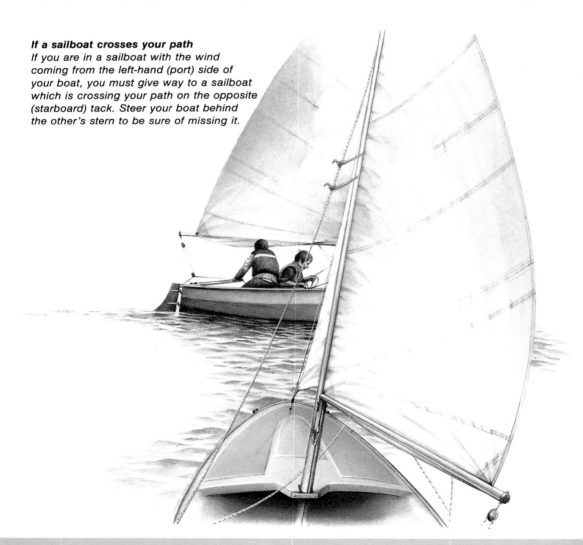

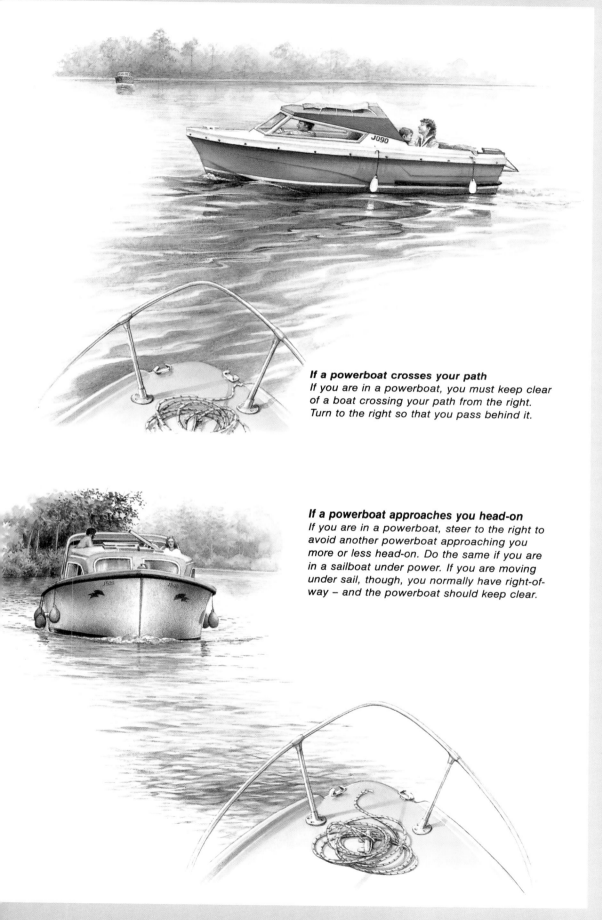

If a powerboat crosses your path
If you are in a powerboat, you must keep clear of a boat crossing your path from the right. Turn to the right so that you pass behind it.

If a powerboat approaches you head-on
If you are in a powerboat, steer to the right to avoid another powerboat approaching you more or less head-on. Do the same if you are in a sailboat under power. If you are moving under sail, though, you normally have right-of-way – and the powerboat should keep clear.

Running aground

A grounded boat must be freed quickly – provided that its hull has not been holed or damaged below the waterline. What to do depends to some extent on the wind direction, the type of keel and – in coastal waters – the state of the tide. If the tide is rising, the boat must be prevented from being driven farther aground. If it is falling, the boat must be moved off fast or it will be left high and dry. The easiest route off is usually the same as the route on.

• On a lee shore (with the wind blowing shoreward) or in a rising tide, drop all sails at once or turn the boat into the wind and let go an anchor to prevent the boat being driven farther aground. On a weather or windward shore (with the wind blowing away from the shore), set the sails so that the wind helps to swing the bow toward deeper water.

• At the same time that you trim – that is, adjust – the sails, start the engine, applying moderate power in reverse. Your own wake rolling under the stern may free the boat.

Using a kedge anchor
• If these actions do not free the boat, try to haul it into deeper water by means of a kedge anchor – a light anchor with a chain and rope attached.

• Secure the end of the rope to a winch or run it through a pulley on the boat.

• Coil the rest of the rope and the chain in a dinghy or rowboat and suspend the anchor over its stern. This saves you having to lift it over the side.

• Row away from the stuck boat into deeper water, paying out the rope as you go, then drop

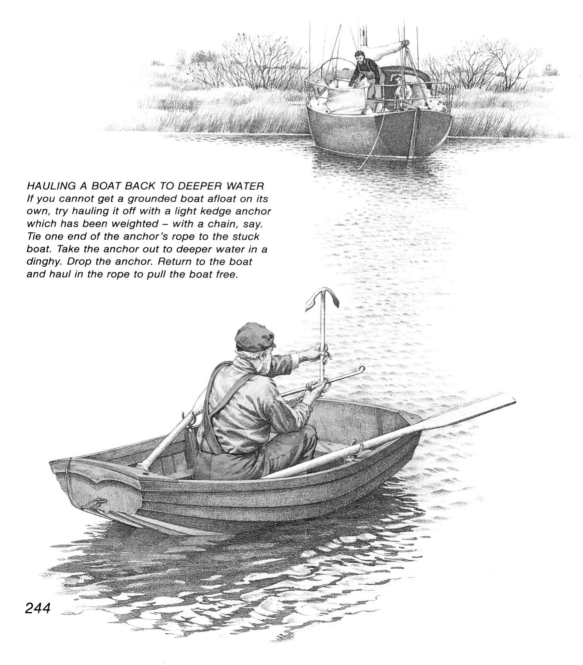

HAULING A BOAT BACK TO DEEPER WATER
If you cannot get a grounded boat afloat on its own, try hauling it off with a light kedge anchor which has been weighted – with a chain, say. Tie one end of the anchor's rope to the stuck boat. Take the anchor out to deeper water in a dinghy. Drop the anchor. Return to the boat and haul in the rope to pull the boat free.

the anchor. Once the kedge anchor is firmly gripped on the bottom, return to the grounded boat and pull in the rope to haul it free.

• If necessary, shift heavy weights onto the dinghy to lighten the load on the stuck boat.

Using the weight of the crew

• Another method of freeing a boat is to get the crew to rock it from side to side. This may break the suction of mud on the keel.

• If the rocking does not work and the boat does not have twin keels (known as bilge keels), it may be possible to free it by using the weight of the crew to heel, or tilt, it to one side; somebody can sit on the end of the boom if necessary. This will help to loosen the keel from mud or sand and may lift it sufficiently to free it.

• In a boat with a full single keel, which is

TILTING THE BOAT FREE
You can sometimes free a stuck boat by getting one or more people to sit on the end of the boom and then swinging the boom out. This will tilt the boat and loosen the keel, and it may lift the keel enough to set the boat free. The boat can then be hauled off with a kedge anchor (see opposite).

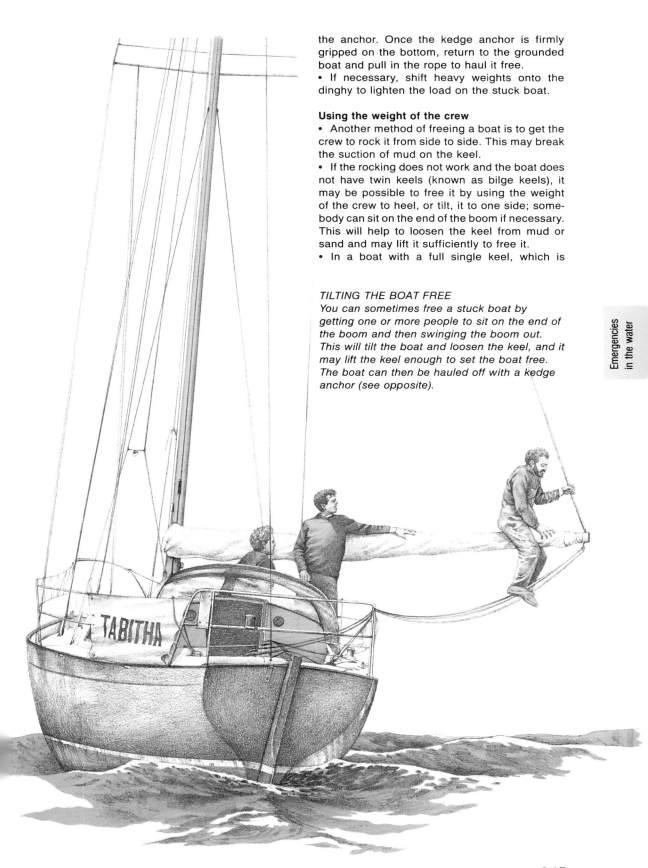

Emergencies in the water

normally deeper toward the stern, try moving all the crew well forward. This may weigh down the bows sufficiently to free the keel.

Leaving the boat high and dry
• If getting off proves impossible, prepare the boat for being left aground until you can get more help or until the next high tide. Normally, a boat will refloat as long after low water as the period before low water that it ran aground.

If a boat runs aground at the height of a spring tide (a high tide occurring near the time of a new or full moon) it could be about two weeks before the water reaches the same level again.

• Leave the kedge anchor in position and put out the main anchor as well.

• A boat with a single keel will heel onto one side as the tide recedes. Make sure it lies with

the keel toward deep water by weighting the deck – with an anchor chain, say – on the side toward the shallows. This will protect the superstructure from waves when the tide returns.

• As the water level drops, wedge sailbags, fenders and other padding under the leaning hull to prevent it being damaged as the returning waves pound it against the ground.

• Secure all loose gear on board. Shut off fuel and water supplies to prevent spillage. Close all seacocks and plug tank ventilator pipes. If possible, off-load batteries onto a dinghy to avoid the risk of acid spilling from them.

• Pump out the bilge so that there is no waste water to weigh the boat down or to affect its balance while it is righting. Batten and seal all hatches to prevent seawater entering.

• If you can stay on board till the tide returns,

WAITING FOR THE NEXT TIDE
If you cannot get a boat afloat, leave it until the next tide. First, though, put out the anchors. If the boat has a single keel, weight it – with a chain, say – toward the shallows, so that it comes to rest with the keel toward deep water. Put fenders and other padding under the leaning hull to protect it. Secure loose gear. Shut off all pipes and pump out the bilge.

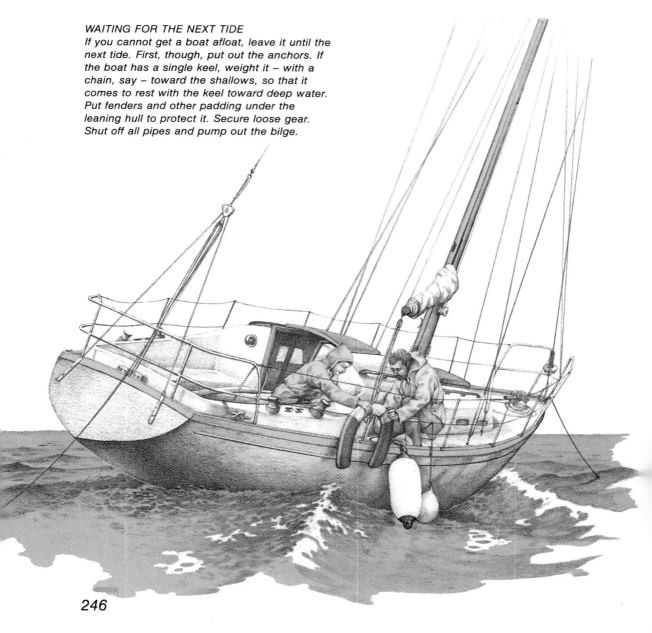

fill bags, pillowcases and buckets with sand. Store them on the boat until it begins to float, then empty them overboard. This will minimize the pounding the boat gets as the water rises.
• Alternatively, a deep-keeled boat can be kept upright by rigging beaching legs (props that fit under the hull on each side). If you have no ready-made props, improvise with a boom or spinnaker pole lashed to the boat's rigging.
• As a last resort, if there is heavy surf and a hard bottom, scuttling the boat will prevent it being pounded to pieces as the tide rises. To do this, leave the anchors in position, move out as much gear as possible, and open the seacocks so that the boat settles on the bottom.
• Later, as the water deepens again, close the seacocks and pump the boat out so that it rises with the tide and floats free.

TIPS FOR STAYING AFLOAT

• Bear in mind the state of the tide and the time of low water. Study charts of the area. Never sail too close to a lee shore.
• Be aware of any change of motion in the boat – such as a shorter rise and fall – that might indicate shallow water. If you are in any doubt, sound the depth with a lead and line.
• Bear in mind, too, the depth and shape of your keel. You may not be able to sail as close to the shore as other boats of apparently similar size.

PROPPING UP THE BOAT
If you have no beaching legs, use a boom as a prop. Tilt the boat with weights toward the shallows. Remove the boom and rest one end on the seabed on the shallow side. On mud or sand, put a plank underneath to stop it sinking in. Then lash the boom to the shrouds both at its top and at deck level. Stop the boom slipping by tying the top to a strong deck fitting.

Emergencies in the water

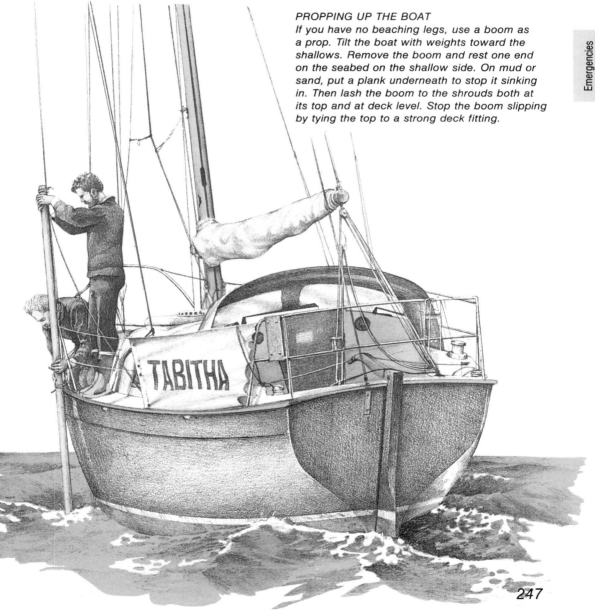

247

Dealing with a hole or leak

Colliding with a rock, a floating log or another boat can all put a hole in the hull of a small boat. But a hole need not mean that the boat will sink at once, or even at all.

Plugging a large hole
• On a sailboat, if there is a hole on or near the waterline, sail the boat on a suitable tack to heel it over slightly and raise the hole from the water. On a sailboat or motorboat, rearrange movable equipment and the crew's position for the same purpose.
• If the hole is below the waterline, use the bilge pump or bail out by hand to control the water level while you make emergency repairs inside and outside the hull.
• Plug the hole first from the inside with any suitable material, such as sail bags, cushions or mattresses. Wedge the plugging in place with something solid, such as a table or seating boards.
• Then, make what sailors call a collision mat. The idea is to spread the mat – which could be a tarpaulin or a spare sail – across the hole on the outside of the hull so that water pressure helps to hold it in place.
• If the hull is so shaped that canvas will not lie flat against it, wrap the tarpaulin or spare sail round a foam mattress or cushion, which is more likely to shape itself to the hull. Then use the bundle as a mat.
• To move the mat into position, tie chains or ropes to each corner. Then tie two or three corners of the mat to fittings on the damaged side of the boat.

• Loop the remaining rope or ropes over the front of the boat and work them along under the hull until the mat is pulled tight over the hole. Tie the ropes to fittings on the undamaged side of the boat. Then make for shore at once.

Repairing a small leak
• If a boat starts taking in water slowly, it may be difficult to find the source of the leak. So make a systematic check of the likely places where water could get into the boat.
• Check all seacocks – the valves that prevent a backflow of water in any pipe that goes through the hull. Seacocks are usually built into the galley, toilet, engine intake and exhaust, bilge pump and cockpit drains.
• Check any fittings which pass through the hull, such as the rudder shaft.
• Check the stuffing box – the greased stuffing compressed round the propeller shaft where it goes through the hull.
• Check the water tank or tanks.
• Check seams in the hull.
• Once you find the leak, plug it firmly with caulking cotton (cotton fiber and sealant), greased rags, underwater resin, towels or any other similar material.
• You can plug a small leak with underwater epoxy glue – available from boating supply stores. For a larger leak, use epoxy with pieces of fiberglass material. Epoxy dries and forms a seal on wet surfaces or underwater within five minutes.
• Make permanent repairs as soon as possible when you get back to shore.

SAFETY IN THE FOG

Fog reduces visibility essential to pilot a boat safely and increases the risk of collision. Some fogs – such as the advection fog observed at sea – form when the cool surface of land or water lowers the temperature of warm air above it. Radiation fogs (ground fogs) – which cover harbors and low-lying coastal areas in early morning – occur when cold air combines with moisture. Advection fogs, which are common to sea coasts and those of the Great Lakes, can persist for days. Radiation fogs usually burn off soon after sunrise.

At the first sign of fog, head to the nearest port or shelter where you can wait for the fog to pass. If fog moves in quickly, plot your position. Then, determine a safe course and destination. In a sailing vessel, avoid a busy channel in the fog. If your boat is small, anchor close to shore, where the water is too shallow for commercial traffic, but not so shallow that you might ground.

Using a bell, a foghorn or a whistle – all required fog-signaling equipment for boats at sea – warn other boats of your position. Make the warning sound appropriate for your boat. Power-driven vessels that are underway must give one prolonged blast (4-6 seconds long) on the foghorn at intervals of no more than two minutes. Power-driven vessels that have stopped should sound two prolonged blasts every two minutes. Anchored power-driven vessels are to ring the bell rapidly for about five seconds at intervals of one minute. Sailing vessels must follow similar, though not identical rules.

Check with the United States and Canadian coast guards about fog-signaling regulations for pleasure boats on inland waterways.

TWO WAYS TO PLUG A HOLE IN A BOAT

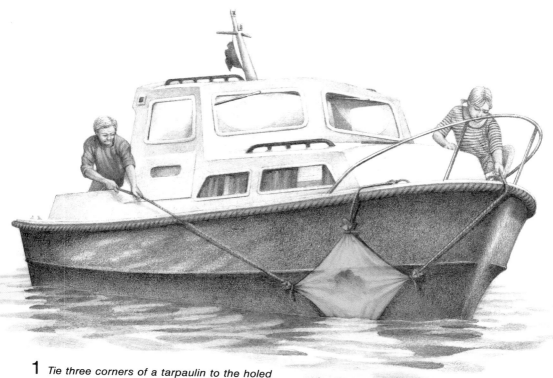

1 *Tie three corners of a tarpaulin to the holed side. Loop the remaining rope under the bow and tie it to the other side. Adjust the ropes' lengths to position the tarpaulin over the hole.*

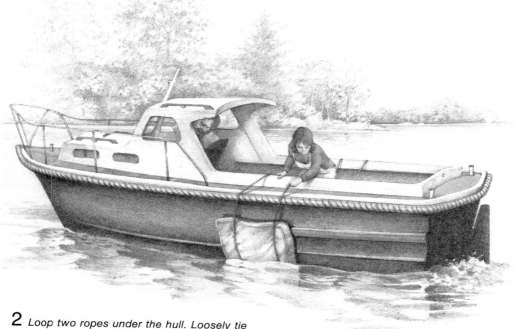

2 *Loop two ropes under the hull. Loosely tie them to fittings. Slide a mattress into place under the rope straps, then pull them tight.*

Emergencies in the water

Fire on board

Because the fittings in most family-size sailboats and power boats are largely made out of wood, and because the boats often contain fuel tanks and gas cylinders in a fairly small space, a fire, once started, can spread at alarming speed. If you are away from land at the time, there may be no easy escape route, either.

For these reasons, fast decisive action is imperative if a fire breaks out on board.
- Shout "Fire" to raise the alarm.
- If the engine is running, turn it off.
- If time permits, call for help by radio, giving the location of your boat.
- Throw burning equipment such as mattresses overboard. Do not, however, try to move a deep fat fryer (see *Fighting a fire*, page 148).
- Never throw water on burning fuel or gas. It can spread the blaze. Instead, use a fire extinguisher containing dry powder or foam.
- In a sailboat, if the wind is light, drop the sails; if the wind is strong, minimize its ability to fan the flames by sailing downwind.
- If the fire is below decks, get everyone out, then stop air reaching it by closing doors, hatches and vents. Fight the blaze from above or from somewhere where you can retreat easily.
- If you cannot extinguish the fire quickly, evacuate the area or abandon ship if necessary.
- After the fire is out, damp down the area thoroughly with water.

GUARDING AGAINST A BLAZE

Most fires in boats happen immediately after refueling. Other fires occur when sparks or naked flames ignite fuel leaks or accumulations of gas from propane stoves. You can cut the risk of fire on board, however, by following a few commonsense rules.
- Make sure that bilges (the space between hull and floor in a boat) and engine spaces have ventilation hoses that reach right to the bottom. The fumes and vapor from gasoline and fuels such as propane are all heavier than air, and so will accumulate at the lowest levels. Each fuel tank should have a vent pipe to disperse gas vapor; the pipe should go out through the hull and be covered with wire gauze.
- Before starting a gasoline engine, open all doors and vents and allow air to circulate for at least five minutes.
- Many boats have a blower to suck the fumes from the bilges. It should be run for five minutes before starting the engine.
- Fit carburetors with drip trays (covered with wire gauze to prevent anything being drop-

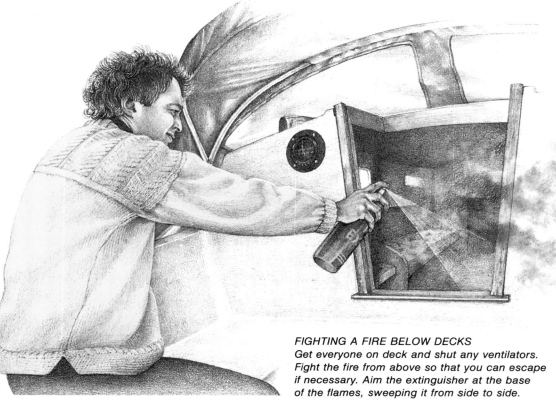

FIGHTING A FIRE BELOW DECKS
Get everyone on deck and shut any ventilators.
Fight the fire from above so that you can escape
if necessary. Aim the extinguisher at the base
of the flames, sweeping it from side to side.

ped in), and clean the trays before starting the engine. That way you will minimize the chances of leaking fuel collecting in the bottom of the boat.

• Fit flame traps in the air intakes.

• Check wiring and plugs regularly and replace faulty parts. Ensure that connectors have the correct fuses; a fuse with too large a capacity will allow cables to overheat.

• Ensure that generators and switches are as far as possible above the bilges to minimize the chance of water causing short circuits.

• Do not strike matches, smoke, or use a kerosene or any other open-flame lamp inside the engine space. Anywhere on board, use only safety matches. Other types of matches, and also lighters, can spark if they are rubbed accidentally or dropped.

• Do not smoke or strike matches within 30 ft. (9 m) of boat during refueling.

• Cover batteries so that tools cannot fall on the terminals and cause a spark.

• Avoid overfilling gasoline tanks – leave some space for the fuel to expand. Check for leakages regularly. The top of the filler pipe should reach to the open deck so that any spillages will run overboard and not down to the bilges. Do not use gas for cleaning. Instead, use clean cotton rags – and dispose of them, and all other rubbish, regularly.

Fire fighting equipment

• Carry one fire extinguisher of at least 3 lb. (1.5 kg) capacity, containing dry powder, carbon dioxide or foam. Do not carry an extinguisher containing the chemical known as halon or BCF (bromochlorodofluoromethane) because it gives off poisonous fumes, which are dangerous in a confined space such as a ship's cabin.

• Carry two extinguishers if there is a galley on board. Keep them in a place accessible from the open deck so that a fire can be fought from a safe position.

• Keep extinguishers regularly maintained to ensure that they are in good working order.

• Keep two bailer buckets with lanyards on deck for hauling up water.

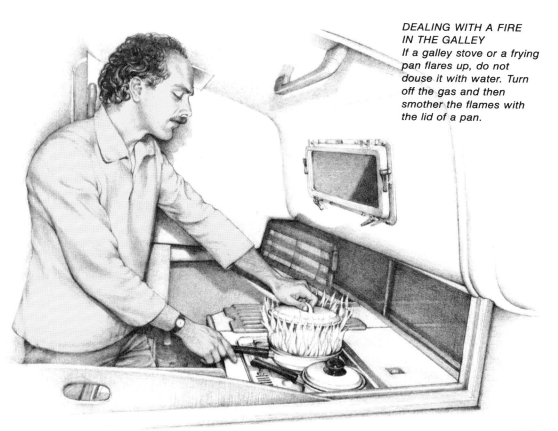

DEALING WITH A FIRE IN THE GALLEY
If a galley stove or a frying pan flares up, do not douse it with water. Turn off the gas and then smother the flames with the lid of a pan.

Emergencies in the water

Deciding what to do in heavy weather

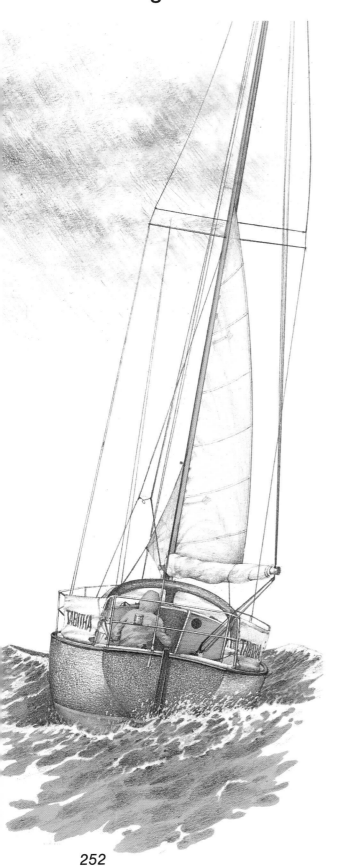

If the water gets rough while you are out in a sailboat or motorboat, you have to decide whether to continue on course (under reduced power or sail so that you can keep control of the craft), head for port as fast as possible, heave to (stop moving), or run before the storm.

If in doubt, it is usually safer to stay on the water rather than to head for harbor and risk being swept and battered against the shore.

Whatever your decision, the boat needs to be rigged for stormy conditions (see *Caught in a storm*, page 258).

Rough water is no place for a novice, though. Before you contemplate taking any boat far from shore yourself, learn about the problems and risks at first hand by crewing for experienced sailors and boat-owners. Local yacht and boat clubs can often put you in touch with knowledgeable skippers. The clubs may also run training courses.

Continuing on course
Carrying on under reduced sail or power is a viable option if the wind is blowing in a direction suitable for the course you want to follow. If the wind is unfavorable, take other action.

Heading for port
Running for shelter is worth considering if the wind is right and the weather is worsening slowly enough for you to be able to beat it to a port or other refuge (such as the sheltered side of a headland). Remember, however, that heavy seas will slow you down.
• A motorboat or a sailboat with an engine is likely to be able to head for port faster than a boat traveling under sail alone. But first check how much fuel is in the tank – refueling from a gasoline can may be impossible in rough water.

Heaving to
• Stopping a boat without anchoring – what sailors call heaving to – is safe only if you are well away from a lee shore: one the wind is blowing toward. But even a boat that has heaved to still drifts slightly with wind and current. It could drift at 2 knots (just over 2 mph or 3.2 km/h) or more, and a storm could last up to 30 hours.
• The advantage of heaving to is that the boat's motion in the water is more comfortable for those on board. Also, little effort is required from the crew once the boat has been prepared.
• The disadvantages are that the boat will move

HOW TO HEAVE TO
To hold a boat more or less in position at sea, pull the front sail (the jib) to the upwind side of the boat and keep steering into the wind. The boat will then sail a roughly crescent-shaped course: forward until it is almost nose-on to the wind, then back and sideways again as the wind pushes more on the front sail.

gradually across the wind and downwind, which could carry it into more dangerous waters, and there is constant strain on the sails and rigging.
• There is also a risk of the boat being swung broadside to the waves and capsizing. This is more likely with a shallow, unballasted hull such as a flat-bottomed centerboard vessel.
• If you decide to heave to, the aim in effect is to sail the boat into the wind at the same speed that the wind is blowing it downwind.
• Back the front sail (the jib) – that is, set it so that the wind is pushing it backward. It then counterbalances the forward thrust of the mainsail.
• Reduce the area of the mainsail so that little sail is exposed to the wind.
• Lash or hold the tiller or wheel to keep the boat pointing toward the wind.

Running before the storm
• Sailing downwind in a storm is a viable option only if you are far enough from land not to be blown onto rocks or the shore. You can reduce sails to a jib only if necessary, or run with bare poles.
• The advantages are that the boat remains under control and maneuverable, and the strain and wear on sails and rigging is reduced.
• The disadvantages are that the crew must be on the alert, with someone constantly at the helm to keep the boat pointing downwind; and the cockpit is exposed to the seas.
• There is also a risk that the following waves will break over the stern. This can be offset by trailing ropes behind the boat, looping the very long ones, so that the waves break on the ropes, and their force is diminished. The drag of the ropes also helps to slow down the boat, making it easier to control. In addition, it helps to keep the stern into the wind, lessening the chance that the boat will swing sideways to the waves and capsize.
• As a last resort, if you are well clear of land and shipping lanes, lower all sails, stow everything securely, shut all hatches and retreat below decks until the weather eases.

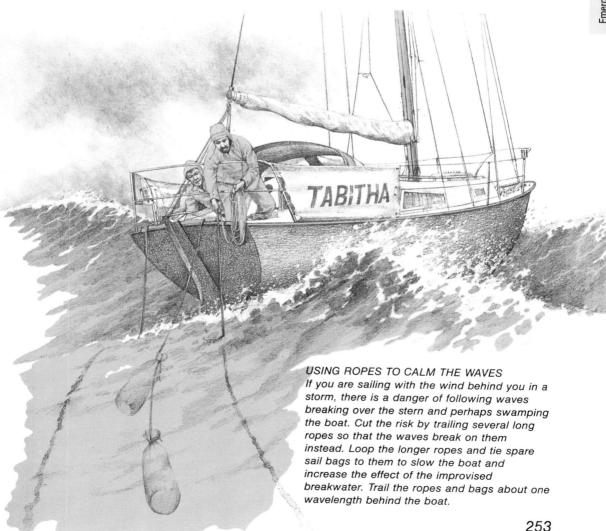

USING ROPES TO CALM THE WAVES
If you are sailing with the wind behind you in a storm, there is a danger of following waves breaking over the stern and perhaps swamping the boat. Cut the risk by trailing several long ropes so that the waves break on them instead. Loop the longer ropes and tie spare sail bags to them to slow the boat and increase the effect of the improvised breakwater. Trail the ropes and bags about one wavelength behind the boat.

Wind and weather

Around North America's coasts, bad weather never arrives suddenly or unexpectedly. There are always warnings, such as changes in wind and clouds and falling barometric pressure – and the more abrupt the drop in a barometer's reading, the more severe the bad weather is likely to be. All the same, the weather at sea may be quite different from weather on land. So listen to shipping forecasts before planning to put to sea.

In the United States, you can get the latest marine weather conditions 24 hours a day on one of three high-band FM frequencies – 162.40, 162.475, or 162.55 megahertz (MHz). In Canada, you can pick up such forecasts on a VHF FM receiver on channels 21B and 83B on the Atlantic coast and the Great Lakes, and on channels 21B and three WX channels on the Pacific coast. Environment Canada also provides continuous weather forecasts on its Weatheradio Canada broadcasts on the VHF band. To get more information about marine weather services, contact the National Oceanic and Atmospheric Administration (NOAA), Silver Springs, Maryland 20910, or the nearest Environment Canada office.

Bad-weather signs

The pictures opposite show the visible clues a sailor or a hiker should watch for. All of them indicate that bad weather is on the way.

Other bad-weather clues can only be felt, not seen, or become apparent only over a period of time. These are the main ones:

- The wind changes suddenly after several days of constant direction.
- The wind increases in the afternoon or evening.

Some weather signs indicate the approach of severe weather – a storm or gale. Mare's tail clouds, and a copper-colored sunset or sunrise are both danger signals. So are a number of other clues:

- A rapidly falling or unsteady barometer.
- Increasing humidity.
- A heavy but inexplicable swell at sea.

TEN WEEKS IN A LIFE RAFT

Playful dorado fish kept yacht designer Steven Callahan alive when he was shipwrecked in mid-Atlantic in 1982. Swimming around his tiny life raft and following it as it drifted across the ocean, the dorados became his only food. The 29-year-old American speared them from the raft and ate them raw.

Solar stills – part of his survival kit on the raft – provided him with 3 pints of water a day (about 1.5 liters), just enough to live on.

The dorados also helped in his rescue. As he drifted near the Caribbean Leeward Islands, the fish attracted flocks of birds – which were spotted by a fishing boat. When the boat picked up Callahan on April 21, 1982, he was about 45 lb. (20 kg) lighter than normal, but remarkably fit after 76 days adrift.

Four years earlier, in 1978, two middle-aged Americans were washed out to sea during a fishing trip after the motor on their boat broke down. They survived the blistering heat of the Gulf of California by making their own still to turn seawater into fresh.

The two men improvised a stove by burning a mixture of gas and oil from their broken-down outboard motor in two open tins. After their matches ran out, they lit the stove by sparking wires from the motor's battery against a gas-soaked piece of cardboard.

They used the stove to boil seawater in a jerrican. The steam condensed as it passed through a hose stuffed in the neck of the can, and trickled into a plastic bottle. The two men were found by a US Coast Guard plane after a week and a half in their open boat – hungry but otherwise unhurt.

HOW TO READ A BAROMETER

The barometer most commonly used by sailors is the aneroid type shown below. Aneroid means "without air."

The pointer moves as air pressure squeezes a vacuum-filled metal bellows inside. The words on the dial – "Fair," "Stormy," "Rain" and so on – are more traditional than useful. What matters more is a change in the reading. Generally, a drop in pressure indicates a storm is on the way. Steady or rising pressure usually means fair weather ahead.

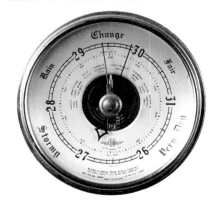

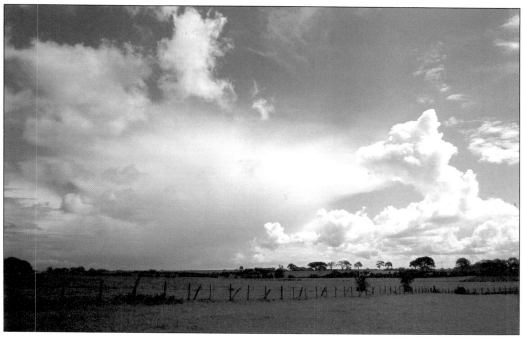

MESSAGE IN THE SKY *Large, anvil-shaped and often fuzzy-edged expanses of cloud, such as that in the centre of this picture, mark the approach of more blustery weather. The change will probably bring showers, and may build into a thunderstorm.*

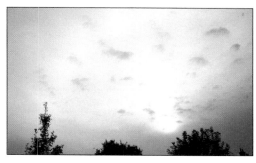

ICE HALO *A halo round the moon, formed when light is refracted by ice crystals, signals rain, or perhaps a storm, within 36 hours.*

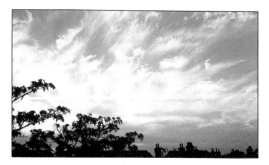

OUTRIDERS OF A GALE *Mare's tail clouds – high wispy streaks across the sky – are often a warning of high winds on the way.*

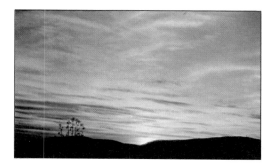

COPPER SUN *A copper-colored sunset or sunrise is a warning of a gale or storm. A yellowish sunset indicates rain and wind.*

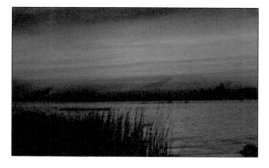

RED SKY AT MORNING *If the sunrise is red, or clear but with a red tinge, the weather is likely to take a turn for the worse soon.*

The wind and the sea

The Beaufort wind scale, devised in 1805 by the British admiral Sir Francis Beaufort (1774-1857), is still widely used in shipping forecasts and by sailors. It enables sailors to estimate the strength of the wind simply by observing its effects and without the need for precise measuring instruments. The scale begins at Force 0, when the wind is less than 1 mph and the sea is flat calm, and rises to Force 12, a hurricane. The chart below shows how to judge the wind on land and sea, and gives the probable maximum wave height for each wind force. Average wave heights are lower.

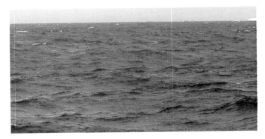

FORCE THREE *A touch of foam on some crests, whitecaps, marks a Force 3 wind – what sailors call a gentle breeze.*

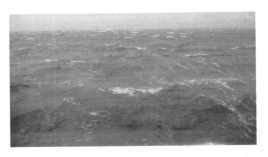

FORCE FIVE *A wind of Force 5 or above can be hazardous even for experienced sailors.*

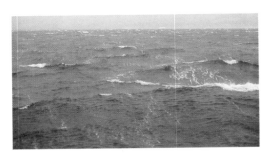

FORCE SIX *In a strong breeze, the waves can be anything from 8 to 13 ft. (2.5–4 m) high.*

THE BEAUFORT SCALE ON LAND AND AT SEA

FORCE ONE: LIGHT AIR

Land: Smoke drifts slightly – but the wind is not enough to move a weather vane.
Sea: Tiny ripples shaped like fish scales form on the sea's surface. No foam crests.

Maximum wind speed: 3 mph (5 km/h).
Probable maximum wave height: Nil.

FORCE TWO: LIGHT BREEZE

Land: Breeze felt on the face. Weather vanes move and leaves rustle.
Sea: Small wavelets form. Crests are pronounced and have a glassy appearance, but they do not break into foam.
Maximum wind speed: 7 mph (11 km/h).
Probable maximum wave height: 1 ft. (30 cm).

FORCE THREE: GENTLE BREEZE

Land: Leaves and small twigs in constant motion. The breeze extends a light flag.
Sea: Large wavelets form. Crests begin to break into foam and there are occasional whitecaps.

Maximum wind speed: 12 mph (19 km/h).
Probable maximum wave height: 3 ft. (1 m).

FORCE FOUR: MODERATE BREEZE

Land: The wind raises dust and loose paper and moves small branches on trees.
Sea: Small waves form and some begin to join together to make longer lines of waves. There are frequent whitecaps.
Maximum wind speed: 18 mph (29 km/h).
Probable maximum wave height: 5 ft. (1.5 m).

FORCE FIVE: FRESH BREEZE

Land: Small trees sway, if they are in leaf. Crested wavelets form on inland waters.
Sea: Moderate-sized waves form into long lines. There are many whitecaps and some spray.

Maximum wind speed: 24 mph (39 km/h).
Probable maximum wave height: 8 ft. (2.5 m).

FORCE SIX: STRONG BREEZE

Land: Large branches move. Telegraph wires whistle. Umbrellas used only with difficulty.
Sea: Some large waves, extensive white foam crests and some spray.

Maximum wind speed: 31 mph (50 km/h).
Probable maximum wave height: 13 ft. (4 m).

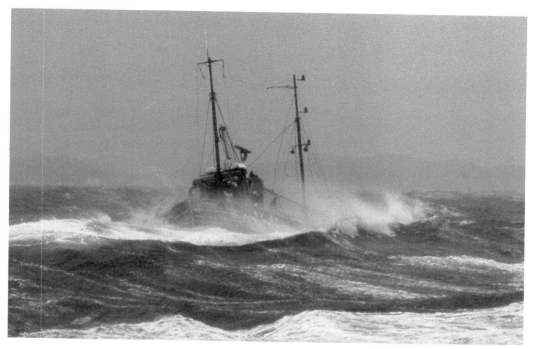

FORCE NINE *The hull of a 60 ft. (18 m) fishing boat is almost concealed by waves and driving spray as it plunges through a strong gale off the Outer Hebrides in Scotland.*

FORCE SEVEN: NEAR GALE

Land: Whole trees in motion. Inconvenience felt when walking against the wind.
Sea: Sea heaped up. White foam from breaking waves blows out in streaks with the wind.

Maximum wind speed: 38 mph (61 km/h).
Probable maximum wave height: 20 ft. (6 m).

FORCE EIGHT: GALE

Land: The wind generally impedes progress. Twigs break off trees.
Sea: Waves are long and moderately high. Spray, or spindrift, blows from their crests. Foam blown in clearly defined streaks.
Maximum wind speed: 46 mph (74 km/h).
Probable maximum wave height: 25 ft. (7.5 m).

FORCE NINE: STRONG GALE

Land: Slight structural damage – chimney pots and shingles are blown off.
Sea: Waves are high, their crests toppling, tumbling and rolling over. There are dense white streaks of foam, and spray reduces visibility.
Maximum wind speed: 54 mph (87 km/h).
Probable maximum wave height: 33 ft. (9.75 m).

FORCE TEN: STORM

Land: Considerable structural damage and trees uprooted.
Sea: High waves, with long overhanging crests, tumble heavily, shocklike. Sea surface appears white. Visibility poor.
Maximum wind speed: 63 mph (101 km/h).
Probable maximum wave height: 42 ft. (12.5 m).

FORCE ELEVEN: VIOLENT STORM

Land: Widespread damage caused.
Sea: Exceptionally high waves, sometimes concealing small and medium-sized ships. Crests blown into froth. Foam everywhere. Visibility poor.

Maximum wind speed: 72 mph (116 km/h).
Probable maximum wave height: 53 ft. (16 m).

FORCE TWELVE: HURRICANE

Land: Mostly confined to the tropics. Widespread damage caused.
Sea: The whole of the sea's surface is white with driving spray. Foam and spray fill the air and visibility is bad.
Maximum wind speed: Over 72 mph (116 km/h).
Probable maximum wave height: Unlimited.

Caught in a storm

The safest strategy for a small boat caught in stormy weather is to reduce power in order to steady the vessel and make it easier to control, and to secure everything movable.

In a sailboat
• Reduce the sail area. Lash down deck gear.
• In stormy weather, it is usually safest to sail as nearly into the wind as possible – provided that this course does not take you into dangerous waters (see *Deciding what to do in heavy weather*, page 252).

• Check the security of lifelines and jackstays (lines to which safety harnesses are clipped). Always put on a life jacket if you are not already wearing one. Be sure to strap on a safety harness, too.
• Pump the bilge dry and check that the cockpit drains are clear.
• Close all other hatches, seacocks, ventilators and exhausts.
• Start the engine (if there is one) to check that it is working.
• Then shut the engine down to conserve fuel in case you need it later.

In a motorboat
• Head quickly for the shore or the nearest shelter.
• Get passengers to squat as low as possible to improve the boat's stability.
• Head into the waves if possible, keeping speed low (to cut down spray and water from

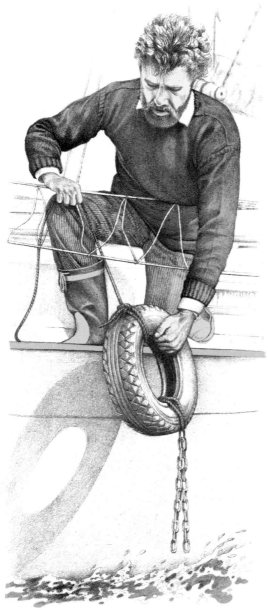

HOW TO USE A SEA ANCHOR
A sea anchor acts as a drag on a boat, keeping whichever end it is tied to pointing into the wind. It is usually trailed from the front.

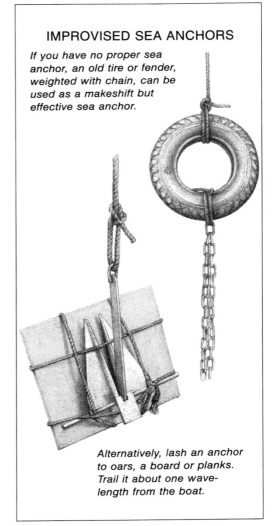

IMPROVISED SEA ANCHORS

If you have no proper sea anchor, an old tire or fender, weighted with chain, can be used as a makeshift but effective sea anchor.

Alternatively, lash an anchor to oars, a board or planks. Trail it about one wavelength from the boat.

the waves). But keep up sufficient speed to maintain full steering power.

• If the engine fails, ride at anchor or put out a sea anchor – a cone-shaped canvas bag that will help to keep the front of the boat pointing into the wind.

• Avoid letting the boat swing broadside to the waves. They could swamp or overturn it.

SAVED BY A CHILD'S CHATTER

On May 3, 1981, the Jeffery family – Les, a 37-year-old airport fire fighter, his wife Virginia, son Darren, and 12-year-old daughter Tracy-Leigh – and a family friend, Stewart Greenough, set out on a cruise off the east coast of Australia in their 47 ft. (14 m) yacht Jedda.

Seven days later, in the early hours of the morning, battered by storm-force winds, they were forced to abandon ship. Roped together, the five tried to transfer from the Jedda to a rescuing oil tanker. But as the ships rolled, they were tossed into the water and pulled right under the tanker by the undertow.

The rope broke and Darren and Stewart were swept away. Their bodies were found later. When Tracy-Leigh surfaced she found herself still tied to her mother and father. Her father was injured and her mother was floating face down – dead. In the darkness the tanker lost sight of the bobbing figures.

Tracy-Leigh knew that once her father lost consciousness he would drown in the huge waves. His only chance was to stay awake, so she talked to him – chattering about anything and everything. As she talked, she clung to her mother's life jacket because her own had been torn away against the tanker's hull.

Her talking worked. By the time a helicopter found them at dawn six hours later, she was exhausted – but her father was still alive.

WAYS OF SIGNALING FOR HELP

The internationally recognized distress signal Mayday (which comes from the French phrase *M'aidez*, meaning "Help me") should be used only when you are in grave and imminent danger and require immediate assistance. If you urgently need help but are not in imminent danger, use the signal Pan Pan (from the French *panne*, meaning "breakdown"). Pan Pan is also the correct signal for man overboard.

Under the International Convention for the Safety of Life at Sea, there are a number of other recognized ways of calling for help. A ship's captain who sees any of these distress signals is legally obliged to respond to them.

• Gun or other explosive signal fired at intervals of about a minute.

• Continuous sounding of a fog signal, such as a foghorn.

• Rockets or shells throwing red stars fired one at a time at short intervals.

• Morse Code SOS (three dots, three dashes, three dots) transmitted by any means available.

• International Code flags NC (flag N above flag C), or a square flag with above or below it anything resembling a ball.

• Red parachute flare or red hand flare.

• Orange-colored smoke.

• Slowly raising and lowering outstretched arms.

• Flames on a vessel – for example, burning tar, oily rags – are an internationally recognized distress signal. (But experts warn this may be dangerous.)

An additional sign – a piece of orange canvas with a black square and circle – can be used to attract the attention of aircraft. Spread the canvas over the cabin or on the deck, or fly it from the mast.

Making a Mayday call

To call for help by radio, tune your transmitter to the international distress frequency: Channel 16 VHF or 2182 kHz MF.

• Repeat the word "Mayday" three times.

• Give the name of the craft three times.

• Repeat "Mayday" once more.

• Repeat the name of the vessel once and then give its position, a brief description of the emergency and the help needed.

• Listen for an acknowledgment that your message has been received before putting out the distress call again.

The phonetic alphabet

Phonetic alphabets use specific words to identify individual letters, in order to help to clarify a radio message. This is a widely used and internationally recognized list.

Alpha	Juliet	Sierra
Bravo	Kilo	Tango
Charlie	Lima	Uniform
Delta	Mike	Victor
Echo	November	Whisky
Foxtrot	Oscar	X-ray
Golf	Papa	Yankee
Hotel	Quebec	Zulu
India	Romeo	

Abandoning ship

A small boat – even one that is badly holed – may take at least five minutes to sink. This gives you time to dress warmly, send out a distress signal and prepare to take to a life raft or the water. Do not abandon ship unless there is obviously no other course open to you. The greatest hazard you have to combat is the cold.

• Put on as many layers of warm, woolly clothing as possible, including a hat – and wear a final layer of waterproof clothing.

• Wear socks and light shoes as well to help to keep your feet warm.

• Put on a life jacket over the top of your clothes.

• Take with you personal and ship's papers, and money, in a waterproof bag if possible.

• Send out a distress signal by radio, giving your position; or fire a distress flare or rocket (see *Ways of signaling for help*, page 259).

• Leave a sailboat from well forward or well aft of the mast to avoid being struck by spars or rigging if the boat heels over.

Taking to a life raft

• If you decide to take to a life raft, make sure that it has a line tied securely to the boat before you throw it overboard.

CHOOSING A LIFE JACKET OR FLOTATION DEVICE

Not even a good swimmer can keep afloat in cold, rough seas for long without a life jacket or a personal flotation device (PFD). By law, all pleasure craft must carry one approved life jacket or PFD for each person on board.

The standard life jacket and the small vessel life jacket are the two main types. Both are designed for use on ships at sea or on major inland lakes and waterways. The standard life jacket is more buoyant than the small vessel type, and it can turn over an unconscious person who is face down in the water to float him on his back. The PFD is suitable for most recreational boating. It is more comfortable than the life jacket, but it has less buoyancy and no turning ability.

When buying a life jacket or PFD, make sure it fits well. A child's PFD should have a safety strap fitting between the legs. The strap holds the PFD in place and keeps the child from slipping out of the head hole.

The label on the life jacket or PFD usually indicates that it has been tested and approved. In the United States, look for the name of the U.S. Coast Guard or the Underwriters' Laboratories on the label. In Canada, the label should read "DOT approved," which signifies its approval by the Canadian Coast Guard and the Department of Transport.

To make sure that you feel safe and comfortable when wearing your PFD, first try it out by swimming in shallow water, using a sidestroke or backstroke. Dry a wet PFD in a well-ventilated place out of direct heat and sunlight. PFDs lose buoyancy and should be tested in the water after a few years' use.

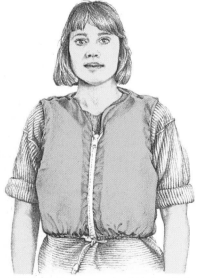

BUOYANCY AID *The vest-style aid is less bulky than a life jacket but not so buoyant.*

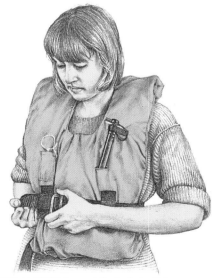

LIFE JACKET *A good life jacket will keep even an unconscious person floating face upward.*

- If the life raft is an inflatable type, it will usually be fitted with an operating line to open the gas cylinder which inflates it. The line also acts as a mooring rope.
- Secure the operating line to the boat, throw the raft container overboard, then pull the line to inflate the raft.
- Board the raft as quickly as possible. The first aboard should be a strong, fit man to help in children or injured or weaker people.
- When everyone is aboard the raft, cut the line. On most inflatable rafts there is a covered-in area, and near its entrance is a safety knife. The knife is specially designed so that it can be used to cut the line without running the risk of causing accidental damage to the raft.
- Do not take off wet clothing. It will give some protection against heat loss.
- Unless you are within easy reach of shore, put out a sea anchor – a cone-shaped canvas bag that acts as a drag in the water. A sea anchor is often part of a life raft's equipment. It helps to keep the raft stable in heavy seas and helps to stop it drifting (see *Caught in a storm*, page 258).
- Try to stay as near to the wreck or its last position as possible. Rescuers will concentrate their search around the boat's last known position, and so you will have a better chance of being spotted and rescued quickly.
- Bail out any water in the raft bottom.
- Have everyone take turns at the lookout to watch for rescuers. But keep the raft entrance closed as much as possible to keep warmth in.
- If the floor of the raft is inflatable, keep it topped up with air to provide insulation against the cold water below. Take anti-seasickness tablets as soon as possible on the raft. Seasickness is common in survival craft and hastens the onset of cold and exhaustion.

If you have to jump into the water

- If there is no time to climb into a life raft and you have to jump straight into the water, go to the windward side – the side facing into the wind – so that the boat will not drift into you once you are in the water.
- Hold your life jacket down and away from your chin by crossing your arms over your chest. Cover your nose and mouth with one hand to keep the water out.
- Look straight ahead and jump feet first with your legs straight and together. Do not look down or you may fall forward and land flat in the water, which is painful and could wind you.
- Your life jacket will bring you up to float at the surface within seconds. If you have an anti-splash hood on the jacket, unroll it and fasten it over your head.
- Get well clear of the side of the vessel, especially if it is a large one. If you do not, you run the risk of being sucked under as it sinks.

Survival in the water

- Do not try to swim for the shore unless land is very near, because you will quickly become exhausted. The shore is often farther away than it looks, and rescuers are more likely to see the wreckage than to spot a lone swimmer.
- If you can, cling to floating wreckage with as much of your body out of the water as possible to cut down heat loss. The greatest loss of body

---

PROVISIONS FOR A LIFE RAFT

What you need on a life raft depends to some extent on the circumstances. If you are not far from shore, for example, you do not need to take food.

Most life rafts come supplied with survival packs on board. But before you go out to sea, make sure that the pack on your life raft has everything you are likely to need if you get into trouble. This is a list of the most important pieces of equipment:

Knife
Waterproof flashlight
Distress signals (flare pack)
Bailer bucket
First aid kit
Anti-seasickness tablets
Oars/paddles
Sea anchor and rope
Water and drinking cup
Length of buoyant rope – about 100 ft.

(30 m) – with life buoy or rescue-quoit attached, for throwing to survivors in the water.

Rescue at sea

When a sailboat or motorboat is lost or in distress at sea, help may be delayed if no one knows anything about the boat. To avoid this situation, a boater is advised to leave his trip plan with friends or relatives.

The plan should include details such as a description of the boat; the type of engine; the number of people aboard; the radio and survival equipment aboard; and the itinerary. Then, if the boat is overdue, those ashore can notify the rescuers, who will know where to look and what to look for.

In the United States and Canada, search and rescue operations are carried out by the Coast Guard, often with the help of local authorities and volunteer groups.

heat is from the head, the neck, the armpits and the sides of the chest, and the groin.

• Stay in a group if there are several of you, to improve your chances of being spotted.

• If you are three or more in the water (all wearing life jackets), huddle together for warmth with arms around each other's shoulders.

• Keep body movements to a minimum to preserve heat. If there is a child, sandwich him in the middle of the group, because children lose body heat faster than adults.

• If you are not in a group (and are wearing a life jacket), conserve body heat by sitting in the water, bringing your knees up and hugging them firmly to your chest. You do not need to paddle; the life jacket will keep you afloat. This is known as the Heat Escape Lessening Position (HELP), because it exposes as little of the body as possible to the water. In water of 50°F (10°C) – typical temperature for most coastal and inland waters of the United States and the milder parts of Canada – the average survival time before death from hypothermia is two and a half to three hours. Using the HELP position can enable you to survive for an hour or so longer, giving yourself more time to be found by rescuers.

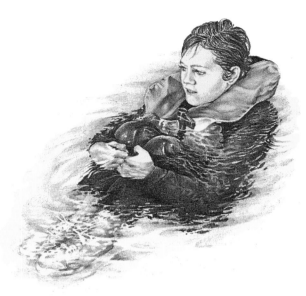

THE "HELP" POSITION
The Heat Escape Lessening Position enables you to survive longer in cold water. Bring your knees up and hug them to your chest. Trust the life jacket to keep you afloat.

ADRIFT IN A SMALL BOAT

Anyone adrift in a small boat – a canopied life raft or an open boat – for any length of time has three crucial needs: protection from the weather; a supply of water; and some means of attracting attention.

Food is less important. Exposure to extreme heat or cold can kill more quickly than starvation. A person can live for four weeks or so without food – but only days without fresh water.

• Limit your boat's movement through the water to make it easier for rescuers to find it.

• To help to keep your boat "parked" in the water, turn the front into the wind and trail a sea anchor about one wavelength away on the side from which the wind is blowing (see *Caught in a storm*, page 258).

• To conserve supplies, do not drink any water for the first 24 hours. Your supply of body fluid will still be adequate.

• After that, unless there is plenty of water from heavy rain, ration water to about 1 quart (1 liter) a day for each person aboard (more if possible in high temperatures). Drink it in small quantities throughout the course of the day. Desalinate seawater if you have desalination equipment.

• Send out distress signals at regular intervals. When using rockets or flares, fire them in groups of two, firing the second in the pair a few seconds after the first goes out. The first may be ignored, but the second will confirm the signal and may help to give rescuers a bearing. But use the flares sparingly, so that you keep a supply for use when help is in sight. When igniting flares, keep them away from your body and the life raft.

• In hot weather, keep as cool as possible. Shade your body and your eyes, if you can. Use sunscreen, if you have any. Avoid unnecessary movement. Soak your clothing in seawater during the day; this minimizes the loss of body fluid through perspiration. Wipe dried salt off your skin; the salt can cause sores. Let clothing dry before nightfall, when it is likely to be cooler.

• In cold weather, keep warm by huddling together and by regularly moving limbs to maintain blood circulation. Wrap up in as much clothing and blankets as possible.

• Collect rainwater or water that condenses on any cold surfaces on the craft – morning dew, for instance.

• Do not drink seawater, or use it to ease parched lips. Its salt content is three times greater than the amount the body can cope with, and it can cause death.

• If necessary, alleviate thirst by sucking a small object such as a button.

• Do not eat unless you have some water to drink with the food. Digestive processes use up precious body fluid.

Safe canoeing

You can canoe with greater confidence and pleasure once you have learned the basics of safe canoeing. If you are a beginner, you must know how to swim and how to handle yourself if you are unexpectedly thrown into the water. Even when you are an experienced canoeist, always travel in a group – three canoes are an ideal number. If possible, stay close to the shore – never venture beyond a point where you might have trouble getting back safely. Even in calm waters, put on a life jacket in case unexpected hazards arise.

Preparing the canoe
• Take a spare paddle and lash it to the thwarts (seats).
• Attach ropes at least 8 to 15 ft. (2.4 to 4.5 m) long to each end of the canoe. Use the ropes to tie the canoe to a dock or to grab if the canoe capsizes.
• Never overload a canoe. Normally, you should keep any load near the middle. But when you expect to be traveling with the wind, place the load toward the stern. When traveling into the wind, put the load toward the bow.
• If you expect rough water, cover your load with a tarpaulin tied down with a strong rope. Tie your pack to the thwarts. Waterproof all equipment such as sleeping bags.
• Attach a float to your equipment to keep it afloat in case your canoe capsizes.
• Push your canoe out from shore to make sure that it is fully afloat before you enter it. The stern (rear) paddler boards first. When boarding, hold onto the far gunwale with one hand and the near gunwale with the other. Swing into the canoe, putting your feet on the center line of the canoe. Sit or kneel in the center of the canoe until the bow (front) paddler boards. Get out of the canoe in reverse order.
• Never wear heavy boots in a canoe.
• Do not stand up or move around quickly in a canoe.
• Wear a helmet if you intend to canoe on rapidly moving water. If you are canoeing in cold weather – early spring, for example – wear a wet suit.
• Make sure your family, friends or the authorities know your itinerary and estimated time of return before you set out.

If your canoe capsizes
• Stay with a capsized canoe if it is still afloat. Use it as a life preserver to support you in the water. Moreover, it will be easier for rescuers to spot the canoe than a swimmer.
• Abandon your canoe only if this improves your safety. If rescue appears remote or there is danger from rapids or numbing cold water, swim for the nearest shore.
• If your canoe is swamped close to shore, sit in the bottom of the canoe and paddle slowly to shore. If your canoe is swamped in deep water, begin bailing immediately.

• To right a capsized canoe, grip the nearest gunwale, rock the canoe to gain momentum, and then roll it over in the water. The canoe will empty as it turns. Board the canoe from either bow or stern and bail out any remaining water.

If your canoe is caught in a storm
Wind is a more dangerous element than rain for canoeists. Storms with high winds will stir up waves that can swamp and capsize canoes.
• Watch for weather changes and head for the shore if a storm threatens.
• Never cross open water in a canoe during a storm.
• Wait out a storm. If a storm persists, canoe in early morning or evening, when the water is calmer.
• If you are caught in a storm, use short, swift strokes at a slight angle to the waves.
• If you are canoeing on rough water, kneel on the bottom of the canoe to improve the balance. If possible, center any load to allow bow and stern to rise above the waves.
• If your canoe is running with the wind on rough water, improvise a sea anchor – for example, a large cooking pail tied by rope to the stern seat – to improve the balance.
• When you reach shore, find a sheltered spot. If there is nowhere to shelter, turn your canoe over and take refuge under it.

Canoeing on rough water
Never canoe a river until you have studied it on a map (see *Tips for Canoeists and Kayakers*, page 264) and noted any rapids, waterfalls, and other obstructions. Remember that, even on rivers you know well, changing seasonal water levels, fallen trees and other obstacles can create unexpected hazards.

Rivers are graded according to an international coding system for rough water. The grades appear as the letters RW (Rough Water) or WW (Wild or White Water), followed by a number in Roman numerals. Grades I, II and III are easy, medium and difficult respectively. Grade III should be attempted only by expert canoeists. Grades IV to VI are taxing even for the experts, although they might be suitable for experienced kayakers. Many rivers in remote regions of North America have not been graded according to the international coding system. It is advisable to talk to someone who has canoed these rivers before attempting them.

Be alert for sudden increases in current – this may mean rapids ahead. Paddle to shore and investigate. Never shoot rapids if there is any doubt you can do it safely.

Beginners should never run rapids. If you are experienced, go through moderate rapids in single file, far enough apart to avoid collisions and for each canoeist to pick his own route. Severe rapids should be left to accomplished canoeists, and then shot by one group member at a time, with the most experienced going first.

Emergencies in the water

263

Kayaking emergencies

A kayak may have a small or large cockpit for the kayaker to sit in. In types with a small cockpit, kayakers often wear a soft, elasticized spray cover – or spray deck – which fits over the lip of the cockpit and keeps it watertight. There is a strap on the front of the spray cover which releases the cover from the cockpit lip when the strap is pulled.

• If you are thrown out when a kayak overturns, grasp the boat and work your way along to one end, where it is easier to hold on.

• If you are trapped in your seat by a spray cover and you cannot right the kayak at once with your paddle, lean forward underwater and pull the spray cover strap. Get out with a forward roll. If necessary, help yourself out by pushing against the boat just behind your hips.

• Once you are out, work your way along to the end of the hull. Hold onto it.

• Hang onto your paddle as well if you can.

• Do not try to right the kayak, but swim with it downstream across any current to the shore.

• If the land is too far, or you do not think you can reach it, stay with the kayak and wait for someone to rescue you. The boat will support you in the water.

If you are caught in rapids
The noise of falling water and possibly a narrowing of the river are signs that you are approaching rapids. A white line of foam or spray may also be visible, or the water may appear to end unnaturally short of the horizon.

• Beach the kayak well before the rapids, then walk along the bank and try to work out a safe route through them. If there is no safe route through, carry the boat round.

• If you are accidentally caught in the rapids, paddle firmly either forward or backward so that your speed is faster or slower than the water. This will help you to retain control of your course. If you let the water take you at its own speed, you will have no control.

• Areas of white, disturbed water and spray indicate rocks, fallen trees or other obstacles, which may or may not be visible. Avoid them.

• Aim for areas of darker, smoother water between disturbed, white-water patches. The channel will be deeper and safer there.

• If the kayak is swung right round by the current, do not try to turn it back again or you may be carried sideways and hit an obstacle. Continue through the rapids backward, paddling upstream and watching over your shoulder.

• Take bends on the outside if possible. The water is deepest there and flows faster, but be careful not to get swept against trees or banks.

• If the kayak turns round quickly and is caught sideways against a rock, do not let it tilt upstream, or water will flood the cockpit.

• Throw your weight against the rock or obstruction to tilt the boat toward it. Hold the rock and use it to lever yourself and the kayak into a position where you can go forward.

• If this does not work, get out of the kayak quickly. Hang onto the rock and wait for rescue.

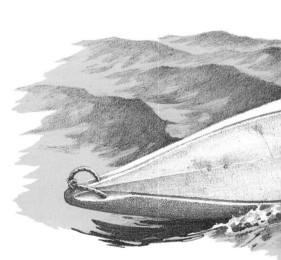

HOW TO GET PAST AN OBSTACLE
If the current sweeps you against a rock, lean downstream to keep water out of the cockpit and push the boat round it with your hands.

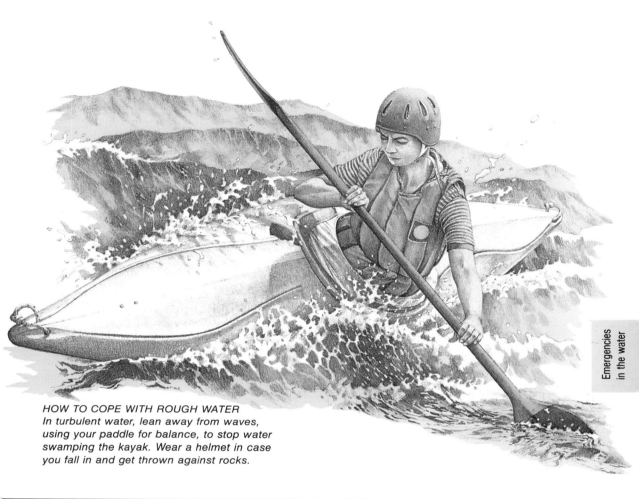

HOW TO COPE WITH ROUGH WATER
In turbulent water, lean away from waves,
using your paddle for balance, to stop water
swamping the kayak. Wear a helmet in case
you fall in and get thrown against rocks.

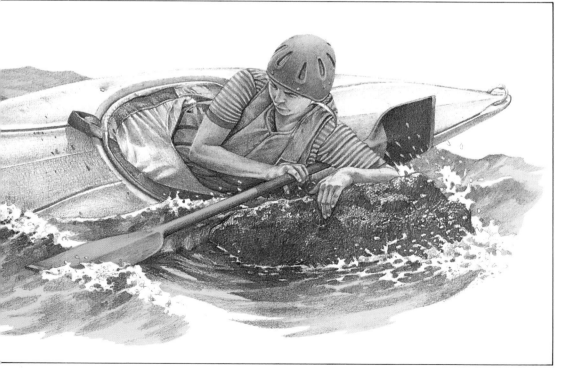

265

Emergencies on vacation and in the country

268   Traveling abroad
272   If your travel firm goes out of business
273   Seeing a doctor overseas
274   Aboard a crashing train or plane
276   Camping out
278   If you are caught in a lightning storm
279   What to do if you encounter a snake
280   Trapped in a bog or quicksand
281   Exposure: the silent killer
282   What to do if you get lost
286   How to use a map and compass
288   Skiing: coping with an accident
290   Crisis underground
292   Survival in the wild

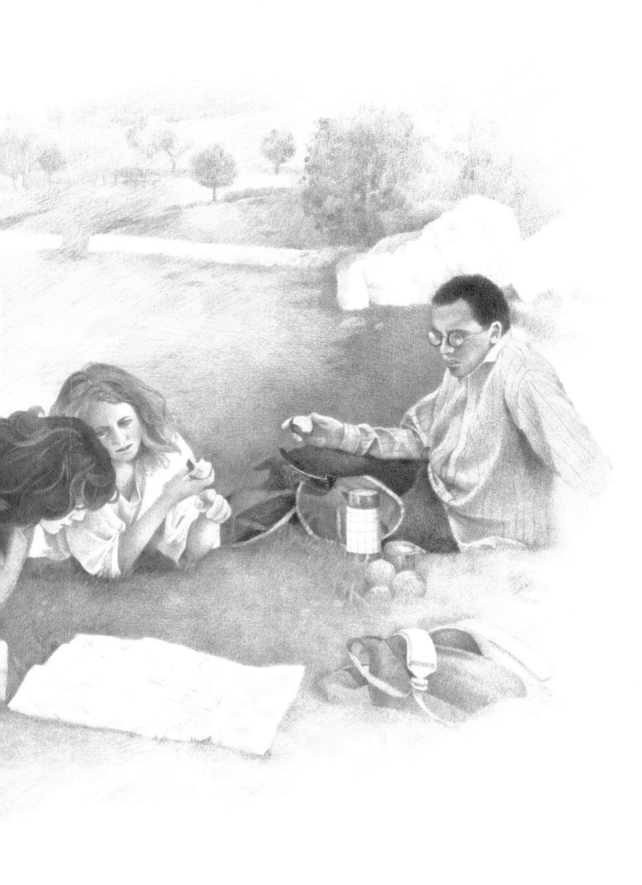

Traveling abroad

Air travel and tour operators have brought some of the most exotic parts of the world within reach of millions of North American vacationers.

But long-distance travel – particularly to tropical or Third World countries – carries special risks and problems as well.

You may, for instance, need to arrange visas or special immunization against tropical diseases. You may need to take with you medicines that are readily available in North America but almost unobtainable in the country you plan to visit. And you will want to see your dentist if you are likely to have difficulty getting dental treatment where you are going.

It is worth thinking, too, about how you should take your spending money – as cash or traveler's checks, for example – about which currency you should take, and about whether it makes sense to take notes and checks in small denominations rather than large ones.

Once you arrive you may also, depending on where you are, have to take precautions against extreme temperatures – heat or cold – or altitude sickness, and to take care about what you eat and drink.

Troubles of this kind are more likely to arise in tropical or Third World countries than in the milder regions of Europe. But some travel problems, such as the collapse of a vacation firm or travel agency, can affect vacationers anywhere (see *If your travel firm goes out of business*, page 272).

Passports and visas

• Make sure your passport or other travel documents will remain valid for the duration of your trip. If there is the slightest chance that you may still be abroad after the expiry date on your passport, get a new one before you leave home.

• Check with the airline or travel agent at the time you book your flight whether you need a visa for the country you plan to visit.

• If you do need a visa, contact the country's embassy or consulate nearest you to find out how to get it. Alternatively, ask a travel agent to make the application for you. Many countries charge a fee for the visa and you may have to supply several passport photographs with your application.

• Allow extra time if you need more than one visa. Your passport will have to go to each embassy or consulate in turn to be stamped with the visa, and some countries can take several weeks to process the application.

• If you plan to visit countries which are politically hostile to each other – Israel and some of the Arab states, for instance – you may save yourself unpleasantness at the frontier by making sure that visas or entry stamps for the opposing countries do not appear in the same passport.

• In circumstances like this, it is sometimes possible to arrange for one or both of the visas to be stamped on separate sheets of paper which can be clipped to your passport and removed after the visit. Ask the consulates or embassies concerned whether they will agree to do this.

• If the offending visa or stamp is the result of an earlier trip, it is also possible simply to surrender your old passport – regardless of how long it has to run – and get a new one.

• If you lose your passport while abroad, try and get a new one immediately. Do not delay, otherwise you may run into trouble with local authorities. An American should apply to the nearest American embassy or consular office. A Canadian should contact the Canadian embassy or consular office or, if there is none, a British consular office, which might provide help.

Immunization

• Find out what the immunization rules are in the country you intend to visit. You can get this information from that country's embassy, consulate or legation. You can also ask your travel agent or airline. Airlines have an interest in keeping you up-to-date about the rules because they can be fined by the government of a country to which they go if you do not have the immunizations that country requires.

• Consult a family doctor. Whatever the formal regulations, it may be prudent to get other shots too, and the doctor can advise you. Knowing your medical history, he or she might also recommend booster shots, alert you to particular health risks, and prescribe preventives such as an antidiarrhea drug or a broad-spectrum antibiotic.

• Check up on immunization long before you travel. For immunization against some diseases you will have to be given two injections at least a week apart and, if you need protection from several diseases, it may not be possible or medically desirable to have all the shots at once.

• You can get all vaccinations (except that for yellow fever) at a doctor's office or clinic, at a health department facility, or at an immunization center. Yellow fever vaccinations are available only at designated centers across the country that have been listed with the World Health Organization. Your vaccinations must be recorded in an international certificate of vaccination, which will be dated, signed by the doctor involved, and validated with an official stamp.

• Immunization may be advisable against any or all of a number of diseases. The main ones are: cholera; hepatitis; poliomyelitis; typhoid; and yellow fever. Smallpox vaccination is no longer necessary for any foreign travel because the World Health Organization has declared the whole world to be free of the disease.

CHOLERA The vaccine gives limited protection. The course is two injections 7-14 days apart.

HEPATITIS (jaundice) Injections give limited protection against hepatitis A and B, which are common in many tropical countries.

POLIOMYELITIS (infantile paralysis) The disease is still common in many parts of the Middle East and North Africa. The vaccine is usually dripped onto a sugar lump which is eaten.

TETANUS If you have never had a shot against tetanus, get one. If you have already been immunized, you will need a booster shot every ten years. Tetanus, often fatal, is caused by bacteria in the soil. They can enter your body if you are cut by a nail in the street or a piece of glass on the beach. The potent toxin they produce attacks nerve cells.

TYPHOID Immunization is advisable for all travelers going to the Mediterranean coastlands, Asia or tropical countries, and is effective for a year. It takes the form of a single injection if time is short, or two injections at least 14 days apart.

YELLOW FEVER The disease, which is confined to the equatorial regions of Africa and the northern, tropical parts of South America, is spread by mosquitoes. Immunization against the disease consists of a single injection which is effective for ten years.

Malaria

Travelers in tropical areas are particularly at risk from malaria, which is spread by the *Anapheles* mosquito. There is no system of immunization, but preventive medicines provide some protection.

• Contact your doctor, who can tell you whether you need protection against malaria. If so, he will prescribe suitable medication. You must start taking an antimalaria drug two weeks before your trip, and keep taking it during your stay in the malarial area and for at least six weeks after you leave it.

• Also get medical advice on a suitable insect repellent to reduce the risk of being bitten.

• Apply insect repellent in the evening, and put on a long-sleeved shirt and long trousers after the sun sets, because malarial mosquitoes fly at night.

• If possible, stay only in air-conditioned hotels. Mosquitoes dislike cool places. If this is not possible, sleep under a mosquito net, and spray your room with insecticide before going to bed. If there is an electric fan in your bedroom, leave it on all night – mosquitoes hate drafts.

Medicines

• If you need prescription drugs regularly, take enough with you to last the entire vacation. Many drugs are unobtainable – or enormously expensive – in other countries.

• For the same reason, consider taking along antidiarrheal medicines and painkillers such as aspirin or acetaminophen.

Money

• If you become ill while you are abroad, you may have to pay on the spot for medical treatment, even if you are covered by Medicare or insurance. Take extra money just in case (see *Seeing a doctor overseas*, page 273).

• Carry minimum amounts of cash on you. Women should carry nothing of value in a handbag. It can easily be snatched.

• Instead, keep passports, travel documents, traveler's checks and other money in a hotel safe.

• If you have to carry valuables on you, use a money belt. Keep a note of your passport number, and its date and place of issue. It will

---

DIARRHEA AND DYSENTERY

Despite precautions, you may come down with traveler's diarrhea – also called La Turista, Montezuma's Revenge, Rangoon Runs, Delhi Belly and other names, depending on where you catch it. It seldom lasts more than three days and is often accompanied by abdominal cramps, loose stools and, sometimes, sweating and vomiting. You can usually treat it successfully yourself.

• Drink enough bottled water to replace lost body fluid. Add a teaspoon of salt to each pint of water. Do not take food or milk drinks.

• Take antidiarrheal medicines.

• When symptoms have settled for a few hours, eat bland food such as dry cookies, jelly, and clear soup. Avoid tea, coffee and acid drinks such as fruit juice because they will further irritate the stomach lining.

Dysentery

Traveler's diarrhea usually creates only a few days' discomfort and inconvenience. Dysentery is much harsher. There are two forms, one caused by bacteria and one caused by an ameba. The amebic form is more serious, but the symptoms of both kinds of dysentery are the same: severe diarrhea and vomiting; stools often streaked with blood, pus or mucus; and gripping pains, tenderness and swelling in the abdomen. The symptoms usually appear 6–48 hours after eating infected food.

• See a doctor if the symptoms are severe, persistent or getting rapidly worse; if the disease was contracted in a country where amebic dysentery is known to occur; or if blood or mucus occur in the stools. Otherwise, treat as for traveler's diarrhea.

speed the process of getting a new passport if yours is lost or stolen abroad.

• Keep a separate note of each credit card number so that you can tell the company at once – by phone or telegram – if you lose it.

• If you take traveler's checks, get them from a firm which has offices in the country you are visiting and which guarantees to replace them within a day or so if they are lost or stolen.

• Buy insurance against the risk of your cash being lost or stolen. But remember, insurance companies will usually refund the lost money only after you have returned home, not during the vacation.

• A travel agent or airline can tell you which currencies (besides the local one) are readily accepted in the country you plan to visit.

• During the vacation, shop around for the best rate of exchange. Hotels often give poor rates compared to banks, for instance. Some gift shops will accept payment in foreign currency at better-than-official rates.

• Buy any international travel tickets you need – particularly air tickets – before you leave home. Immigration authorities in many Third World countries insist on travelers having a ticket to take them out of the country. If, on arrival, you do not have a return or onward ticket, you may be detained and then deported on the next flight out of the country. You may have to pay for the ticket in foreign currency at a worse exchange rate than you might have received in different circumstances.

• If you are visiting a country with a high rate of inflation, such as Israel or some South American countries, take U.S. dollars in small-denomination bank notes and traveler's checks. Exchange rates in these countries can change on a daily basis, so converting only small amounts in the local currency each day can make your money go significantly further.

• Many Third World nations have strict regulations governing how much of their local currency can be taken into or out of their country. Check with the country's embassy or consulate before you leave on your trip.

• Toward the end of your vacation, reduce the amount of local cash you have. It may not be possible or permissible to change local currency back into dollars before you leave, and the currency may have little value back home.

Clothing

• In hot and humid climates, clothes should absorb sweat, be loose-fitting, and reflect the sunlight. They should, therefore, be lightweight and light in color.

• Cotton is the best material for hot-weather clothing. It is capable of absorbing 50 percent of its weight in water. Avoid drip-dry clothes and man-made fibers, particularly next to the skin. They have little ability to absorb moisture, encouraging prickly heat (see page 107).

• Take a lightweight hat and sunglasses for protection against hot sunshine and glare. In areas where snakes are likely, wear boots, not open sandals.

• In frigid climates, layers of loose-fitting clothes trap pockets of insulating air and allow you to add or subtract a layer if you become too cold or too hot.

• Wool is best for underlayers and headgear. If woolen clothing bothers your skin, wear cotton under wool. Outerwear should repel wind and water. Some fabrics not only do this, but also let body moisture escape, keeping inner clothing dryer.

• If you plan to spend much time outdoors in subzero temperatures, take long thermal underwear; woolen gloves (or better still, mitts) to wear under a pair of water-repellent gloves or mitts; waterproof footwear that is roomy enough for two pairs of socks; and a down-filled or similarly insulated parka with a hood.

How to treat motion sickness

Seasickness, car sickness, air sickness – all are the same affliction, and about nine out of ten people suffer from it at some time or other. The symptoms include nausea, vomiting, sweating, faintness, pallor and diarrhea.

• If you feel sick, put your head back and hold it still. Lie flat, if you can, without a pillow.

• Use motion sickness medication.

• If you travel by air, try to get an aisle seat in the middle of the plane, over the wings.

• Get some fresh air – go up on deck if you are

PREVENTING MOTION SICKNESS

If you have been prone to motion sickness or fear you may succumb to it on an upcoming trip, see your doctor. Depending on the state of your health, he or she may prescribe a drug to prevent or relieve such sickness. The drug could be in the form of pills – antiemetic, antihistamine, or a combination of both – or scopolamine skin patches to be worn behind the ears.

Since such medications can cause drowsiness, impair driving performance and add to the effects of alcohol, do not drive or operate machinery until the effects of the medication have worn off. This may be from four to six hours after taking a pill.

Pregnant or breast-feeding women, the elderly, and those with a medical disorder or taking medicines should consult a doctor before using any motion sickness drug, even an over-the-counter product.

on a boat, or keep the car window open and make regular stops.

• Look out of the front of the car. Watching to the side at objects flashing past windows can make nausea worse.

• Do not attempt to read or write during a car journey.

• Eat small, easily digested meals before and during your journey.

• Take small amounts of fluid regularly to avoid dehydration.

• Stay away from smokers – particularly if you are a nonsmoker. The smell may make you feel more queasy.

Food and drink

Numerous tropical and subtropical diseases are transmitted by food and drink which have been infected by bacteria or contaminated by flies or unhygienic handling. The diseases include cholera, hepatitis and dysentery. You can minimize the risks by following the guidelines suggested here.

• Avoid drinking milk or water from the faucet, unless they have been thoroughly boiled. Black tea or coffee, for instance, is likely to be safe to drink.

• Avoid unbottled cold drinks, ice cream and ice for the same reason. Freezing does not kill bacterial contamination – it merely suspends it until the ice melts. Cold carbonated drinks in bottles are, however, usually safe.

• Avoid uncooked foods such as shellfish, shrimps, salads, locally prepared mayonnaise, raw vegetables and peeled fruit. They may have been fished from or washed in contaminated water, made with contaminated milk, or contaminated by handling. Fruit you peel yourself, however, is safe to eat.

• Avoid eating food that has not been thoroughly cooked – preferably boiled or baked – just before serving. Underdone pork in particular is unsafe.

• Do not eat leftovers or any foods that may have been out on a buffet table for a long time. Avoid cold hors d'oeuvres and dips.

Altitude sickness – how to treat it

Climbing too high or too quickly in the mountains, or traveling in an unpressurized aircraft, can cause altitude sickness because of the reduced level of oxygen in the air.

A mild attack of altitude sickness brings breathlessness, palpitations, headache, loss of appetite and insomnia. The symptoms of severe altitude sickness – which can cause serious lung damage if left untreated – are dizziness, nausea, vomiting, convulsions, severe thirst, weakness, drowsiness, blurred vision and hearing difficulties.

People usually begin to be afftected on mountains over 10,000 ft. (3,000 m), but the symptoms can occur at as low as 6,500 ft. (2,000 m).

• If you get a mild attack of altitude sickness,

HOW TO AVOID SUNBURN

• Avoid the sun as much as possible, especially between 10 a.m. and 2 p.m. If you must spend time in the sun, keep well covered, and limit yourself to no more than half an hour the first day, an hour the second and so on, adding 30 minutes each day.

• Use a sunscreen with an SPF (Sun Protection Factor) of 10 to 15, preferably one that contains PABA (para-aminobenzoic acid) and benzophenone. Apply it 30 minutes before you go into the sun and reapply every two hours or after you swim or perspire heavily.

• Remember that burning rays can penetrate clouds, water and loosely woven clothing. Even when you are in the shade, rays reflected from sand, water and snow can burn you.

---

avoid all strenuous exercise until you become acclimatized. Go to bed and rest. The symptoms usually disappear on their own in 24-48 hours.

• If the symptoms do not ease in that time, or if they are severe, get medical help.

• Take a few breaths from an oxygen canister, if one is available. It will relieve a mild attack, and may help even in a severe attack.

• If no medical help is available and severe symptoms persist, the only solution is to descend to a lower altitude at once. The symptoms will ease automatically as you lose height.

• Spend a few days at a lower level before trying to climb again. Ascend in easy stages, acclimatizing at each level before going higher.

When the sun is an enemy

Too much exposure to the sun can cause painful burns, premature aging of the skin, and even skin cancer. Darker skins respond more readily to sunlight than fair skins, by producing a brown pigment (melanin) which screens out harmful rays. Freckled skins are particularly prone to solar burns because their melanin does not spread evenly. Severe cases of sunburn need treatment (see page 135).

Greater care is needed as you get closer to the Equator, and in mountains, where thin air filters the sun's rays less than the more absorbent atmosphere at lower levels.

Too much heat – in or out of direct sunlight – can induce heat exhaustion, heat cramp and, more dangerous, heatstroke, which can kill (see *Heat exhaustion and heatstroke,* page 106).

The main defenses: wear a hat that shades the back of the neck and drink plenty of water. In extreme conditions take salt tablets as well.

Emergencies on vacation and in the country

If your travel firm goes out of business

Vacationers traveling on package tours could find themselves stranded abroad if the tour operator or airline they are booked with goes belly-up during their vacation. But there are ways to minimize the impact such a bankruptcy could have on your pocketbook and travel plans.

• Deal with a business that belongs to the American Society of Travel Agents (ASTA) or the Alliance of Canadian Travel Associations (ACTA). Such a firm will have met strict requirements to become a member and must follow an equally strict code of ethics.

• Buy your tour package from a travel agent who participates in the ASTA Tour Protection Plan. Then, if the tour operator collapses, your deposit will be safe, provided the operator is also a plan participant. But the plan covers your deposit only, not any other losses you may suffer as a consequence of such a collapse.

• The best way to cover yourself against the costs of a botched vacation is through insurance. Some travel firms include cover for these expenses as part of a standard insurance package they offer travelers. The insurance policy will explain exactly what costs are covered. Alternatively, get advice from an insurance broker, your travel agent, or one or more insurance companies.

• Keep receipts for all expenses you incur. If you have to organize any part of your trip on your own, keep all booking documents and ticket stubs. You will need them to claim a refund from the insurance company.

• Take extra money or make sure you will have enough extra credit limit on your credit cards for any travel emergencies. Even if you are fully insured, you may have to pay certain bills on the spot and claim the money back later. Your hotel, for example, may demand payment for your room and meals – even though you have already paid the travel firm.

If your airline goes out of business

If you travel on a package tour, the tour operator remains responsible for looking after you should any airline it uses go out of business. It is the operator's responsibility to find a replacement airline or to compensate you if it cannot. If you have bought your ticket direct from the airline, however, you may have to find some other way of reaching your destination. You are very unlikely to get the full cost of your ticket back from the failed airline.

• Take your ticket to another airline flying the route you want to travel, and ask the airline to book you onto one of its flights. Airlines that are members of the International Air Transport Association (IATA) will usually accept tickets issued by other member airlines, and may accept tickets from nonmember airlines as well. But they are not obliged to.

• If you cannot persuade another airline to accept your existing ticket, you will probably have to pay for a new ticket yourself. If you are insured against this possibility, though, you will be able to claim all or part of the cost of the new ticket from the insurance company later.

If you miss your plane

If you arrive at the airport and discover that you have missed your plane, go immediately to the airline check-in desk for help. Whether you will be able to get on another flight depends on what type of ticket you have.

If you have paid full fare, your ticket will be valid for a year and will not restrict you to a specific flight. A charter, special excursion or cheap ticket is likely to have a number of conditions attached to it. Restrictions such as "Valid only for flights and dates shown" will be written on the ticket.

• Show your ticket to the person at the check-in desk and explain what has happened. Ask to be put on the next available flight.

• If you have an unrestricted ticket, the airline is obliged to put you on the first flight with seats available, possibly with another airline.

• If the next few flights are fully booked, ask for a connecting flight to another airport and get a flight to your destination from there.

• If you have bought a cheap ticket, the airline will probably do its best to help, but may not be able to do much for you if, for example, the flight you just missed is a special charter, and your ticket restricts you to that flight and the return charter a week later. And you will lose out on the return part of your ticket as well, unless you can find a way to get to your vacation destination on your own.

• When you buy a special charter or similarly restricted airline ticket, ask about insurance that will cover at least part of the cost of alternative arrangements if you miss a flight you were booked on.

• The only reliable way to avoid the risk of missing a flight and perhaps having to buy a new ticket is to give yourself plenty of time to reach the airport.

If your journey is held up

If bad weather, technical faults or labor disputes delay your journey overseas, the airline, rail, ferry or bus company you have booked with will often offer refreshments during the delay. The company may also provide hotel accommodation if you are forced to wait overnight.

On a package tour – where you have booked with a tour operator rather than directly with a transport company – the same principles apply. The operator will usually look after vacationers held up at docks or airports. But it is not obliged to unless its booking conditions contain a promise to do so.

If the booking conditions do not contain such a promise, consider buying insurance to cover the costs of delays. Many firms include this cover in their standard package.

Seeing a doctor overseas

There is not much to be said for being sick at any time, in any place. But falling ill in some exotic vacation spot halfway round the world can be much more frightening than falling ill at home, with a family doctor just a phone call away and a reputable hospital nearby.

In some parts of the world, you could have problems finding an English-speaking doctor whose medical training, skills and standards are comparable to those you would expect at home. If you are traveling outside North America to a foreign-language country, be sure you know where you are likely to find reliable, English-speaking medical help. Ask your doctor for advice, or better still, write to the International Association for Medical Assistance to Travelers (see box).

The cost of medical treatment in some places can be surprisingly high. For example, a doctor who visits your Paris hotel room and gives you a shot for an infected throat might charge you as much as $100.

Even though you are covered at home by a government or private health insurance plan, do not count on it reimbursing you fully for medical or hospital expenses you incur abroad. Most plans set a strict fee schedule, and if your away-from-home medical bill exceeds some limit in your insurance plan, you may be out of pocket.

The safest way to guard against the expense of an accident or illness while you are traveling is to buy travel medical insurance before you leave home. Such an insurance policy will meet costs beyond those covered by your regular health scheme. It will also cover the cost of getting you home if you are ill, and can even cover nonmedical costs for such things as car repairs after a crash or making alternative travel arrangements.

Major bills – for a stay in hospital, say – may be settled by the insurance company direct. Smaller bills, however, for a visit to a doctor or a dentist, or for medicine, will usually have to be paid on the spot, and the money reclaimed after you return home.

Getting medical treatment

• If you need medical help while you are staying in a hotel, ask the manager or someone at the front desk to get in touch with the physician on call. For certain problems, a specialist can often be called. Hotel management can also arrange to get you to a hospital if need be.
• If you are staying in lodgings other than a hotel and cannot locate a doctor, telephone the police or the nearest hospital and ask them to recommend a physician who will see you within a specified time, depending on the urgency of your problem.
• You can get advice and help at Travelers' Aid booths in major railroad stations, bus terminals and airports in many North American cities. Personnel can direct you to the nearest doctor or medical facility and may even arrange an appointment for you. Similar societies operate in some countries abroad. Although the "aid" is generally free, a contribution is always welcome from those who can afford it.
• In a medical emergency, ask the police to help you get to a hospital, or call an emergency number for an ambulance. In large American and Canadian cities, the emergency number is 911. There are similar numbers to call in many other countries.

Medical insurance

Insurance against medical emergencies abroad can be bought through travel agents, automobile clubs and credit card companies, or direct from insurance firms. It is often included in a package covering trip cancellation and lost or stolen baggage and money. The policy will make clear which risks are covered, and for how much. Some travel insurance packages now include unlimited medical cover for little more than the standard premium.

• Make a copy of the policy or certificate to leave at home, and take the original with you on vacation as evidence that you are covered (a photostat copy may not be acceptable). Show it to the hospital or doctor you see, if you want to delay paying the bill until you get home.
• When you buy the policy, check how soon you have to notify the company if you need to make a claim. The policy may require you to phone or send a telegram as soon as possible – not when you get home.
• If you have to pay on the spot, get a receipt and send it to the insurance company with your claim form when you get home.

> ## WORLDWIDE HELP FOR AILING TRAVELERS
>
> Membership in the nonprofit International Association for Medical Assistance to Travelers (IAMAT) entitles you to an annually updated pocket directory of some 500 IAMAT centers around the world (even in some remote spots). You can call these centers to be referred to an IAMAT-approved, English-speaking doctor who will not charge you more than IAMAT's published fee scale.
>
> You will also get charts and pamphlets covering a range of health matters of concern to the traveler.
>
> Membership is free, but you will be asked to consider a donation. In the United States, write to 417 Center Street, Lewiston, New York, 14092. The address in Canada is 188 Nicklin Road, Guelph, Ontario, N1H 7L5.

Emergencies on vacation and in the country

273

Aboard a crashing train or plane

Train and plane crashes often seem more terrifying than a car crash because they involve such large numbers of people.

In fact, your chances of being injured in a train or plane are far smaller than your chances of being hurt in a road accident.

If your train crashes

There is unlikely to be much warning before a train crash, but you might feel the emergency brakes go on and, in the seconds before impact, be able to take up a safer position.

• Get clear of windows and doors. Throw yourself to the floor, if necessary. Hang on to anything fixed to prevent yourself being thrown out of the car.

• Brace yourself against anything solid.

• Tuck your chin onto your chest to protect your neck against the risk of whiplash injury.

• If you are sitting with your back to the engine, away from windows and doors, stay put.

• If you are not sitting with your back to the engine, away from windows and doors, move into this position if you can, but do not risk being caught unsupported when the impact comes.

• Do not try to jump out of the train, even if it careers for some distance off the tracks. While you remain in the train, the car will absorb some of the crash impact. If you jump out, your body hitting the tracks will receive the full force. There may also be a danger from a live rail or other hazards – broken equipment, for example. A broken train battery could create a pool of acid which would be indistinguishable from a rain puddle.

• Once the train has come to rest, assess the situation. In a busy area, or if the train is in a tunnel, it may be best to stay put until official help comes. Wandering outside the train may expose you to further dangers, particularly since you are likely to be in a state of shock after a crash.

• If there is a live rail, do not get out of the train until you are told by rail staff that the current has been turned off.

• The windows of modern cars on long-distance trains have double-thick, shatterproof glass, which may not break even if the car turns over. If an accident blocks all regular exits, and you need to get out through a window, find one specially designed as an emergency exit. It will have a release handle, and the instructions for opening it will be posted nearby.

If a train door swings open

Some railroad cars in Britain and other countries have compartments, each with its own outward-opening door. Leaning out of a moving train to close such a door is dangerous – you could be jolted out of your train or hit by one coming in the opposite direction.

• If you find a door open on a moving train, do not try to shut it. Move well away from it, and get others to do the same.

• Notify a guard or, if this is not possible, pull the emergency cord. Do not do anything else; let the train staff deal with the problem.

If your plane crashes

Being frightened of flying is a common and understandable problem among air passengers. Doctors believe that the fear is often related to the fear of being helpless if things go wrong, or the fear of being in a confined space. If the fear is serious, ask your doctor's advice. Otherwise, keep reminding yourself that air travel is safer than motoring.

The riskiest part of any journey by air is the beginning and the end; six out of ten plane crashes happen on takeoff or landing.

So listen carefully when the cabin crew brief you on emergency procedures at the start of the flight, and make yourself familiar with safety features such as exits before the plane leaves the ground.

• Identify the emergency exit nearest to your seat. Memorize its position and how to open it – the instructions will be on the door. In the aftermath of a crash, you might have to find and open it in thick smoke.

• Read the emergency procedures card in the seat pocket in front.

• In the event of an emergency, follow the instructions of the cabin crew. They are highly trained in emergency procedures.

TRAPPED UNDER A BURNING ENGINE
On February 26, 1984, a Pittsburgh-bound freight crashed into the rear of another freight stopped ahead. At impact, conductor Charles Hazlett, 51, jumped from the engine cab to the catwalk. The derailed engine, its front end engulfed in the flames from a ruptured tank car, tottered for a moment and then tipped onto its side.

Beneath the overturned locomotive, Hazlett lay flat on his back, his foot pinned by a handrail, and his face just inches below the blistering hot side of the engine. Over the roar of the blaze, he could hear the gurgle of leaking diesel fuel and feel it soaking his jacket and trousers.

His only hope, risky as it seemed, was to immerse as much of his body as he could in the cool liquid. He knew the fuel was not as flammable as gasoline, especially when chilled – and the ground was frozen.

He began digging a hole, tearing fist-size ballast rocks from the rail bed. As the hollow filled with diesel, he heaped stones around him almost to the side of the engine, leaving enough of an opening to let in fresh air being drawn past him by the flames. Then, his face buried in his arms to avoid the nauseating fumes, he prayed.

Hazlett's perilous fuel bath insulated him from the searing heat long enough for rescuers to locate him and, after heroic efforts, free him and get him to a hospital.

• If instructed, remove eyeglasses, dentures and high-heeled shoes. Also remove sharp objects such as pens and pencils from your pockets.

• If there is smoke in the aircraft, protect your nose and mouth with a handkerchief. Wet the handkerchief, if possible. Keep near the floor when moving to the emergency exit.

• Escape slides inflate automatically when the door is opened. Jump onto the slide in a seated position.

• When you reach the ground, move well away from the aircraft. Do not attempt to go back for personal belongings.

• If you or someone else has been injured, tell one of the crew. They are trained in first aid, and have the equipment necessary for dealing with victims.

HOW TO STAY COMFORTABLE IN THE AIR

• Choose your flight schedule carefully. If you are traveling east or west across time zones, plan to arrive at your destination late in the afternoon or early in the evening by local clocks so that you can get to bed shortly after arrival.

• Plan to arrive early at the airport and give yourself plenty of time to get there. More heart attacks occur at airports than during flight. This is due chiefly to passengers panicking on late arrival (see *If you miss your plane*, page 272).

• If you have a choice of seats, try to get as far forward in the plane as possible. The ride will be more comfortable there, which is why first-class compartments are always at the front. Noise and vibration tend to be worst near the tail. There is no evidence, though, that where you sit makes any difference to your safety in the event of a crash.

• Wear casual, loose-fitting clothes and shoes for the flight. Sitting upright for long hours may cause stomach, ankles and feet to swell, and make tight clothes uncomfortable.

• Carry a comfortable sweater to slip on or off. Temperatures may change even on a short flight. On a longer flight, climatic conditions may vary enormously. When it is winter in North America, for instance, it is summer in Australia. Think about climatic changes at refueling stops, and dress appropriately for the weather. Note the local time at these stops; a desert airport at night can be surprisingly chilly. Pack toiletries in your carry-on luggage, so that you can freshen up en route.

• Avoid smoking, or, if you are a compulsive smoker, cut it down. Smokers are more affected by high altitudes than nonsmokers, because tobacco smoke hinders the body's ability to absorb oxygen. In flight, the oxygen level in the air inside the plane – which is usually pressurized to the equivalent of an altitude of 6,000-7,000 ft. (1,830-2,130 m) – is lower than when on the ground.

• If you experience popping in the ears, do not worry. It is perfectly normal and occurs as air in the middle ear adjusts to the air pressure in the cabin. To clear your ears on the ascent, swallow; on the descent, shut your mouth, hold your nose and try to blow out gently. Try to avoid flying if you have a heavy cold or sinus problems, but if you have to fly, use a nasal decongestant.

• Make a point of drinking plenty of liquid during a long flight. Aim to consume 4-5 pints (2-3 liters) of liquid every 24 hours. At high altitudes, the aircraft cabin air is extremely dry, and you lose fluid which must be replaced if you are to avoid increased fatigue and dehydration. The best drinks are water and fruit juice.

• Avoid alcohol, because it dehydrates the body. Coffee and tea also tend to dehydrate, so drink them sparingly.

• Aircraft meals help to relieve the boredom of a long international flight. But try to time your meals so that they conform to your normal eating pattern. If your internal clock says it is 2 a.m., it is best to avoid a meal because your gastrointestinal system has largely shut down for the night. If you do want something, drink water or fruit juice.

• Sleep as much as you can on a long flight. Even dozing or taking short naps will help to minimize jet lag – the disorientation caused by crossing several time zones.

• Travel sickness (see page 270) is rarely experienced today on large jet aircraft. They rapidly penetrate bad weather and cruise high above it, so the effects of motion and acceleration are minimal.

• If you are prone to travel sickness, try to get a seat away from the windows and in the middle of the aircraft, where there is the least motion.

• If you use travel-sickness pills, take the first dose 30 minutes before takeoff, and others at recommended intervals thereafter. Remember, though, never drink alcohol if you are taking pills such as antihistamines. They also cause drowsiness, and should be avoided if you plan to drive at the end of the flight.

Emergencies on vacation and in the country

Camping out

Modern tents are compact, strong and light. But they can be as vulnerable as any other shelter – to wind, rain, snow and fire.

If you are caught in a burning tent
• Get out fast if your tent catches fire. As you go, beware of pieces of burning fabric – brush them off if they fall on you, and smother the flames with clothes or a sleeping bag, which will not be damaged if you work quickly.
• Once outside, collapse the tent poles and, if necessary, the main guy ropes. Then stamp out the flames.
• If your tent has no waterproof flooring, grab it by the end furthest from the fire, and pull it clear of your equipment inside.
• If the fire is too fierce to approach, though, let it burn. Equipment can be replaced; your life cannot.

• If the cause of the fire is a blazing stove near the tent, push or kick it clear before collapsing the tent poles.
• When the fire is out, pour water over the area around the blaze to stop undergrowth catching fire.
• Try to keep the fire away from any foam rubber or plastic mat being used as a sleeping pad. Many of these materials give off poisonous fumes when they burn.

If the tent leaks
• If rain or melting snow finds its way into the tent, try to block up the holes by pressing warm candle wax or sticky tape onto the fabric from the inside or outside. Alternatively, run a finger down the inside of the tent from the site of the leak to divert the drips.
• If the leaks persist, protect clothes and sleep-

EMERGENCY EXIT

1 *A sleeping bag can become a dangerous trap in a sudden crisis – if a campfire sets fire to the tent, for example. To get out of a sleeping bag safely and quickly, do not waste time trying to unzip it. First, sit up and push the sleeping bag down around you as far as your waist.*

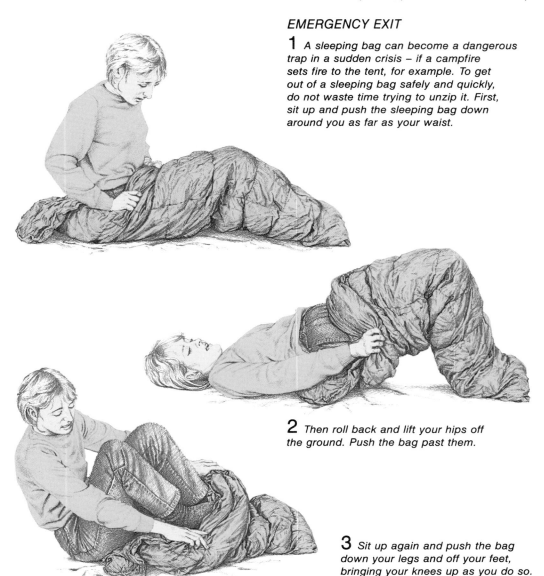

2 *Then roll back and lift your hips off the ground. Push the bag past them.*

3 *Sit up again and push the bag down your legs and off your feet, bringing your knees up as you do so.*

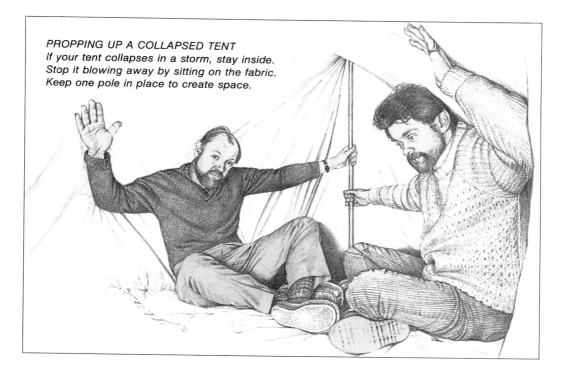

PROPPING UP A COLLAPSED TENT
If your tent collapses in a storm, stay inside. Stop it blowing away by sitting on the fabric. Keep one pole in place to create space.

ing bags with a waterproof jacket or a large sheet of plastic.

If the tent is flooded

The safest course of action in a flood depends on what your sleeping bag is made of. A down-filled bag loses its insulation properties if it gets soaked. The safest course in this situation is to abandon tent and bag and make for somewhere dry.
• If there is no shelter nearby, make a platform – of branches, say – and sit out the night in your driest clothes.
• In very cold weather, preserve body heat by not using the sleeves of the top one or two layers of clothes. Instead, button or zip the clothes up; then work them down over your head and body. Fold your arms under the cocoon, tucking your hands into your armpits.
• Sleeping bags that are filled with synthetic material retain warmth even when wet. The safest course then is to prevent any further water coming in – perhaps by digging a channel around the tent to divert the flow. Mop out the tent, wring out the bag and stay put.

If the tent blows down

• Repitching a collapsed tent in high winds is very difficult. In severe weather, if there is no other shelter – a car, say – stay inside the tent.
• Use the weight of your body on the edges of the tent or on the sewn-in groundsheet to stop the tent being blown away.
• Make some space inside by propping up the fabric with a backpack or one of the tent poles.

PITCHING CAMP

Setting up a campsite carefully can minimize the risk of things going wrong.
• Pick a site on firm, flat ground away from river banks and dried-up water-courses.
• Pick a spot that is sheltered from the wind. Test the site for concealed stones by lying down on the ground.
• Pitch the tent so that its doorway faces away from the wind. Pull the fabric taut so rain will run off, but not so taut that you strain the fabric and stitching.
• If rain is expected, dig channels under the edge of the tent roof and across any slope above the tent to carry water away.
• When high winds are likely, rest heavy stones on the pegs and flaps.
• Always keep some ventilation – especially if, in bad weather, you decide to do your cooking inside. If you start to feel drowsy, or a stove burns with a yellow flame rather than a blue one, it may mean that there is insufficient oxygen. Get out into the open at once.
• Anchor a stove to the ground with tent pegs to stabilize it while it is in use. When it is not being used, store it and any fuel containers away from the tent. Do your cooking outside if at all possible.

Emergencies on vacation and in the country

If you are caught in a lightning storm

When lightning comes to earth, it tends to strike the highest point around and to travel to earth along the line of least resistance.

Tall, isolated trees and buildings are particularly vulnerable. But people can be targets too, either because they are themselves the tallest object in the area, or because they are in contact with, or close to, something struck by lightning. Every year in North America, at least one hundred people are killed by lightning.

• If your skin tingles and you feel your hair stand on end during a thunderstorm, it means that a lightning strike may be imminent.

• If you are in an open area, drop to the ground. This lessens the risk that you will be struck.

• If you are near tall objects, such as trees or boulders, get away from them quickly if you can.

• Make for low, level ground and kneel down.

• If you cannot get away from tall objects, kneel on something dry – a wooden board, for example. Keep your feet on the dry material and off the ground. It is important that the material you kneel on should be dry. Wet objects provide no insulation and thus no advantage, because water is a good conductor of electricity.

• When you kneel, keep your feet and knees close together. Bend over and lower your head – which is the most vulnerable part of your body – to your knees.

• Do not put down a hand to steady yourself. This will make double contact with the ground and expose you to greater risks.

If someone is struck by lightning

A lightning strike is not necessarily fatal. If the lightning has already struck a nearby tree or house and spent its force, a person may escape with only shock and minor burns.

Lightning is most likely to kill if it strikes the head and passes through the torso on its way to earth. In such circumstances it is more likely to cause heart failure or asphyxiation.

Lightning may also cause severe burns, broken bones – because of muscular spasms caused by the shock – and cuts. In addition, the victim's clothing may catch fire and metal ornaments or watch straps may melt.

• If the victim's clothing is on fire, lay him down on the ground at once to keep the flames away from his face. Otherwise he could die from lack of air or from burns caused by breathing in the flames.

• If necessary – if, say, he is panicking and not responding to your instructions – trip him or knock him over, taking care as you do this not to get burned yourself.

• Put out the flames quickly by dousing them with water or wrapping the person in a heavy coat or blanket.

• Treat as for electric shock (see page 93).

• Get medical attention immediately – even if the victim appears to be unhurt.

• Reassure him and keep him warm and comfortable until help arrives.

SAFETY DURING A THUNDERSTORM

Your chances of getting struck by lightning during a thunderstorm are extremely small. Nevertheless, lightning is not an entirely predictable phenomenon, and it is worth taking precautions to cut the risk still further.

• Get off high ground, such as the brow of a hill, and away from tall trees.

• Do not take cover in cave mouths, rockface overhangs or recesses under boulders. They create spark gaps across which lightning can arc on its way to earth, striking anyone there. A deep cave is, however, safe; go right to the back.

• Keep well away from metal fences and other metal objects. Lightning does not have to strike directly to kill. Subsidiary flashes can arc out sideways from the main spark across several yards. In addition, the enormously high temperature of the bolt heats the air along its path explosively, causing shock waves. At a distance, these shock waves are audible as thunder. But close by, they are powerful enough to crush the lungs.

• If you are swimming or in a small boat, make for the shore at once. If you are in a larger boat, the crew should go below deck and the helmsman should avoid touching anything metal.

• Never fly a kite, ride a bicycle or ride a horse in a thunderstorm.

• If you are driving, stay in your car. It is one of the safest places to be. If lightning does strike, it will flash over the surface of the vehicle – which is virtually a metal cage – and run harmlessly to earth.

• In general, buildings offer good protection, but avoid isolated barns, sheds and huts.

• At home, unplug the TV. If you have a roof antenna, disconnect it, too.

• Outdoors, rubber-soled shoes or rubber boots may offer some protection, but they are no guarantee of safety.

• The traditional belief that you should close your windows during a thunderstorm is of only limited value. It is unlikely that lightning would strike through an open window or any other opening.

• Lightning may enter a house through anything that conducts electricity. Do not handle electrical appliances during a storm, and stay away from all parts of the plumbing system. It is also not advisable to use the telephone during a thunderstorm.

What to do if you encounter a snake

Most snakes are timid creatures that attack only when startled or cornered. Even a poisonous snake will usually slither away before you get near it. But if you are bitten, you have a good chance of surviving. Although about 10,000 people are treated for snakebite each year in North America, only a dozen or so die. Nevertheless, snakebite victims can suffer crippling injuries to their limbs.

Snakes are cold-blooded creatures that seek hot places when it is cool. They will bask on sun-bathed rocks and ledges. When it is hot, they are found under rocks, logs, or leaf piles. They also occupy caves, crevices, shady ravines, swamps or rivers.

Although many of the snakes you might encounter are harmless, all should be treated with extreme caution. If poisonous snakes are found in your area, learn to recognize them and to know their behavior and habitats.

• If you go walking in areas where snakes are likely, keep to paths and wear hiking boots and long pants to protect your feet and ankles – the commonest targets of a striking snake.
• In the woods, never step over logs without first looking on the other side. If you plan to sit in the shade, first examine the ground carefully for snakes.
• In rocky areas, watch for snakes lying on ledges above or below your path. Never place your hand on a surface that you cannot see.
• If you see any snake, stop at once and move quickly to at least 20 ft. (6 m) from it.
• If you do get bitten, clean the wound and bandage it firmly. Keep the injured limb low (see *Snakebite,* page 125).
• If you have killed the snake, bring it to the hospital. Be careful: a dead snake can still bite from reflex. If possible, decapitate the snake and bury the head under a log or a rock.

POISONOUS SNAKES

Most poisonous snakes in North America are pit vipers. In the United States, they include rattlesnakes, copperheads, and cottonmouths. All have arrow-shaped heads and indentations between their slitlike eyes. Rattlesnakes have rattles at the tips of their tails. Both the copperhead *and the rattlesnake are widely distributed. The cottonmouth is found mostly in the South. The deadliest snakes are the coral snakes, which range from North Carolina to California. They have wide bands of red and black separated by narrow rings of bright yellow encircling their bodies.*

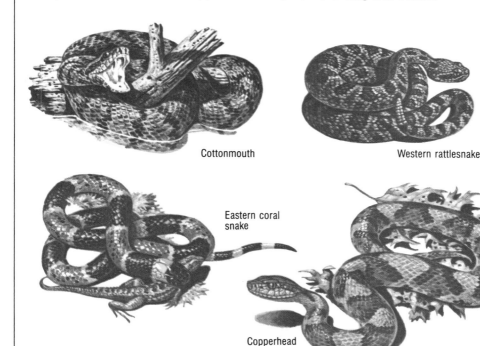

Cottonmouth

Western rattlesnake

Eastern coral snake

Copperhead

Trapped in a bog or quicksand

Hazardous bogs and quicksands are found on both high and low ground. And they can be lethal to the unsuspecting walker. The principle of surviving is the same whichever you fall into: spread your body weight as widely as possible, and move very slowly.

• As soon as you realize that you are stuck in a bog or quicksand, discard your backpack or anything else that might drag you down.

• Fall as gently as you can onto your back, spreading your arms wide as you drop. Spreading your weight in this way will enable you effectively to stay afloat on the surface.

• Make all your movements – including getting your feet back to the surface – deliberate and extremely slow. You have to allow time for the mud or sand to flow around your limbs as you move. Quick movements only create pockets of vacuum in the mud or sand, which will tend to suck you deeper.

• If you are with a companion, lie still. Wait until he or she throws you a line or holds out a pole to you.

• Use long, firm pulls to haul yourself out of the mire. Frantic jerks will be less effective and will tire you more quickly.

• If you are alone, stay on your back and use your arms and legs as paddles with a breast-stroke movement to propel yourself very slowly toward the edge.

• Use roots or large clumps of grass, if there are any, to pull yourself along.

• Do not hurry. It may take an hour or more to cover only a few feet in safety. If you need to rest, spread your arms and legs wide, and lie still. You will float.

DANGER SIGNS

Bogs are poorly drained, low-lying depressions – some may have been ponds or shallow lakes – that slowly fill up with decomposed plant life. Their surfaces are often expanses of bright green sphagnum moss that cover lethal mire.

If you have to cross boggy terrain, always keep to the highest ground where taller trees or bushes grow. Tread only where scrub is growing – vegetation indicates drier ground.

If you are in any doubt about which way to go, throw heavy stones ahead of you as well to check the firmness of the ground. At the edge of a doubtful patch, try stamping hard. If the ground ahead quivers, the patch is probably water-logged; avoid it.

A quicksand is a pocket of loose sand which has been saturated by water seeping upward from an underground source. This forces the grains apart, creating a souplike mixture in which even objects as large as trucks can sink. It is often difficult to spot, for a firm crust may cover the fluid below.

When exploring any unfrequented beach or unknown sandy area, carry a stick or pole as a probe, and toss stones ahead of you to test the ground.

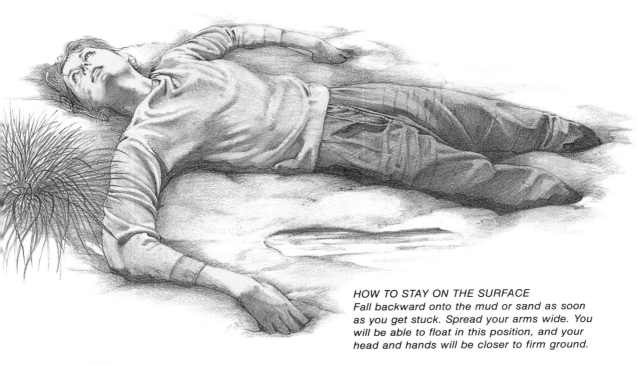

HOW TO STAY ON THE SURFACE
Fall backward onto the mud or sand as soon as you get stuck. Spread your arms wide. You will be able to float in this position, and your head and hands will be closer to firm ground.

Exposure: the silent killer

Anyone who is exposed to extreme cold without adequate protection may suffer from a drop in the body's normal temperature, which can be fatal if left untreated. Doctors call the condition exposure or hypothermia.

Exposure is blamed for the deaths of more than 900 people a year in North America. But mountain rescue experts say that exposure could be the indirect cause of many more deaths because it saps the victim's strength and clouds his judgment, increasing the chances of some other accident, such as a fall.

Most cases occur in temperatures ranging from 30 to 50°F (−1 to 10°C), when climbers or hikers are less likely to be well prepared for sudden, bitingly cold winds and rain. The severity of the condition varies with age and general health. But exposure can kill even a vigorous, healthy person in less than four hours.

Warning signs

Feelings of cold and numbness, accompanied by shivering, are among the first signs of falling body temperature. Other symptoms are: slurred speech, stumbling, lethargy, erratic behavior and irritability.

What to do

• If you notice any of the warning signs in yourself, change into dry clothes if your clothes are wet. Cover your head, face and neck as well as your body to minimize further heat loss. About 50 percent of the heat lost by the body escapes through the head and neck.
• Find shelter fast and get into a sleeping bag. For added warmth and protection, wrap the bag in a survival blanket or a large sheet of plastic.
• Consume warm, sweet drinks and food.

How to help a victim

• If you notice the symptoms of exposure in somebody else, do not force the victim to keep moving or to walk quickly.
• Stop. If the victim's clothing is wet, remove it and replace it with dry. Wrap the victim in a blanket or place him in a sleeping bag – with a companion for extra warmth.
• In severe cases, remove the victim's outer clothing. Remove your own outer garments and get into the sleeping bag beside the victim. Skin-to-skin contact should bring the victim's temperature back to normal.
• Protect the victim against the weather with a tent, a plastic sheet or any makeshift shelter. Use clothes, grass or anything else available to insulate the sleeping bag from the ground.
• If the victim is conscious, give him warm drinks and food.
• Do not offer alcohol or massage: both tend to dilate the blood vessels near the skin. This draws body heat away from deeper organs at a time when it is crucial to warm the core of the body, not the surface.
• If the victim loses consciousness, put him in the recovery position (see page 136). Never give an unconscious person anything to eat or drink. It could choke him.
• Once the worst symptoms have passed, treat the victim as a stretcher case. Even if he appears fully recovered, do not move him without covering his head, neck and face.
• If you reach a house and the victim is conscious, put him in a warm, but not hot, bath. Keep the water at a temperature that is comfortable to the elbow.
• When the victim begins to sweat, dry him, put him in a warm bed and keep him rested.
• Do not put an unconscious person in a bath. Instead, once you are indoors, take off any wet clothes he is wearing and put him in a warm bed. Place hot-water bottles (wrapped thickly in towels to avoid burning him) around his torso.

HOW TO AVOID EXPOSURE

• Get a good night's rest before spending a day outdoors. Victims of exposure often admit to having felt off-color on the morning of the incident. Common causes are arduous overnight traveling – and drinking sprees – before setting out.
• Eat a good breakfast with plenty of fluids before you leave. Eat high-energy snacks such as chocolate frequently during the day.
• Always carry a plastic bag – large enough to hold a person inside a sleeping bag – inside your backpack.
• Wear warm clothing that gives full protection against the wind. Outer clothing should be fully waterproofed.
• Carry a spare set of dry clothing.
• When walking, take off excess clothing if you get hot. It is important not to get soaked in sweat, because water draws warmth from the body faster than air.
• Never carry more weight than you can comfortably bear. In cold weather, it will make you more vulnerable to fatigue and exposure. For the same reason, go at a comfortable pace.
• Be alert to the risk of exposure from windchill. Near-freezing temperatures on windy days can be as chilling as below freezing temperatures on wind-free days. For example, a 34°F (1°C) temperature with a 25 mph (40 km/h) wind has the same effect as a 7°F (−14°C) temperature in calm conditions. Before going out on winter days, check the weather reports for the windchill factor. Windchill becomes dangerous when temperatures below 19°F (−7°C) combine with winds above 6 mph (10 km/h).

What to do if you get lost

What you should do if you get lost in the country depends largely on the circumstances. At night or in cold weather, the priority is to find warmth and shelter. On a sunny day, the priority is likely to be to find a main road or a telephone.

If you get lost on a clear day
• Once you suspect you are lost, stop and take stock of your situation. Going on blindly may only make the situation worse.
• If you have a map, check the key so that you know what its symbols stand for. You will probably have at least a rough idea of where you are.
• Look around you for landmarks that match the map.
• Try to find on the map the last position you were sure of, and try to trace your route since then by remembering any buildings, streams or other landmarks you have passed.
• Examine the contour lines on the map to get an idea of the lay of the land in the area where you are lost. Widely spaced contour lines (which join places of equal height) indicate gentle slopes. An absence of contour lines indicates a plain or a broad ridge. Contours bending in a loop mark the spur of a hill or a valley.
• Check the scale of the map, too. It is usually given as a ratio – 1:50,000, say. This means that 1 cm on the map equals 50,000 cm (0.5 km) on the ground. On this scale, 1¼ in. on the map is about 1 mile. The scale of American topographic maps – 1:25,000 – gives greater detail. On this scale, 2 cm on the map equals 0.5 km on the ground; 2½ in. is about 1 mile.

• Use your finger as a rough guide to estimate distances. The index finger of most adults measures about 1 in. (25 mm or 2.5 cm) from its tip to the first joint.
• Turn the map until the symbols on it are lined up with the landmarks they represent. Decide on the direction you want to travel to reach a main road or settlement.
• Check that there is nothing – a cliff, say, or a wide river – to bar the way to your chosen destination. If there is, work out a way to get round it.
• Look on the map and on the ground for a landmark to aim for. Check your progress on the map by watching out for more landmarks on either side of your path as you walk (see *How to use a map and compass*, page 286).

If you have no map
It is still possible to find your way to safety even if you have no map and no compass.
• Consider first retracing your steps to the last main road you passed.
• If going back is not practicable, look around you. If you can see a road – or something that indicates its presence, such as a building or power lines – head for the road.
• If you can orient yourself by any landmarks, so that you know roughly where you are, aim for a nearby road, path, railway line or stream that you know will lead you to safety.
• Ideally, head for a feature, such as a road or stream, that you know cuts squarely across your line of travel. That way, you will still be able to find it even if you stray slightly off course.

HOW TO CALL FOR HELP IN THE WILD

People on foot in open country are extremely difficult to spot from a distance or from the air. But there are a number of ways of improving your chances of being found.
• The internationally recognized mountain distress signal is three gunshots, whistle blasts or light flashes – use three of anything, as long as it is loud or bright enough to attract attention. Follow the signal with a brief pause and then repeat as often as necessary.
• If you have wood and matches, light some fires. Once the fires are ablaze, add damp wood or grass to make plenty of smoke.
• Wear brightly colored clothing and a brightly colored hat.
• Lay objects on the ground – branches, stones or clothing – to form the words HELP or SOS. Make the letters as large as possible – at least 20 ft. (6 m) long. If there is snow on the ground, tread out

trenches in snowdrifts to form the same words.
• In addition, wave a large flag made out of the most brightly colored clothing you have.
• If you are being rescued by helicopter – on a mountain, say – let off a flare if you have one or light a small smoky fire near the pickup point when the helicopter approaches. The smoke will show the pilot the direction of the wind, and help him to hold his position accurately while he is hovering.

Using a homemade heliograph
Heliographs – devices which use reflected sunlight to flash messages from one person to another – have been used by military signalers since ancient times. They are easy to make at home before you travel – though they can be improvised on the spot – and, on a clear day, can attract attention from a distance of several miles. This is how to make and use one.

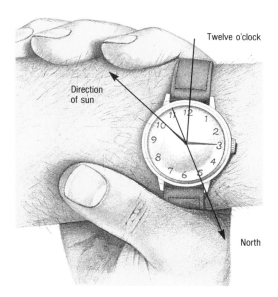

Twelve o'clock

Direction of sun

North

HOW TO FIND NORTH WITH A WATCH
Point the hour hand at the sun (ignore the minute hand). In the Northern Hemisphere, south is halfway between the hour hand and the 12.

• If no reliable landmarks are visible, decide what direction to head in, then orient yourself by using the sun.
• The sun rises in the east and sets in the west. At midday it is due south in the Northern Hemisphere.
• You can use your watch to determine direction in the wild. Hold the watch level, pointing the hour hand toward the sun. (Ignore the position of the minute hand.) If you are on daylight saving time, first turn the watch back an hour to standard time. Divide the angle between the hour hand and 12 o'clock in half with an imaginary line. If it is 4 p.m., for instance, the line will pass through 2 o'clock. The imaginary line will point due south in the Northern Hemisphere.
• If the clouds are too dense to find the sun, look for moss on trees and rocks. Since moss grows best in the shade, the most luxuriant growth will be on the north or north-east side in the Northern Hemisphere. This will give you a rough idea of your bearings. But confirm your direction from the sun as soon as there is a break in the clouds.
• If you have to stay put for a time, you can work out your bearings by placing a stick upright on flat ground. Mark the tip of the stick's shadow on the ground every hour or so. A line drawn through the marks will point due east and west.

If you are caught in bad weather
• If you have survival equipment – such as a survival blanket or a plastic bag or tube large enough to sit inside with your whole body and head protected – consider staying where you are and sitting out the bad weather.
• If you have no survival equipment and the weather turns bad with driving rain or high winds, the priority is to get down from high ground. It does not matter if you arrive in the wrong valley – so long as you do it in one piece.
• Check for danger spots on a map, if you have

Emergencies on vacation and in the country

• You need a flat sheet of metal which is bright enough to show a reflection on both sides. A tin lid rubbed clean will work, or even a piece of tinfoil will do.
• Make a small hole through the centre of the lid. Look through the hole until you see the person or place you want to signal to.
• Now, holding the lid steady, look at the reflection of your own face in the back of the lid. You will see a spot of light on your reflected face from the sunlight shining through the hole.
• Tilt the lid until the spot of light in the reflection disappears into the hole. When it does, the flash is on target.
• Rock the lid slowly to generate a series of flashes.
• Time the flashes, if possible, to match the international mountain distress signal – three flashes in a row, followed by a pause, followed by another three flashes, and so on.

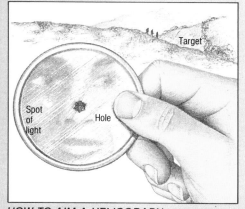

Target

Spot of light

Hole

HOW TO AIM A HELIOGRAPH
Sight through the central hole on your target. Then tilt the lid so that the spot of light on your reflected face vanishes into the hole.

one. Steep slopes, for instance, are indicated by contour lines that are drawn close together. Plot a route around them.
• Use the direction of flow in streams to tell you which way leads downhill. But do not follow streams too closely; on hills, water sometimes carves deep ravines that could be dangerously steep. Instead, keep the stream within earshot and aim to follow its line.
• Avoid areas in a depression where there are tufts of spiky, light green grass. Tufts of this kind often indicate a bog or swamp.
• As you come down the hill, watch out for places that might offer or lead to shelter – a farmhouse, say, or a track. Make for them.

If you are lost in mist or fog
• If mist closes in, line a map up with a compass and decide which direction to go in.
• Sight along the bearing you want to follow, using a straightedge or a compass, and pick out some visible marker along the line – a rock, say, or a branch or fern.
• Walk to the marker, then use your compass again to identify another marker in the same direction.
• Repeat the procedure until you walk out of the mist.
• If you have no map or compass, stay put until the mist clears.

Caught in a whiteout
When the light reflected by snow is the same color as the sky, the landscape loses all form. It has no horizon, no height, no depth and no shadows. Climbers and explorers call this weather condition a whiteout.
• Stop and wait for the whiteout to pass if you can. In a blizzard, find a snowdrift, scoop out a depression in the snow and burrow into it for shelter (see *How to make a snow-hole shelter*, page 297). Alternatively, enlarge the depression that often forms in snow around the base of a tree and shelter in that.
• If you have a survival blanket, wrap it around you. Use a pad – a backpack, say, or branches – to insulate your body from the cold ground.
• Put on as many layers of clothing as you can. Take your arms out of the sleeves of the top jacket or coat. Button or zip it up, then work it down over your head and body as you would a tube. Cross your arms underneath the jacket and tuck your hands into your armpits to help conserve warmth.
• If you have to move during a whiteout, toss snowballs ahead of you as you walk. Watching where they land and how they roll will show you the direction of any slope. If they vanish altogether, you could be on the edge of a cliff.

Lost at night
• If there is a moon, moonlit grass or snow can give good visibility. In these circumstances, try to reach a road or any house or barn.

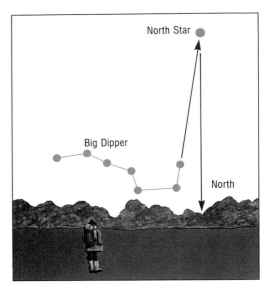

HOW TO FIND NORTH BY THE STARS
Look for the Big Dipper, which can be at any angle in the sky. Its end stars point at the North Star, which marks true north.

• If you have no compass, use the stars as a guide. In the Northern Hemisphere, find the North Star, which is due north, by sighting along the outer edge of the Big Dipper's bowl.
• In latitudes below 40 degrees north (approximately that of Philadelphia and Denver), the Big Dipper sometimes slips below the horizon. Below this latitude, look for the W shape of the constellation Cassiopeia, whose center star points in the general direction of the North Star. Remember also that the North Star is at the end of the Little Dipper's handle.
• If visibility is too poor to travel by and you are on a mountain, find what shelter you can in the lee of a wall or a rocky outcrop, and wrap yourself in a survival blanket if you have one.
• Members of a group can help each other to stay warm, even if they do not have survival blankets, by sitting or lying huddled together. The middle position is the warmest, so change over from time to time.

If a child gets lost
An adventurous toddler or child, absorbed in his exploration of a beach, a picnic spot, a hillside or a fairground, can easily get lost.
• At the start of the outing, impress on the child the dangers of wandering out of sight. But fix some prominent place where you can meet should he or she nevertheless get lost.
• As soon as you notice the child's absence, make a quick search of the area where he or she was last seen.
• Go to the prearranged meeting place. If possible, have somebody wait there while you look around.

- If there is a public address system – as there often is at a fairground, say – find the people in charge of it and ask them to describe the missing child over the air.
- If all this fails, phone the police as soon as possible. Be ready with a detailed description of the child – his name, height, age, coloring, and what he was wearing.
- Once you contact the police, stay where you have arranged to meet them – even if there is a delay before they arrive.

How to avoid getting lost
Anyone who ventures into rough country on foot can minimize the risks of getting lost or stranded by following a few simple guidelines.
- Tell someone where you are going and when you expect to arrive. Check in when you do arrive, so that your contact does not call out rescue services unnecessarily.
- Estimate how long your journey will take. A fit adult can reckon to walk over open country at about 2 mph (4 km/h), not counting rest stops.
- Add 30 minutes to your estimate for each 1,000 ft. to be climbed along the route (50 minutes for each 500 m).
- Telephone for a local weather report before you go, and dress accordingly.
- Walk in groups of at least four people. Then if one person is hurt – with a sprained ankle, say – another can stay with him while the other two go for help.
- If you have no hiking experience but would like to learn to use a map and a compass, consider joining an orienteering club. Contact the national office for the address of a club near you. Write to the United States Orienteering Federation at Box 1444, Forest Park, GA 30051. In Canada, the address of the Canadian Orienteering Federation is 333 River Road, Vanier, Ont., K1L 8H9.

What to take with you
- Carry a large plastic tube or bag big enough to envelop a person in a sleeping bag.
- Carry or wear: a waterproof (not just rainproof) jacket and waterproof trousers; stout, comfortable boots; a spare sweater; and a warm hat and gloves. Also carry: food, including chocolate and dried fruit; an up-to-date large-scale map of the area and a compass; matches; a first aid kit; whistle and flashlight; and pencil and paper.
- In addition, take a first aid kit which includes a survival blanket that is large enough to envelop completely a person in a sleeping bag. (See *What you need in a first aid kit*, page 44).
- For extended journeys, take a more comprehensive survival kit as well (see *Individual survival pack*, page 301).
- If you change your plans after setting out, try to telephone those expecting you. If necessary, contact the police to make sure that emergency services are not alerted.

PESTICIDE POISONING
Spraying with pesticides and fertilizers usually takes place in spring and autumn. Yard and roadside treatments may be done with hand-held equipment or by tractor, but frequently planes or helicopters are used to spray crops.

Even in light winds, spray and dust can sometimes drift out of the area being sprayed and pose a threat to nearby workers, hikers and picnickers. Some pesticides are toxic and can cause harm if inhaled or if they contact the skin.
- If you see a tractor or plane spraying, move well away from the area.
- Do not let dogs run on fields which are being sprayed with pesticide or sprinkled with fertilizer. They may pick up the chemicals on their paws, or swallow them.
- If the spray or dust falls on you or someone else, assume – for the sake of safety – that the spray is harmful.
- Get out of the spraying area.
- Seek medical help immediately. Tell the doctor or ambulance crew the name of the pesticide being used – if you know it – or what crop is being sprayed. This will help doctors to decide which is the most appropriate treatment.
- If you do not know what chemical is involved, tell the doctor where the field is. With the help of local police, he will be able to find out who owns the field and which pesticide or fertilizer was being used.
- Remove any contaminated clothing, and wash thoroughly any areas of skin that have been exposed to the chemicals. Use soap and water if possible.
- If chemicals have entered the eyes, flush them with clean water, under a running faucet if possible, for at least ten minutes.
- Keep warm by wrapping up in a clean blanket or coat.
- If you have not been exposed to the spray yourself but are helping someone who has been, put gloves on before you touch his contaminated clothing. Otherwise the chemicals will get onto your skin too. If you do not have any gloves, wrap your hands loosely with, say, a sweater.
- If the person who has been sprayed loses consciousness, place him in the recovery position (see page 136).
- If he stops breathing, give artificial respiration (see page 50). If his face has been exposed to the spray, clean the area around his mouth and nose first, and protect your mouth with a handkerchief.

Emergencies on vacation and in the country

How to use a map and compass

With an accurate map and a compass, plus a pencil and a straightedge (a ruler, or even a notebook or the edge of an orienteering compass), it is possible to navigate with a fair degree of precision across unfamiliar country. And if you get lost, you can quickly rediscover where you are, provided there are some identifiable landmarks in sight.

Finding your position on the map

• Fold the map flat so that the arrows on it which identify north are visible. Large-scale maps (1:25,000 or larger) of the kind used by walkers normally have two arrows. One shows true north (the direction indicated by the North Star); the other shows magnetic north (the direction to which a compass points).

• Lay the orienteering compass on the map, and then turn the map until the compass needle and the arrow pointing to magnetic north are aligned.

• Once the map is lined up, look around you for clear landmarks – for example, a building, a power line, or a known peak. Find the same landmark on the map.

• Lay the straightedge on the map so that it touches the landmark symbol. Sight along the edge and turn it – *without turning the map* – until it points directly at the corresponding landmark on the ground. Draw a line along the straightedge from the map landmark back toward the position of your eye.

• Repeat the procedure with a second landmark. Your position is approximately where the two lines on the map cross. Use a third landmark, if one is visible, as a check.

• Once you have worked out where you are, use the map to work out where you want to go. Lay the straightedge along your intended line of travel and – again without turning the map – sight along the edge at the landscape ahead.

• Choose some easily recognizable natural or man-made feature along the line and use it as a beacon. When you reach it, use the map to replot your line of travel – avoiding any obstacles such as cliffs and bogs – then pick another marker to walk to.

• Whenever you use a compass, make sure it is well away from metal, which could affect it, and away from the magnetic fields generated by electric current, such as in power lines.

• It is possible to use a compass instead of a straightedge to plot the direction, or bearing, of each landmark from your position, and to use a straightedge only to draw the lines on the map. But it is easier, and just as accurate, to use a straightedge for both jobs.

• If you use the compass method, remember to draw each line in the *opposite* direction from the bearing you measure. If one landmark is, say, exactly NE of you, draw the line SW from the corresponding spot on the map. To calculate a ''back-bearing'' in this way, add 180 degrees to the bearing if it is less than 180 degrees; subtract 180 degrees if it is more.

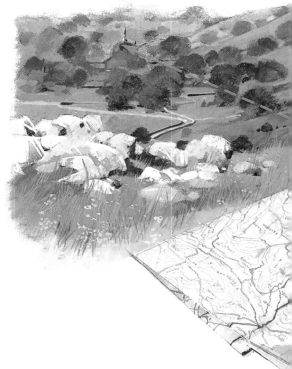

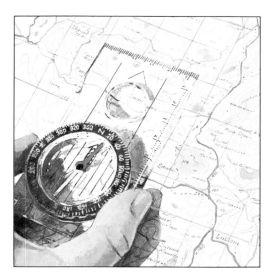

Lining up the map with a compass
Find on the map the arrow showing the direction of magnetic north – it is in the margin at the bottom of the map. Turn the map until the arrow and the compass needle are exactly in line.

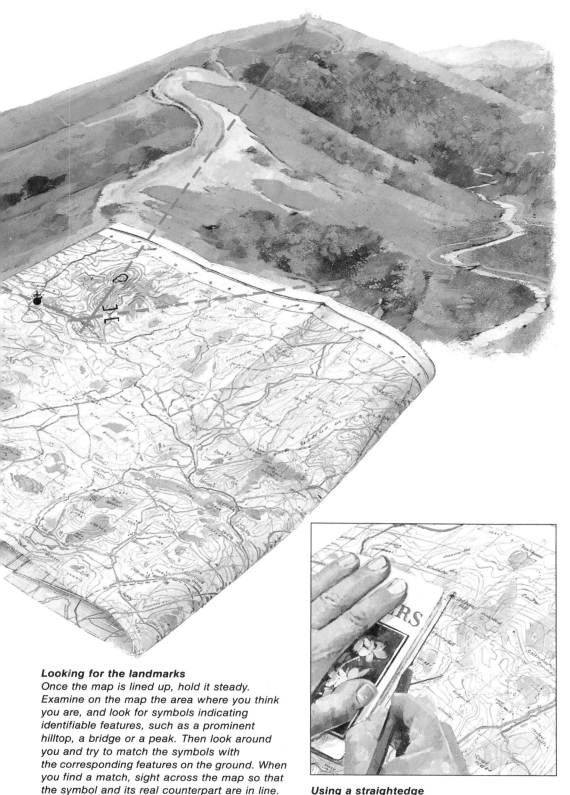

Looking for the landmarks
*Once the map is lined up, hold it steady.
Examine on the map the area where you think
you are, and look for symbols indicating
identifiable features, such as a prominent
hilltop, a bridge or a peak. Then look around
you and try to match the symbols with
the corresponding features on the ground. When
you find a match, sight across the map so that
the symbol and its real counterpart are in line.
Your position is somewhere along that line.
Repeat the process with other landmarks and
your position is where the lines meet:
somewhere in the triangle they usually form.*

Using a straightedge
*Any straightedged object can be used as a
sighting instrument. Look along it the way a
golfer sights along a putter, or hold it and the
map up to eye level without turning the map.*

Skiing: coping with an accident

Ski resorts are well equipped to cope with accidents. If you break a leg on a well-used slope, emergency services are unlikely to be far away. But if you go skiing alone far from the normal routes, a broken leg may threaten your life unless you can reach shelter on your own.

• If you do break a leg, stop any bleeding by making bandages from torn strips of cloth. Use shirtsleeves or underclothing. But do not use an outer garment; you must keep warm.

• Apply snow to the wound to reduce swelling.

• Put splints on either side of the leg, tying them above and below the fracture (see *Splints*, page 127). The task may be painful, but it must be done: tackle it with patience and determination. For splints, use ski poles or any branches available.

• Do not try to walk across the snow. You are likely to sink in and do more damage. Instead, lie flat on your stomach on one or both skis and propel yourself with your hands.

• Follow a zigzag or diagonal path downhill, heading for anywhere help may be available.

• The best way to avoid the risk of having to find your own way to safety with a serious injury is never to ski alone. If you do plan a trip away from well-used routes, even with companions, consider setting your ski bindings looser than usual. It is easier to put a ski back on if you fall than to deal with a badly twisted ankle or a broken leg.

How to help an injured companion

• If a companion breaks a leg on a remote slope, apply emergency first aid (see page 98).

• Make an improvised litter using skis, ski poles, and jackets or scarves (see page 115). Do not use the victim's jacket for this purpose; he needs to be kept warm.

• Tow the litter slowly and carefully – on foot unless you are an expert skier. Head for the nearest well-used route.

ORDEAL IN THE MOUNTAINS
In late April 1986, Robin Sachs, 31, set out alone on a ten-day cross-country solo skiing expedition through Yosemite National Park in California. His hefty pack contained trail foods, a first aid kit, shovel, cooking fuel, clothing and sleeping gear.

On the first day Robin decided to take a short-cut down a rocky, snow-free slope. He attached his skis and his poles to his pack and began backing down the slope. But the rocks were thinly covered with ice. He tried to climb back to the ridge, but couldn't. Instead, he began to slide backward, tumbling down the slope more than 100 ft. (30 m).

After Robin had clawed his way to a stop, he felt his left leg and found a fracture and, worse, a dislocation of his left ankle. Every movement caused intense back pain, and he could not stand. Moreover, his pack was about 100 ft. (30 m) below him, and his skis 100 ft. up the slope. To survive he knew he had to keep his wits. He made a splint for his ankle with branches and a strip of his sleeping pad. Despite crippling pain, he made his way up the slope to recover his skis and one pole, and then down the slope to retrieve his pack.

For the next ten days, Robin traveled slowly toward a camp 10 miles (16 km) away where he hoped to find help. He used his skis as a makeshift toboggan for his pack, sometimes waddling behind it, sometimes sitting on it and pushing with his ski pole. At night, he built snow shelters with his shovel.

On the tenth day, Robin encountered another skier who went for help. Although Robin had to

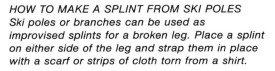

HOW TO MAKE A SPLINT FROM SKI POLES
Ski poles or branches can be used as improvised splints for a broken leg. Place a splint on either side of the leg and strap them in place with a scarf or strips of cloth torn from a shirt.

spend two more nights in a snow shelter before being rescued by a helicopter, he survived because he had kept a clear head during his ordeal.

If you lose your skis

• Skis spread your body weight over the snow. If you lose them in a fall, but are unhurt, do not make for home simply by walking across the slopes. Walking through deep, soft snow will quickly exhaust you. If possible, improvise snowshoes. They spread your weight, and help to save energy too.

• Find two bushy pine branches, the thicker the needles the better. Place them on the snow with the natural curve down at the center, rising forward and behind. The wider end of the branch should be toward the front and the stem behind your heel.

• Strap the branch onto your foot using improvised binding. Strips of cloth, laces or soft pine twigs will all serve for binding.

• Move downhill with care, and cross slopes diagonally or following a zigzag course. Use your ski poles for support as you walk.

If your bindings break

Ski bindings can fail, making conventional skiing impossible. If this should happen, you can still get down a slope safely – and more quickly than would be possible on foot – by making an improvised hobbyhorse.

• Bind your skis together, using strips of cloth for lashing, and tie the ski poles across the back end of the skis.

• Sit astride the skis with the tips behind you. Hold onto the ski poles and lift them.

• Follow a zigzag path down the slope, controlling your descent with your feet.

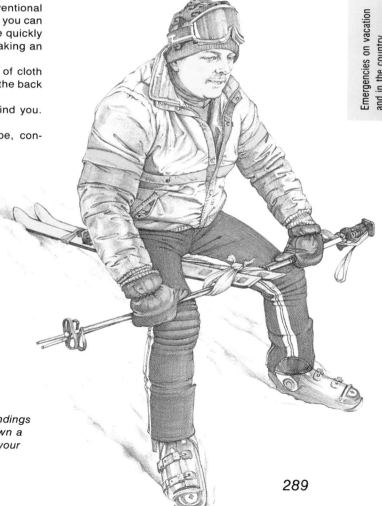

HOW TO MAKE A SNOWSHOE
If you have to walk through soft snow, make improvised snowshoes by tying bushy branches, stems backward, to your boots.

HOW TO TOBOGGAN ON SKIS
On firm snow, make skis with broken bindings into a hobbyhorse to help you to get down a slope more easily. Sit well back and lift your toes so that you plane over the snow.

Crisis underground

Exploring caves can be extremely dangerous for the casual or ill-equipped. On average, the United States National Cave Rescue Commission is called out to help cavers in trouble about 40 times a year. In 1986, there were 16 deaths in the United States as a result of caving accidents.

Mine workings are particularly dangerous because they often contain unmarked vertical shafts, whose entrances can easily be mistaken for deep shadows on the floor of a tunnel. Miners also used to store waste rock on timber platforms in the ceilings of tunnels. When the timbers rot, the rock can be left jammed precariously overhead and can be dislodged without warning by noise or an unwary hand.

Old mines may also contain dangerous or even lethal concentrations of foul air or poisonous or explosive gases. Because of these hazards, never explore a man-made hole in the ground, or any hole which looks man-made.

If you get lost in a cave system
• If you think you might be lost, stop at once. Try to work out where you might have gone wrong. Calculate the time you have spent underground so that you can estimate how long it ought to take you to get back.
• Mark where you are. Scrape a mark in mud on the floor or pile rocks to make a small cairn. If this is impossible, scratch on the wall with a knife or make a mark with soot from a candle flame.
• Try to retrace your steps.
• Keep looking back to recognize passages. A passage viewed from one direction on the way into a cave system can look very different on the way out.
• Leave markers as you go.
• Rest often to save energy. Switch your light off whenever you stop, to prolong the life of the batteries. Warming the batteries against your body will also make them last longer.
• If your path takes you deeper into unfamiliar territory, return to the last point you were sure of by following your markers, and try another route. Keep trying until you find the right one. Even in a honeycomb of passages you will gradually narrow the options.
• Shout, or blow a whistle, if you hear sounds that may be other people in the cave.

If you get stuck in a passage
• Relax completely. Taut muscles and fast, panicky breathing inflate your body and make escape more difficult. Go limp.

SAFE CAVING

• The only safe way to go caving is with experienced and properly equipped cavers, usually members of a specialist club. In the United States, contact the National Speleological Society, Cave Avenue, Huntsville, Ala. 35810, for groups in your area. In Canada, there are groups in Alberta, British Columbia, Ontario and Quebec, but no national office. Provincial tourism offices should be able to put you in touch with them.
• Never go caving with fewer than four in a group. If there is an accident, one can stay behind with the injured person while two go for help.
• If you leave markers such as cairns on the way in as a precaution, remove them on the way out. Follow the National Speleological Society's motto: Take nothing but pictures, leave nothing but footprints, and kill nothing but time.
• Tell someone of your plans so that help can be raised quickly if necessary.
• If you have to raise the alarm, call 911 or the local police. In the United States, if the local rescue organization needs help, it will contact the National Cave Rescue Commission.
• Check weather reports before you go. Rain can flood some caves very quickly.
• Wear warm clothing topped by a coverall – caves are chilly, muddy and usually damp all year round. Wear heavy boots with lug soles and a good helmet.
• Take with you: a miner's electric lamp, a carbide lamp, a flashlight or candles with matches; high-energy food – such as chocolate, glucose, fudge or raisins – and water; a map of the cave system; a first aid kit; a whistle; a watch with a luminous dial; and strong climbing rope.

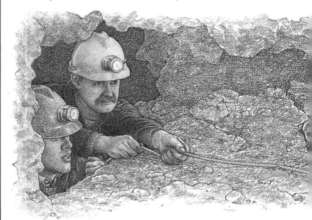

HOW TO GET OUT OF A TIGHT SPOT
If you get stuck underground and can find nothing to hold on to, get your companions to tie a loop in one end of a line. Put your foot in the loop and bend your leg. Tell the others to pull the line taut and anchor it, then push your leg down hard and heave your way out.

- Once you are breathing normally, try to wriggle out slowly. Tackle the task patiently, keeping as relaxed as possible.
- Use your whole body. It is often easier to push your way out with your legs than to pull with your arms.

If your light goes out

Inside a cave system, the blackness is total. And without light it is easy to become completely disoriented.

- Stop immediately. Crouch down and put one hand on the ground directly in front of your feet, the other hand directly behind you.
- Keep your hands still and turn round, using your hands as markers, so that you are facing toward the way out. Do not turn any more or wander about.
- Sit down and wait for at least ten minutes to let your eyes adjust as much as possible to the dark. If you are not far from the entrance, a glimmer of light may become visible as your eyes adapt.
- While you are waiting, try to recall the caves and passages you came through.
- If there is a glimmer of light from the opening, crawl toward it slowly, on hands and knees, testing the ground in front of you as you go. Keep feeling in front of your face and body, too, to check for projecting rocks and boulders.
- If there is no light at all, but the route you took was straightforward – few bends, no passages branching off, a floor without hazards – retrace your steps on all fours, keeping the route in your mind's eye. Feel your way along the wall of the cave.
- If you have come through a hazardous or complicated system, wait for somebody to come and rescue you. Your chances of finding your own way out safely are minimal.

A STONE'S THROW FROM SURVIVAL
Twenty times, a hundred times, a thousand times, Larry Ritchey threw a stone tied to a rope up into the patch of light that was his only chance of escape. Each time, it fell back.

Ritchey, a 35-year-old salesman, had been on a hiking expedition in the Cascade Mountains in Oregon one November weekend in 1982. Suddenly, as he picked his way through deep snow, the ground gave way beneath him. He plunged 14 ft. (4.3 m) into a subterranean stream flowing through a cavern about 10 ft. (3 m) wide. The stillness of the air showed that there was no exit to the surface via the stream. And the rock walls were sheer. There was no chance of scrambling out.

Ritchey tied the stone to the end of his 30-ft. (9-m) climbing rope and tossed it up through the hole in the cavern ceiling in the hope that it would catch on something. Again and again he threw, working his way round and round the lip of the hole. Three times the stone seemed to hold fast and then pulled loose as he tried to climb. But he never gave up, even after five days of failure. By the end of the fifth day he had no more food, the water was rising about him, and he was showing signs of hypothermia.

At last the stone caught again. This time it held. Ritchey hauled himself painfully back to the surface. He trudged and staggered 10 miles (16 km) to a road and flagged down a car.

A search had been organized once Ritchey was overdue, but his shouts would never have been heard over the crashing of the stream, even had the rescuers come near him. What had saved his life was his own endurance – and the adage he had kept repeating to himself: "If at first you don't succeed..."

Emergencies on vacation and in the country

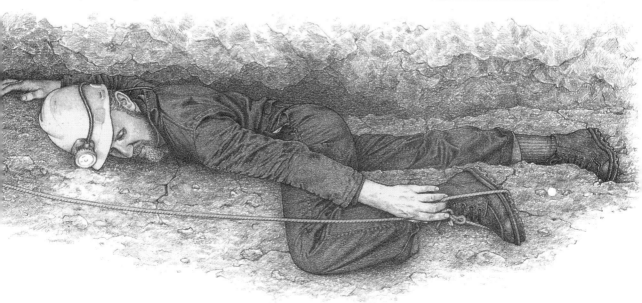

Survival in the wild

An injury, a breakdown, bad weather or sheer bad luck can turn an adventurous expedition into a fight for life. It can happen anywhere: on a mountain, in a tropical rain forest or a barren desert. Wherever it happens, there are four immediate priorities. In order of importance they are: shelter; a signal; water; and food.

The ten pages that begin here describe how survival experts cope with these priorities in a variety of circumstances. All the techniques mentioned have been used in real-life emergencies. Some techniques, however, are hazardous and should be used only when their risks are outweighed by other dangers.

The first steps

• Wherever you are, the first step is to get out of the cold, heat, wind or rain so that you can make plans with thought and care.

• Next, let other people in the vicinity know where you are by setting up a conspicuous signal. You can use anything at hand for signaling. Spread out bright clothing that contrasts with the environment. Light a fire to make a smoke signal. Use a gun or a whistle if you have one. The internationally recognized distress signal is three blasts followed by a brief pause, followed by another three, and so on. Improvise mirrors to reflect the sun, or, at night, flash lights. There is no point in foraging for food and water before this task is done. Search parties may be in the vicinity already – and may miss you if no signal is set up.

• Finding water is more important than finding food. An average person who is lost in the wild can survive for only a few days without water –

and then only in a temperate climate. During the time spent finding and improving a shelter, setting up a signal and so on, you will have used up a significant amount of body fluid, which has to be replaced.

• Finally, find food. Under average conditions, an adult male can survive for at least a week without food before serious physical deterioration sets in.

• Nevertheless, start foraging early. Where necessary, test nearby vegetation for edible foods (see *The edibility test*, page 296).

Making and using a fire

Survival in the wild may depend on your ability to light a fire. Warmth, cooking, boiling water, drying clothes, signaling, protecting yourself against animals and insects – all are essential needs. On any excursion into remote or difficult terrain it is vital to take an adequate supply of matches or a lighter. Waterproof matches are available; otherwise carry ordinary matches in a waterproof container.

Finding dry tinder and kindling

• Tinder must be bone-dry. Sources of tinder include dry grasses, stems, straw, leaves, twigs, bark fragments and splinters of wood. In wet weather, look especially under the bases of trees and under rock overhangs for the driest material.

• Even in wet weather, birch bark peeled from a tree makes good tinder since it contains highly flammable oils. The resinous pitch in pine knots has the same flammable properties.

• Where no natural dry tinder can be found, shred fragments of clothing. Tufts of absorbent

---

PREPARING FOR A JOURNEY IN THE WILD

No amount of preparation can remove all the risks from a journey through remote or rugged country. But preparation can considerably lessen the chances of things going wrong and improve your chances of survival if they do.

• Learn to use a map and compass until you can navigate with confidence.

• Before setting out, inform relatives, friends or the police of your route, departure time, estimated time of arrival, and the number in your party. They can raise the alarm if you are held up. Never travel alone.

• Talk over your plans with people familiar with the area you are going to. They will often be able to give you valuable advice about local conditions.

• Wear clean, loose-fitting clothes that protect you against the weather. What you wear will depend on the climate.

• Next to the skin, wear fabrics that will absorb sweat. In general, cotton and wool are better than man-made fibers, but synthetic "thermal" material is also good. Cotton is good in warm climates because of its sweat-absorbing properties, but it is not suitable for cold-weather conditions because it dries out slowly.

• In warm climates wear lightweight pants. For cooler climates choose pants made of wool or corduroy. Do not wear blue jeans. When the fabric is wet it loses all its heat-retaining properties.

• Wear one or two pairs of wool socks. They absorb sweat and cushion the feet.

• Roughly 50 percent of the heat that escapes from the body is lost from the head and hands. Wear a hat and gloves to help conserve heat in cold weather.

• Carry a survival kit (see pages 300-301).

cotton, unraveled bandages from a first aid kit and fluff from pockets all serve as tinder.

• Blow gently on glowing tinder, and add bits of kindling sparingly as it ignites. Remember that split branches burn better than whole ones. Stack fuel loosely so that the air continues to circulate as you build the fire. Once the fire is going, add whatever wood is at hand.

Lighting a fire with a car battery

If you are stranded in a car but have no matches, there are two main ways that you can use the car to get a fire going. Never be tempted, however, to use gasoline to light a fire or to keep one going. Gas burns explosively, and the flames or the blast can kill.

• If the car has a cigarette lighter, twist a piece of paper into a taper, or use a piece of dry, frayed cloth or dry bark (birch bark is best).

• When the cigarette lighter is red-hot, pull it out and touch it to the taper to light it. Then use the taper like a match to light the fire.

• Alternatively, if the car has no built-in lighter, use the car battery to light a fire.

• Disconnect the battery and remove it from the vehicle. Keep the battery upright when you lift it out to avoid splashing any acid onto yourself.

• Use jumper cables. Or take two pieces of

HOW TO USE A BATTERY TO LIGHT A FIRE

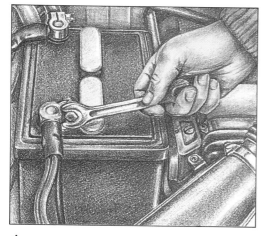

1 *Disconnect the terminals on the battery, and lift it out of the car. Take care not to touch both terminals at once with the wrench.*

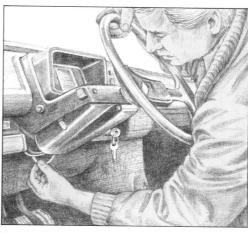

2 *If you have no spare wire or jumper cables, take out two pieces of insulated wire – the longer the better.*

3 *Bare the ends of the wires, attach one end of each to a terminal, and touch the free ends together. Catch the sparks in tinder to ignite it.*

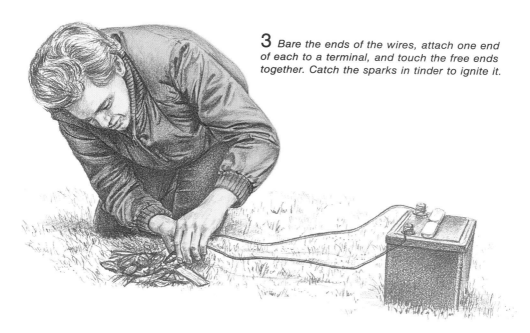

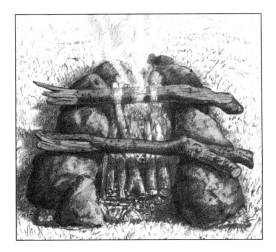

HOW A TRAPPER'S FIRE WORKS
The fireplace's funnel shape, which can be made out of logs, stones, earth or turf, acts like a natural flue. Use green logs or a metal grille to support cooking pans over the embers.

unessential wiring – from an interior light cable, for example.
• Connect one cable or wire to each terminal. Then, carefully, touch the free ends together and catch the sparks in a pile of dry tinder.

How to build a fire
Before you light any fire, clear the ground around it of anything that might burn, and have something handy to put it out if necessary: water, perhaps, or branches to beat it out.

One particularly effective and simple fire is a type sometimes called a trapper's fire. It makes an excellent cooking fire.
• Use logs, earth or stones to form a funnel shape about 12-18 in. (30-45 cm) long. The wider end should point directly into the wind and be about 12 in. (30 cm) across. The narrow end, pointing away from the prevailing wind, should be about 3-4 in. (7.5-10 cm) across.
• Light the fire at the wider end.
• The hottest part of the fire will be a little downwind of the embers. So by moving pans toward or away from the narrow end, you can control the cooking temperature fairly precisely.
• Another way to make the funnel is to slice through the turf with a knife and roll back the turf on either side of the cut. The turf then forms the walls of the funnel, and the grass can be rolled back into place later, when you leave.

Keeping a fire going through the night
• To keep a wood fire burning overnight, reduce the draft of air by banking around the edges with earth or stones. Add slow-burning hardwoods or green logs.
• For maximum warmth at night, lie between the fire and any natural barrier such as a bank,

MAROONED IN AN ALASKAN WINTER
The Wortman family – 53-year-old Elmo, a disabled carpenter, and his three children – were on their way home from a visit to the dentist on February 13, 1979, when they were shipwrecked on the hostile coast of Alaska.

The family, who had traveled by boat to the nearest dentist, across the border in Canada, were washed up on a bleak snow-covered island, injured and without food or shelter. They had matches with them, protected in glass bottles by Elmo in the last moments before the boat went down. With these, they were able to start a fire. Using salvage from the boat, the children – Cindy, 16, Randy, 15, and Jena Lynn, 12 – built a shelter. They rested two poles on a pair of large rocks and draped a sail over them, covering top, back and floor. The opening faced the fire to keep the crude shelter warm.

The Wortmans ate clams, mussels and seaweed scavenged from the shore.

With logs and some of the salvage from the boat – electrical wire, rubber tubing and plywood – they later improvised a raft, and managed to reach a trapper's cabin on a neighboring island. From there, all were rescued on March 10 – weak and frostbitten but alive.

rock wall or big log. This will reflect the heat back at parts of the body not facing the fire.
• If necessary, improvise a heat-reflector by rolling boulders or logs into position.
• Huddle together with any companions for extra warmth and to conserve heat.

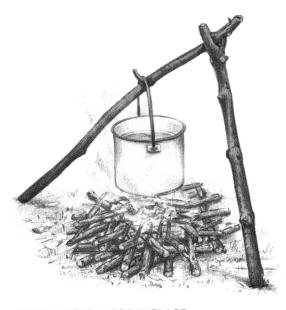

HOW TO HOLD A POT IN PLACE
Stick a forked branch firmly into the ground, and prop another stick against it to hold a cooking pot securely in place over a fire.

Cooking in the wild
• Cook on glowing embers, not on flames.
• Cook all food – especially meat and fish – thoroughly before eating. This is particularly important in hot and humid conditions where bacteria thrive. Cooking destroys harmful bacteria and also neutralizes some poisons.
• Boiling is usually the safest method of preparing food for eating. Boiling will also soften tough meat.
• If you are in doubt about whether any particular species of animal or plant is safe to eat, use the edibility test (see page 296).

How to cope with stomach upsets
You may succumb to severe stomach pains in the wild. Common causes are eating a poisonous plant, or drinking contaminated water.
• If you think that food or water is the cause of the pain, and you have no medicines for it, try to make yourself sick. Either put a finger down your throat or drink clean salt water.
• Alternatively, eat some carbon or chalk. Either is capable of absorbing poisons. Chalk may be available from nearby rocks; carbon can be any piece of charred wood from a fire.
• Crush the pieces and eat one or two tablespoons of the powdered chalk or carbon. Wash the powder down with plenty of clean drinking water.

If you suspect that water is contaminated
• Dirty or contaminated water should be boiled. To be completely safe, the water should be boiled for at least ten minutes. Alternatively, it can be purified with water-purification tablets.
• Filtering water will not purify it, but it will often improve the water's appearance and taste.
• If no proper filters are available, you can make your own equipment. For the container, use a canvas bag, a polyethylene bag, a large tin, a knotted shirtsleeve – or even a sock.
• Fill the bottom of the container with a layer of fine gravel. Above it place alternate layers of crushed carbon and sand – as many as will fit. Make each layer about 1 in. (2.5 cm) thick. If no sand is available, use fine gravel instead.
• Make small holes in the container's base. Pour the water through, catching it in a cup.
• If you decide to filter the water, do the filtering before you boil or treat it chemically – not afterward. The filter may otherwise contaminate the water again.

Using snow or ice
Where there is snow, there is water. But snow needs to be melted and purified before consumption. To melt snow, pack it firmly in a container – this will save fuel. Never eat raw snow itself, because air pollutants in it can cause diarrhea and dehydration.

In general, ice is more valuable than snow, because it takes 50 percent less fuel to melt it. When heating snow, much fuel is wasted warming the air trapped among the flakes.

Surviving in the jungle
Getting stranded in jungle is, in some ways, less of an ordeal than fighting to survive in other environments. Food and water, for example, are

HOW TO FILTER WATER

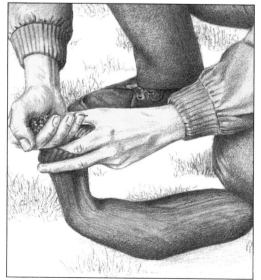

1 *Any tubular container with holes at the bottom – a clean sock, say – can make a filter. Put 1 in. (2.5 cm) of gravel in the bottom.*

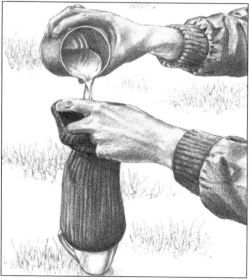

2 *Add layers, alternately, of sand and carbon (crushed burned wood), then pour the water through. Boil the water afterward to purify it.*

usually plentiful. And trees offer both fuel for fires and protection against the elements.

The worst enemy is generally anxiety: you cannot afford to be squeamish about anything that walks, crawls, swims or flies.

• Use what natural shelter you can find, or build a simple lean-to off the ground.

• For building a shelter, bamboo is an invaluable plant and found widely in tropical rain forests. It has innumerable additional advantages. You can make anything from a spear to a full-scale raft with bamboo. The canes can be used as firewood, and the tender shoots are both edible and nutritious.

• Filter and boil all water. Cook all food. Germs, like the vegetation, thrive in humid forests. When collecting food, beware of any brightly colored plants, especially red and orange ones. They are often poisonous.

• Wash yourself whenever possible to discourage insects and prevent skin infections.

• Wash your clothes every day to stop sweat from rotting the fabric.

• Use fire to get rid of bugs and other insects. Use an insect repellent, too – it also helps to ward off leeches.

• When traveling through thick jungle, movement is bound to be slow. Do not try to rush. It often helps to move backward – if you get tangled in climbing vines, say.

• To find your way out of the jungle, locate any flow of water and head downstream. Follow a spring to a stream, a stream to a river, and a river to the sea if necessary.

• Sooner or later you will almost certainly come across other human beings, for waterways are the main lines of communication in tropical rain forests.

TWENTY-EIGHT YEARS IN THE JUNGLE
One night in January 1972, two hunters on the Pacific island of Guam came across a mysterious figure. He was wearing trousers and jacket made of tree and bark fiber, and he was heavily bearded. Brought in at gunpoint, he turned out to be Shoichi Yokoi, a former sergeant in the Japanese army. He had been hiding out in the jungle for 28 years – ever since the end of the Second World War.

Yokoi had fled into the jungle when U.S. troops recaptured the island in 1944. Fearing capture,

---

THE EDIBILITY TEST

If you are stranded in remote country, you may be forced to live off the land, and that will mean trying to survive mostly by eating plants. The range of poisonous and non-poisonous plants is vast, and you may get confused trying to remember the different species. In an emergency, it is possible to find out which is which by cautiously using yourself as a guinea pig.

Do not try this technique at home, however, and particularly do not encourage children to try it. Use it only in an emergency when the risk of making yourself ill is outweighed by the risk of starving.

• One person should test only one plant at a time, and each plant should be tested by only one person. And remember that just because you see birds or animals eating a plant, it does not mean that the plant is safe for humans.

• Choose a species which seems to grow plentifully in the area. But do not experiment with fungi. Unless you know that a fungus is edible, make no attempt to eat it or to prepare it for eating. Even boiling fungi does not always remove dangerous toxins.

• Having selected a plant, look for the color of the sap by squeezing the leaf or stem between your fingers.

• Discard any plant that has a creamy or milky sap – it is probably poisonous. (An important exception to this rule is the dandelion: the whole plant is edible and nutritious. It also helps to stop diarrhea.)

• Rub the juices or sap around the tender parts on the inside of your bottom lip. At the same time, place a small piece of the plant – fingernail-size or smaller – on the tip of your tongue. Wait for 4-5 minutes. If you detect any stinging, burning or putrid sensation, discard the plant.

• If you detect none of these sensations, take a larger piece of the plant, roughly 2 in. (5 cm) square. Chew it and swallow it. Wait for two hours. If you experience any stomach upset or feeling of nausea, discard the plant – it is probably poisonous.

• If you detect none of these symptoms, take a larger portion of the plant, roughly 6 in. (15 cm) square, chew and swallow it, and wait a further two hours. If you feel no ill effects, the plant is probably safe to eat.

• Having identified the plant as probably safe, boil it and throw away the juices. Then, as a final precaution, boil it again before eating.

• As the days pass, repeat the test with other plants – trying out roots, fruits, berries and flowers as well as leaves and stems – so that you build up, in time, a varied diet.

he had burned his service uniform and improvised clothing with the materials at hand. For shelter he dug out a cave in a bamboo thicket and left it only at night.

Through the entire period he survived on a diet of nuts, breadfruit, mangoes, papaya, fish, shrimps, snails, rats and frogs. When discovered by the hunters he was on his way to a river to set his traps for fish.

Yokoi was in good physical health (though bewildered by the world of TVs and space travel to which he was returned). His largely salt-free diet had, however, left him slightly anemic. Salt is present in roasted meat, but not in boiled food. In an emergency, it can be obtained by boiling seawater and collecting the salt crystals left behind.

Surviving in the mountains

• Look for shelter in caves and overhangs. Besides offering protection from the elements, they almost always contain some water or moisture. But avoid them during a thunderstorm. They are dangerous if lightning strikes.
• Avoid any area which threatens landslide or avalanche, such as a slope with rocky debris.
• If you are trapped in a remote valley, the higher ground on either side may be safer than the basin.
• Use spare clothes or a bright groundsheet to mark your position.
• Try to attract attention by using a whistle or by calling out – sound travels far in mountains. Give the international distress signal – three blasts of a gun, a whistle or anything that is loud enough to attract attention. Then pause and follow with another three blasts, and so on. This is more likely to be noticed than random shouts.

How to make a snow-hole shelter

• If you are in snow, and bad weather or fading light prevents you from traveling for the time being, you can make your own shelter in the form of a snow hole.
• Use natural snow cavities where possible. The heavily snow-laden branches of a tree, for example, may provide a promising shelter which needs little extra work. Otherwise, dig into the side of a drift.
• Test the drift for depth: about 5-6 ft. (1.5– 1.8 m) is best.

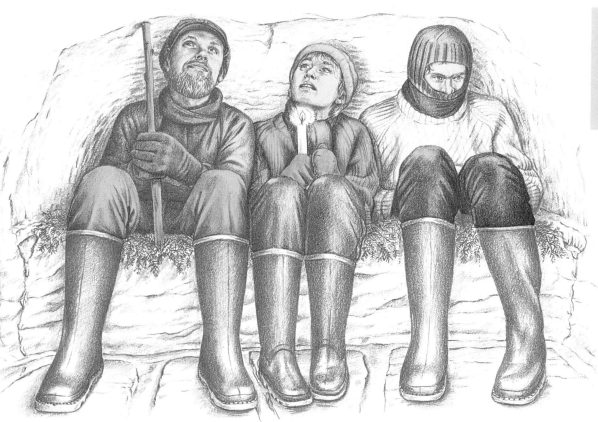

USING A SNOW HOLE FOR SHELTER
Once you have dug a snow hole, get inside and block the entrance tunnel. Keep a stick or pole handy to poke ventilation shafts through the roof, and keep them open. Burn a candle if you have one. Put evergreen branches on the bench to insulate yourself from the snow.

• Once you have found a suitable spot, mark your position conspicuously. Dig out a small entrance low down, tunnel in about 2 ft. (60 cm) and scoop out a cavity. It should be large enough to hold you in a sitting position. If there are more than three of you, it may be necessary to dig more than one hole, but otherwise share. Company and additional body warmth will make the ordeal easier to endure.

• Dig with a shovel or an ice ax, or improvise using cooking pans, for example, or branches. Your hands alone will not be enough.

• Pierce an air shaft through the roof with a stick for ventilation. You may need more than one shaft if several people are in the hole. Keep the stick handy to clear the shaft in case it gets blocked by snow.

• Shape a rough bench for yourself within the cavity. Scoop out a small trench where the bench meets the back and side walls. This will prevent any melting snow from flooding your seat. Line the bench with bushy branches.

• Scoop out a well in the floor in front of your feet. Cold air travels downward, and the well will help to ensure that the chilliest air collects below the level of your body.

• Once the snow hole is ready, get inside, block up the entrance and stay put until morning or until the weather clears and you can move on.

• Avoid falling asleep in a snow-hole shelter unless you are properly equipped with a sleeping bag and plastic survival bag. Keep your spirits up by singing, telling yourself stories – whatever it takes to keep you alert.

• Light a candle, if you have one. It will provide warmth and help to keep your spirits up.

BOYS AGAINST A BLIZZARD
Training, preparation and a determination to stay alive saved the lives of three teenage climbers who became trapped by a terrifying blizzard on *Mount Hood in Oregon. Once Gary Schneider and Matt Meacham, both 16, and 18-year-old Randy Knapp realized they could go no farther during their New Year hike in 1976, they dug a snow hole and settled in to wait out the storm. They were well equipped and had plenty of food, and they kept wriggling their toes and rubbing their feet to keep the circulation going.*

They were rescued after two weeks when the storm died away. Each had lost about 28 lb. (13 kg) in weight, and Randy and Matt had minor frostbite. But all were well enough to go back to school within a couple of weeks.

Surviving in the desert
The vital need in a desert is to avoid dehydration. If you are stranded in a car, use its shelter to keep cool during the heat of the day. If you are on foot, find whatever shade you can – in a cave, say, or in the shadow of rocks.

• Improvise a headdress – for example, a hat with a handkerchief hanging from the back of it – to protect your head and the back of your neck from the sun. It is important to cover the back of the neck as well as the head to guard against heatstroke (see page 106).

• Set up a signal for rescue parties (see page 292), then take cover from the sun. Keep to the shade throughout the day. Move only at night.

• If you are stranded in a car, never leave it and try to walk out. Stay with the vehicle.

• An adult in the shade can make do on 2 quarts (2 liters) of water a day. Try to drink in the early morning and evening. Drinking during the heat of the day can lead to excessive perspiration and loss of body salts.

• To obtain drinking water, collect water in a solar still or use a dew trap.

• Look, too, for underground moisture in the beds of dried-up streams or rivers. Dig in damp patches or around the bases of plants.

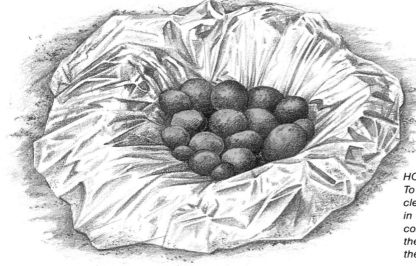

HOW TO MAKE A DEW TRAP
To collect dew in the desert, pile clean, smooth stones on plastic in a shallow hole. Each morning, collect the dew that drains from the stones into the plastic before the sun gets up and evaporates it.

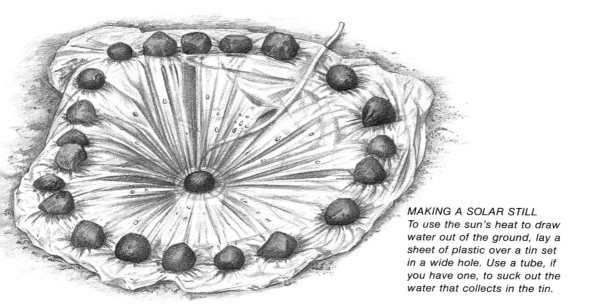

MAKING A SOLAR STILL
To use the sun's heat to draw water out of the ground, lay a sheet of plastic over a tin set in a wide hole. Use a tube, if you have one, to suck out the water that collects in the tin.

• Watch the behavior of wildlife also. Wherever there are insects, flies, animals and birds, there is moisture somewhere nearby.
• For food, look for any vegetation around. Most desert plants have some edible part to them (see *The edibility test*, page 296).

Making a dew trap
During the night, water collects on shiny surfaces such as windows and metal, or on smooth stones and pebbles. The dew can be collected by wiping the surfaces with a cloth early in the morning and wringing it out into a container. It can also be collected in a dew trap.
• Dig a shallow hole and line it with plastic sheeting or some other nonabsorbent material.
• Pile clean, smooth stones onto the sheet. The dew which collects on the stones will drain into the plastic sheeting.
• Early in the morning – before the sun evaporates the dew – remove the stones and collect the water.
• Sterilize the water before drinking it. The stones may be contaminated.

How to make a solar still
Another way to collect water in the desert is to suck it out of the ground with a solar still. A well-constructed still will collect up to 3 pints (about 1.5 liters) of water a day.
• Dig a hole at least 3 ft. (1 m) across.
• Place a clean can, or any other container with a wide neck, centrally in the bottom of the hole.
• If there are any leaves or shrubs near, put them loosely in the base of the hole. This will increase the water yield.
• Spread a sheet of plastic over the hole and anchor it round the edge with stones or other heavy objects. Place a stone in the center of the plastic so that its lowest point is right over the container, but not touching it. Condensation will collect on the underside of the plastic, trickle down the sheet and drip into the can.
• If you have a length of plastic tubing, place one end in the can and the other on the surface, protruding from under the sheeting. You will then be able to suck the water from the can without disturbing the still.
• There is no need to sterilize water from a solar still as long as the can and the plastic are clean. The process of distilling the moisture from the ground makes it safe to drink.

Protection against bears
Bears are the most unpredictable and hazardous animals you are likely to meet in the wild. The black bear – the commonest and smallest species of bear – roams forests, swamps and mountains in virtually all wilderness areas of North America. It is not always black; its colors may range from dark brown to pale cinnamon, often with a white patch on the chest. Adult black bears weigh up to 300 lb. (136 kg) and some are 3 ft. (92 cm) high at the shoulder.
The grizzly bear is bigger than black bear – some weigh as much as 500 lb. (227 kg). This heavy-limbed creature is found in the wilderness areas of Alaska, the Yukon, the Northwest Territories, British Columbia, Alberta and Montana. Its color ranges from off-white or yellow to black.
The grizzly bear can be distinguished from the black bear by the hump on its shoulder. Its behavior is more unpredictable than that of the black bear and it is more likely to attack campers if it is taken by surprise.
A bear will usually keep away from you unless it feels threatened or cornered, or it wishes to protect its cubs. Unfortunately, this natural shyness is easily overcome when the bear's

appetite is aroused by the smell of food. Bears have become more fearless – and, therefore, more dangerous – in national parks where the public insists on feeding them despite warnings against this.

By following the tips suggested here, you can protect yourself in areas where bears range.
• Be alert to surprise raids by hungry bears while preparing your meal. Always cook and eat outside your tent.
• Burn fat and leftovers after eating. Bury scraps well away from your campsite. Wash dishes and utensils thoroughly.
• To prevent food smells wafting through the woods, store provisions in containers with tight lids. Put the containers in your pack and then hang it on a branch at least 10 ft. (3 m) high and 6 ft. (2 m) from the trunk. Although a bear can climb trees, it is unlikely to risk falling from a branch that cannot hold its weight.

• When you walk through the woods, make noises and talk loudly. This may be enough to drive a bear away.
• Never wear perfume, scented deodorants or hair spray in the wild – sweet smells attract bears.
• If you see bear cubs, move away quickly and quietly – a protective and potentially aggressive parent may be lurking nearby.

If you are threatened by a bear

If you encounter a bear in the wilds, use the utmost caution. You are in danger if you are within 150 ft. (46 m) of the animal. Do not consider running away – the bear can probably run faster than you.
• Keep calm. Make no sudden moves that might trigger an attack.
• If the bear does not move and you see a nearby tree that you can climb easily, move

---

MOTORIST'S SURVIVAL KIT

A survival kit kept in the trunk of the car is a valuable piece of equipment for any motorist preparing for a long journey in remote country.

The contents suggested here are not expensive to assemble: many of the items can be old or used materials from everyday life. You may never need to use the kit – but

on the one occasion when you do, it could prove absolutely invaluable.

The clear polyethylene bag can serve as the container for the kit. It is important that the bag should be clear, because in an emergency you will not want to waste time rummaging through an opaque container for an item which is needed immediately.

Item	Uses
Large, clear polyethylene bag	Keeping things dry and together; shelter; flotation aid; cordage (when torn into strips); solar still; water container; emergency windshield.
Nylon clothesline 16 ft. (5 m) long	Tow rope; lashing.
Blanket	Warmth; stretcher; cordage or bandages if torn into strips.
Sweater and socks (in various colors)	Warmth; improvised filters; distress signals.
Flexible water can	Water container; flotation aid.
Cans of food	Nourishment; cooking utensils (when empty); signaling (using lid as mirror – see box, page 282); improvised stove.
Waterproof matches	Lighting fires.
Water purification tablets	Disinfectant.

slowly toward it. Drop your backpack before going up – this will make your ascent easier and may distract the bear while you climb.

• Grizzlies will climb only 10 ft. (3 m) up a tree. Black bears are more likely to pursue you on the ground than up a tree. However, be prepared to climb as high as you can to avoid a bear.

• If the bear charges in your direction and there is no time to climb a tree, play dead – lie down and roll up in a ball with your hands over your neck. Keep your backpack on for extra protection. At first, the bear may swat and maul you, but it will lose interest if you lie still.

• After the bear leaves, be sure that it is far away before moving again. If the bear hears or sees any movement, it may attack again.

Protection against insects

If you are stung by an insect, the consequences are unlikely to be serious. However, a sting may cause an allergic reaction, and a bee or wasp sting inside the mouth is dangerous to anyone. For first aid, see *Insect stings and bites*, page 110.

• To minimize the chance of getting bitten by insects such as mosquitoes and flies, use a repellent cream or spray. One of the best active ingredients is diethyl toluamide, which is found in many commercial preparations.

• Apply the repellent all over the body. Check the directions on the repellent to see if you can apply it to your clothes as well. Repellents are washed off the skin in time by perspiration, but they last longer when applied to material.

• Avoid camping at the edge of a river, lake or stream. Waterside campsites are prone to constant attack by flies during the summer.

• Avoid campsites surrounded by tall damp grass that may harbor flies. Pitch your tent upwind – on higher terrain, if possible.

INDIVIDUAL SURVIVAL PACK

Even a pocket-sized survival kit can carry enough equipment to stop a problem becoming a crisis. It should be carried as a backup kit and separately from a backpack – in a jacket pocket, say. Then, if you get parted from your gear for any reason, you can use it to find your way back to safety – or to stay alive until rescuers find you.

Item	Uses
Small waterproof tin with tight lid	Container for survival pack; cooking utensil; signaling device (when used as a mirror – see box, page 282).
Small compass	Direction finding.
Waterproof matches	Lighting fires.
Small, square candle	Light; warmth; fire-lighting aid.
Absorbent cotton	Swab; packing; tinder.
Knife	Cutting; opening tins; cooking.
Thin nylon line	Repair of equipment; ties for shelter.
Survival blanket	Warmth; shelter.
Water purification tablets	Disinfectant.
Whistle	Signaling.

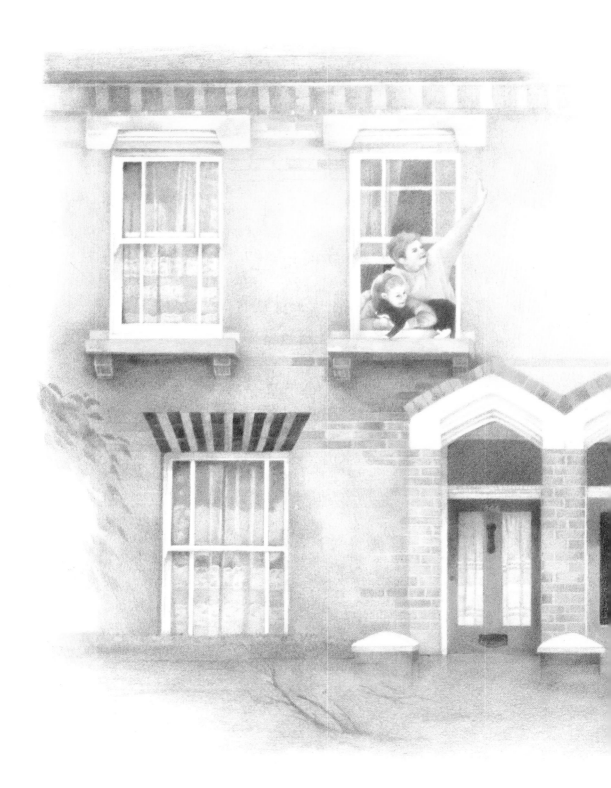

Natural disasters

304   Caught in an avalanche
305   Escaping a volcanic eruption
306   How to stay safe in a hurricane
307   Earthquake!
308   Trapped in a forest fire
309   What to do if you are caught in a flood

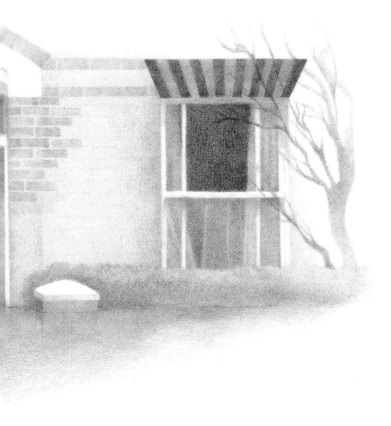

Caught in an avalanche

A snow slope that starts to slide may come down slowly like a flow of wet concrete, sometimes halted by obstacles in its path.

Alternatively, it may hurtle down the mountainside as a "slab" avalanche of broken chunks, preceded by a mighty blast of air.

In either case, the priority is the same: get out of its path.

• Assess the situation. Your first instinct may be to run downhill, but the avalanche is traveling downhill too – and it may be moving at as much as 100 mph (160 km/h).

• It is usually safer to head to the side. You may be able to get out of the path of the avalanche, or to reach higher ground.

• Get rid of any encumbrances such as a backpack, skis and ski poles. They will make it more difficult for you to move if the snow engulfs you.

• Do not try to escape by skiing unless you are on the very edge of the avalanche's path where a sprint will see you clear.

• If you cannot escape and the avalanche overtakes you, clamp your mouth tightly shut and hold your breath. This will prevent snow from entering your throat and lungs, and so minimize the risk of suffocation.

• Hang on to the downhill side of any fixed object – a rock pinnacle, for example. Even if you are engulfed for a time, the avalanche may eventually flow past and come to rest farther down, leaving you free.

• If you are swept downhill, fight to stay on top of the avalanche. Swim against the tide and toward the nearest side, using breaststroke, dog paddle or backstroke.

• While swimming, you may need to use your arms to fend off rocks and snow slabs, but above all keep fighting for the surface.

If you are buried by an avalanche

• To find out which way up you are, collect saliva in your mouth and dribble it from your lips. If the spit travels toward your nose, for example, you will know you are upside down.

• When you know which direction to aim for, try to break out of the snow.

• Summon every effort to break out immediately the avalanche begins to slow up, because avalanche debris begins to set hard within minutes of coming to rest.

• Wrap both arms around your head to create as much of a breathing space as possible.

• If you cannot break out, conserve your oxygen by moving as little as possible and breathing slowly. It is possible to survive under snow for some time until rescuers reach the scene.

SAFETY IN AVALANCHE COUNTRY

• When skiing or walking in mountainous areas, listen regularly to weather reports. Conditions can change very suddenly and it is better to cancel or cut short a planned excursion than to endanger your life and the lives of your rescuers.

• Never venture onto a mountain slope soon after a heavy snowfall. Avalanches often happen after successive falls of snow have built up in layers. The upper layers may then become unstable, and the weight of a single skier – or even the vibrations of a shout – may be enough to trigger a slide.

• Be particularly careful during intervals of warm weather or once a general thaw has set in during the spring.

• Be alert for the first signs of an avalanche: sounds of cracking ice; snowballs rolling down the hill; a dull roaring sound; or clouds of white dust farther up the hill.

• Obey all warning notices and avoid crossing risky slopes.

• If you have to cross a dangerous slope, do not go alone. Travel in a party and cross one at a time so that there is always someone to go for help.

• Continue to cross singly until all are safely over. Just because one person negotiates the slope successfully does not mean that the slope is safe.

• On long ski tours or walks in high hills, always take a professional guide. Touring parties should work to a timetable so that the alarm can be raised quickly if they do not reach their destination.

Precautions against avalanches

Helicopters, dogs and mountain rescue teams provide emergency services in areas where avalanches are common. For skiers and walkers, there are specific aids that may save life if disaster strikes.

• The quickest and most effective means of locating someone buried in an avalanche is a transceiver. This small, portable electronic homing device can be worn by skiers, and it emits a signal. When an avalanche accident occurs, survivors or rescuers can switch on their own transceivers to locate the buried transceiver immediately.

• Skiers should be equipped with shovels as well as transceivers. Speed is essential to save someone buried in the snow. The usefulness of a transceiver is limited if rescuers lose time because they have to dig the victim out of the snow with bare hands.

Escaping a volcanic eruption

Whether dormant or active, a volcano may erupt without warning. In a violent cataclysm, clouds of ash darken the sky, shattered rocks hail from above and molten lava floods down the slopes. Clouds of poisonous gas may also be released from the crater or from fissures on the flanks of the mountain.

A volcanic eruption is a catastrophe on such a large scale that it may seem impossible that any action one person could take would make any difference. Luck, of course, plays a large part in determining who survives and who does not, but decisive action may tip the balance of luck in your favor.

• If you are near a volcano and you notice any of the warning signs of an imminent eruption (see box, this page), leave at once. Travel is likely to become much more difficult – because of panicking refugees and the breakdown of transportation services – if or when an eruption begins.

• If you are caught in an eruption, leave the area immediately.

• Use any transport available. Be prepared, though, for wheels to stick in deepening ash. You may have to abandon the vehicle. If necessary, run, heading where possible for the nearest road out of the area.

• If you are threatened by lava flows, climb to high ground.

• Try to protect your head during an eruption. Flying rocks are a serious hazard, and a hard hat or crash helmet is ideal. However, any kind of headgear, padded out with newspaper, will provide useful protection.

• Improvise a protective mask against toxic fumes, using whatever piece of clothing or material is at hand. A wet scarf or handkerchief over nose and mouth will help to filter out volcanic dust and gases.

• Put on close-fitting goggles, such as swimming goggles, if you have some, to protect your eyes from the volcanic ash.

• Wear the thickest clothing possible for protection.

• Avoid taking cover in any buildings unless you find that you are under imminent threat from advancing lava. Though walls may survive the impact of flying debris, roofs are likely to be crushed.

• Be wary of finding yourself caught in the path of what scientists call a *nuée ardente* (glowing cloud) – a red hot cloud of dust and gases which can roll down the side of the volcano at more than 100 mph (160 km/h). In these dangerous circumstances, your only hope is to get underwater. If there is a stream, river or lake nearby, jump into it and hold your breath underwater. A small *nuée ardente* normally passes over in less than 30 seconds.

• If a period of calm follows a volcanic eruption, continue your escape from the area. It is likely that further – and more violent – eruptions may follow.

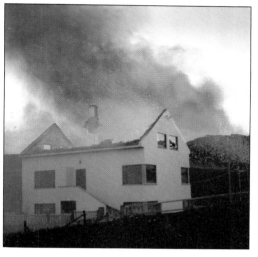

FIRE AND ICE *Ash and rocks caved in the roof of this house during an eruption that partly buried a fishing port on the island of Heimaey off Iceland in 1973.*

WARNING SIGNS

A volcanic eruption may occur at any place where the earth's surface is deeply fissured. Hawaii is part of a well-defined volcanic belt around the Pacific. Two North American examples are California's Lassen Peak, and Washington's Mount St. Helens, which erupted in 1980. There are also a number of active volcanoes in Alaska. Most volcanoes are in areas that are usually prone to earthquakes.

Some volcanoes are constantly rumbling, but even a volcano dormant for centuries may suddenly burst into life. The warning signs preceding a major eruption may last for weeks, and can include:

• Increasing seismic activity, ranging from barely noticeable tremors to substantial earthquakes.

• Loud rumbling noises from the volcano or the ground.

• The smell of sulphur coming from local rivers. The water may also feel warm. .

• A cloud of steam hovering over the mountaintop.

• Falls of acidic rain, which may sting unprotected skin.

• Fine pumice dust hanging in the sky like heavy talcum powder.

• Periodic emissions of hot ash and gases from the volcano's throat.

If a nearby volcano issues any of these warning signs, leave the area at once.

How to stay safe in a hurricane

Hurricanes are the world's largest and wildest storms. Racing winds of up to 190 mph (300 km/h) can destroy houses, tear down power lines and uproot trees. Hurricanes – known in some parts of the world as typhoons and cyclones – also bring torrential rain and may cause tidal waves which crash inland, washing out roads and flooding large areas.

You are unlikely to be caught entirely unawares by a hurricane. Warning announcements on radio and television give time to make preparations. If you live near a coast or a river, or in a low-lying area, you may be ordered to evacuate. Check with your local civil defense about evacuation routes and shelters.

• When a hurricane is imminent, board up all windows and glass doors. Anchor outdoor furniture and equipment or bring it indoors.

• If your house is inland, solidly built, and on high ground, you may decide to stay home. When the hurricane begins, move to the side of the house away from the wind and keep away from windows and doors.

• If you must evacuate, drive out of the storm's path or head inland – hurricanes weaken as they pass over land. Keep away from shores, rivers, and low-lying areas that may be swept by tides or floodwaters. Head for high ground. Get as high above the possible flood level as you can.

• When leaving home, take stocks of food and drinking water. Avoid foods that need cooking, refrigeration or dilution. Supplies of power and water may be disrupted for days.

• If a hurricane strikes before you can escape, stay indoors. The wind and rain make travel virtually impossible, once the storm begins.

• If the hurricane begins while you are driving, take shelter in the largest and most solidly constructed building available.

• Do not go outdoors until authorities announce that the storm has ended.

• If you are caught on high or open ground as the winds reach hurricane force, lie flat on the ground. Crawl on your stomach into the protecting shelter of anything – a belt of trees or an outcrop of rock – that will break the full force of the wind. If you are sheltering close to trees, take care in case there are falling branches or the trees are in danger of being uprooted.

• Shortly after the winds reach their fiercest, there may be a period of calm. This occurs as the eye of the hurricane passes overhead, bringing a clear sky and respite from the winds. Stay in a sheltered spot. In less than an hour the hurricane will resume, this time with the winds blowing from the opposite direction. If you are sheltering behind a rock or trees when the eye reaches you, move to the other side during the period of calm.

What to do if a tornado strikes

Tornadoes are whirling funnels of air which descend from the base of a storm cloud. They are usually about 80-160 ft. (25-50 m) across.

Where the funnel touches the ground it causes great destruction.

The winds in the funnel may be spinning at more than 200 mph (320 km/h). But the tornado itself moves forward at about 30-40 mph (50-65 km/h), so the storm is over in a matter of minutes.

No region in the world suffers as many tornadoes as the continental United States. Every year there are roughly 800 tornadoes and an average of 120 fatalities. In 1985, five giant tornadoes hit the Ohio-Pennsylvania border as well as parts of southern Ontario, injuring 1,000 people and killing 88.

• Buildings in the path of a tornado can explode, because the normal air pressure inside is much higher than the exceptionally low pressure in the storm's center.

• If your house is in a tornado's path, open all the doors and windows on the side away from the approaching storm to help equalize the air pressure inside and out.

• Keep the windows and doors tightly closed on the side from which the tornado is approaching. If the wind gets in, it may lift off the roof or blow out the walls.

• Take other precautions as for hurricanes.

WHERE HURRICANES HAPPEN

Hurricanes form over tropical and subtropical seas. The storms go under different names in different parts of the world: typhoons in the Pacific, cyclones in Australia and hurricanes in the Atlantic. But they are all essentially the same.

Around the calm eye, winds race at 75-190 mph (120-300 km/h), and the area they cover is an average of 100 miles (160 km) across. Outside the spinning mass of air, gale-force winds – over 40 mph (65 km/h) – may sweep an area four times as great. Most violent storms tend to occur in well-defined regions: the southwest Indian Ocean; the Bay of Bengal; the Arabian Sea; off the north coast of Australia; in the west Pacific; and in the West Indies and Gulf of Mexico.

Hurricanes are common in the southeastern and southern United States. There the hurricane season lasts roughly from June to October, and as soon as the weather bureau issues an alert, a comprehensive disaster organization goes into action. The hurricane is located and its movement forecast. Threatened areas are identified and the inhabitants are warned in repeated radio and television broadcasts.

Earthquake!

An earthquake is unlike a hurricane or flood in that no reliable advance warning can be given, although small tremors in an area prone to earthquakes may be a sign that a larger shock is coming. The immediate risk during a quake is from falling debris.

• If you are indoors when tremors begin, do not rush out into the streets.

• Take cover beneath a strong desk, table or bed. If no heavy furniture is available, stand in a doorway – the frame will provide some protection against the earthquake.

• Keep away from windows. The vibrations of the shock or movement in the building could shatter them.

• If you are outdoors when the earthquake strikes, keep away from tall buildings, trees, power lines and any other high structure which might collapse.

• Run into an open space as far from any high structure as possible. If there is no such space, take cover in a doorway.

• Do not take refuge in cellars, subways or tunnels. The exits could become blocked by debris, or the tunnels could cave in.

• If you are in a car, stop the vehicle and dive for the floor, crouching below seat level if possible.

• If you are in a large outdoor area and the earthquake is severe enough to throw you off balance, lie flat.

• When the initial tremor is over, stay put. Several further tremors may follow the first one at unpredictable intervals. Wait until police or rescue teams give the all clear.

• In the aftermath of a major earthquake, fires may start from overturned cookers and broken power lines, and pollution could result from shattered sewage pipes. Water is likely to be in short supply, too, or cut off entirely because of broken mains.

• Check your own home for signs of damage, and listen to radio or TV broadcasts for official instructions and warnings.

• If you have to go outside, keep well away from houses or any other structures which may have been weakened by the shocks. They could collapse without warning.

Earthquake zones

Certain areas of the world are more prone to earthquakes than others. The main areas are: the Pacific coast of North and South America; Japan; Southeast Asia; Indonesia; the east coast of China; central Asia; and a band that stretches across the eastern half of the Mediterranean from Italy to Iran. But nowhere in the world is entirely safe from earthquakes. In some cities in very unstable areas, such as Tokyo and San Francisco, some modern buildings are constructed on earthquake-resistant foundations. Most building codes in the United States and Canada require the construction of earthquake-proof structures.

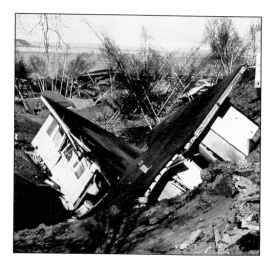

WHEN THE EARTH MOVED   *A bungalow, half swallowed by the earth, and trees tipped at crazy angles testify to the force of a quake which devastated Anchorage, Alaska, on Good Friday 1964. The earthquake measured 8.6 on the Richter scale.*

FAMOUS EARTHQUAKES

In North America, the most earthquake-prone region stretches from California to Alaska along the Pacific coast. Two of the region's most severe earthquakes occurred at San Francisco in 1906 and at Anchorage in 1964.

The San Francisco earthquake killed 800 people and wrecked many buildings, but it was the ensuing fire that destroyed a large part of the city. The earthquake, which lasted only 67 seconds, was caused by movements in the restless San Andreas Fault – the geological rift that runs through California.

The Anchorage earthquake was one of the strongest that ever hit North America. The initial tremors lasted three minutes, causing $311 million worth of damage. In some places, the quake pushed the surface rocks upward more than 30 ft. (9 m). It also set off a tsunami – a great sea wave – that flattened coastal towns. Not all earthquakes have been confined to the west coast. In the winter of 1811-1812, violent tremors shook the midwestern United States. The force of the earthquake changed the course of the Mississippi River in some places. On the east coast a 1755 tremor shook Boston and was felt as far away as Nova Scotia.

Trapped in a forest fire

A forest fire can spread at enormous speed, defying every attempt to contain it. In a large blaze, burning leaves and twigs, blown ahead of the flames, can enable the fire to leapfrog across the countryside faster than a galloping horse, and to jump even wide natural barriers such as rivers and roads. So, before you try to outrun the fire, quickly assess the situation. There may be better courses of action.

• Aim for a road or a river – these are the best escape routes. Otherwise, head for a plowed field or an expanse of rocky terrain – anywhere which has little vegetation.

• Remember that forest fires travel faster uphill than downhill. If possible, try to choose a downhill escape route.

• If the flames block your escape route, get into the middle of the largest open area you can reach.

• If you have the choice, go through a stand of hardwood trees rather than evergreens, which burn quickly. Avoid areas of dry or dead vegetation – they may be tinder-dry and virtually explode on contact with the flames.

• If you are in a car, stay in it. The risks of the gasoline tank exploding are less than the risks of being burned by the fire's fierce heat or suffocated by smoke.

• If you are on foot, get as low as you can when the flames come close. Thick smoke and lack of oxygen can suffocate.

• If there is a stream or pond, wade or swim as far as possible from the fire. Immerse yourself in the water.

• Cover your head and body with a blanket or coat, wet if possible, to protect your skin from the hot air.

• Stamp out nearby sparks or smother smoldering clothes after the main fire front has passed.

• Once the main fire has gone past you, look for a way out upwind through areas where the blaze has died away.

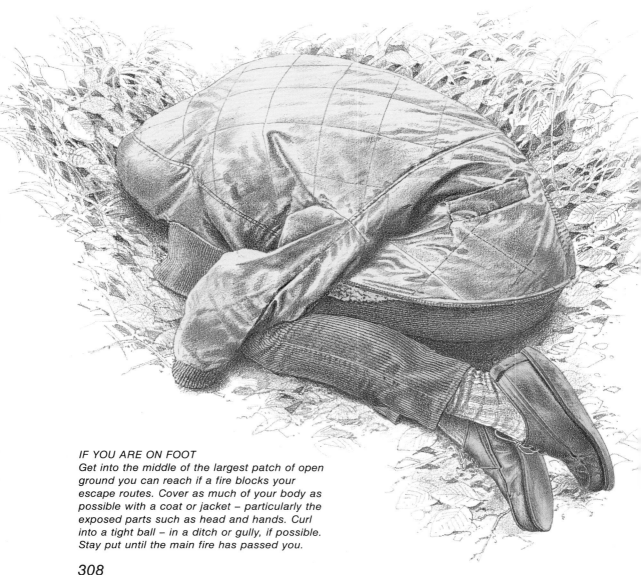

IF YOU ARE ON FOOT
Get into the middle of the largest patch of open ground you can reach if a fire blocks your escape routes. Cover as much of your body as possible with a coat or jacket – particularly the exposed parts such as head and hands. Curl into a tight ball – in a ditch or gully, if possible. Stay put until the main fire has passed you.

What to do if you are caught in a flood

Major floods tend to occur in river valleys, on coastlands and in other low-lying regions. If you live in an area prone to flooding, keep alert after spring ice breakup, or during and after storms and periods of prolonged rainfall. If there is a flood threat, local emergency officials will report developments on radio and television and advise you on what to do – in extreme cases, be prepared to evacuate your home.

• If a flood threatens your home, turn off the gas, and switch off electricity to lessen the risk of fire from flooded wiring.

• To keep water out of your home, first block all gaps under the outside doors. This is best done by lining the outer edge of the threshold with sandbags. Local authorities may provide bags. If not, you can make your own by using any plastic bags filled with soil, sand or gravel.

• Sandbag ground-floor windowsills on the outside in the same way if the water seems likely to rise that far.

• If the floodwater continues to rise, take any food in the house upstairs. If you live in an isolated area it may be two or three days before anyone can reach you. The essentials are drinking water, food, warm clothing and a portable stove for heating water. Take a fresh, disposable cigarette lighter or dry matches with you. Make sure that you have a battery-operated radio and a supply of spare batteries.

• If you have time, take up carpets and collect all valuables, putting them on an upper floor for safety. Try to move your furniture, electric appliances and other belongings upstairs, too.

• If possible, remove weed killers and pesticides to prevent water pollution.

• If there is no time to spare, place valuables for safety on any raised surface such as a table, cupboard or shelf.

• Always keep some form of identification for each member of your family, as well as personal and family documents, with you.

• In a very severe flood, you may be forced onto the roof and have to improvise a raft for escape. As the waters rise, gather up any equipment which can be used to signal for help, such as a flashlight, whistle, flags, bright-colored sheets or blankets, oily rags (for flares) and a mirror.

• Before going on the roof, eat and drink as much as you can to build up your energy reserves. Put on your warmest clothing and footwear – they will help to preserve body heat even if you are immersed in water.

• Take ropes or bedsheets to tie yourself to the chimney stack, to prevent you from slipping down the roof.

• To improvise a raft, assemble whatever buoyant materials are at hand: an air mattress, wooden beams, chests, planks or even a wardrobe. If you have no rope for lashing a raft together, use bedsheets. Use the raft only as a last resort, and test it to see that it floats before climbing aboard. Take some sort of paddle with you, and your signaling equipment.

KEEPING WATER OUT OF THE HOME

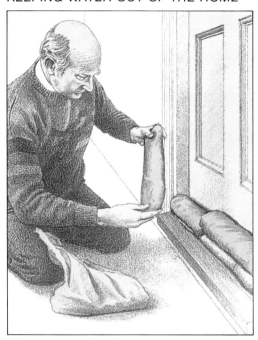

1 To stop water getting into a house, lay sandbags along the outside thresholds of the doors. If necessary, improvise by rolling up plastic shopping bags partly filled with soil.

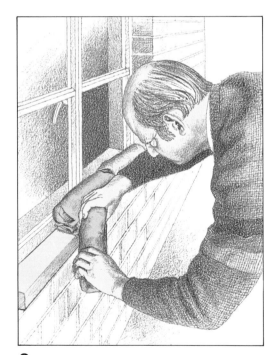

2 If the flood seems likely to rise as far as the windows, pack more bags along the sills outside. If you run out of bags, pack any gaps tightly with strips of old carpet or blankets.

Natural disasters

How to cross a flooded stream

If you are trapped by a stream in flood, take the utmost care when attempting a crossing. Even a small stream, swollen by fast-flowing water, may be strong enough to sweep you away.

• Make absolutely sure that the crossing is necessary before starting. It may be possible to make a detour to a bridge or to go upstream where the watercourse may divide into smaller tributaries which are easier to negotiate.

• Remove your socks, then put your boots or shoes back on to give you a firm footing on the streambed. Once across, you will be able to empty your footwear of water and replace your socks to keep your feet warm and dry.

• If you are carrying a backpack, adjust it so that it rides high on your back. Do not discard the contents. The weight will provide stabilizing ballast when you cross. As a precaution, however, undo the waist strap so that you can jettison the pack quickly in an emergency.

• Use a walking stick, or any other strong staff available. A stick about 6 ft. (1.8 m) long is best. It will improve stability, and you can also use it to probe for depth. Hold it on your upstream side so that the current does not tug the base away from you.

• Aim either straight across or diagonally downstream. But walk sideways, facing upstream so that your knees are braced against the current. If you face downstream, your knees may fold under the pressure of water from behind.

• Sidestep through the water, shuffling one foot at a time and moving each leg only when you are sure that the other is firmly planted.

• Do not cross your legs as you sidestep – you may lose balance.

Crossing with a rope

The safest way to cross a flooded stream, if you are not alone, is with a rope.

• One person should cross the stream holding

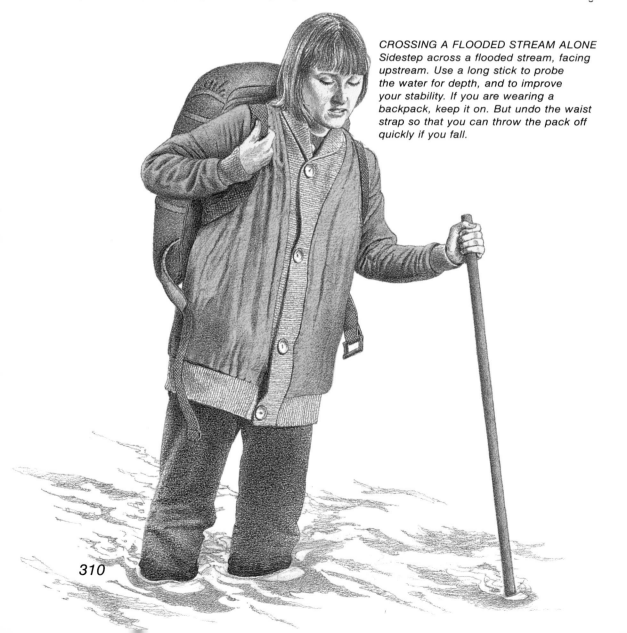

CROSSING A FLOODED STREAM ALONE
Sidestep across a flooded stream, facing upstream. Use a long stick to probe the water for depth, and to improve your stability. If you are wearing a backpack, keep it on. But undo the waist strap so that you can throw the pack off quickly if you fall.

one end of the rope. If the rope is long enough, he should tie it around his body. His companions should secure the other end of the rope by tying it to a tree or rock. If this is not possible, hold the rope so that if the first person slips he can be pulled back.

• When the first person reaches the far bank he should secure his end of the rope.

• The others should cross one by one, holding onto the rope with one hand and using a staff to steady themselves.

• If the rope is not long enough to cross the stream, the group should tie themselves together in a line. Each should have a stick. Only one person should move at a time. While he is moving, the others should be braced against the current in case he slips.

Crossing in a group

Three or more people who have no rope can help each other by crossing in a group.

• Form a file, one behind the other, in a direct line down the current, all facing upstream. Each person should hold the waist or shoulders of the one in front. First, the leader takes a small step sideways, then the second, then the third and so on. While one person is moving, the others should be braced in case he slips.

• Alternatively, the whole file can move as one person. Everyone behind the leader should hold the person in front, and all take a step sideways at the same time.

• Three people can also cross with linked arms. The middle person faces upstream, and the other two face each other sideways on to the current. Only one person moves at a time.

Choosing a crossing point

• Look for a section where the stream has broadened out. The flow should be slower and shallower there.

• Avoid crossing at a bend. Although the current may be slow and the stream shallow on the inside of the bend, the water will be deeper and more powerful toward the outside bank.

• Large rocks and boulders can provide valuable handholds as you wade past them. But do not try to use them as stepping-stones – the surface may be slippery or the base unsteady.

• Avoid crossing near submerged trees, high or slippery banks, and above rapids or weirs.

• Avoid stretches where a stream approaches a lake or valley basin. In flood, the stream will deepen and flow most powerfully here. It is best to head upstream until you come to a point where the flow is divided.

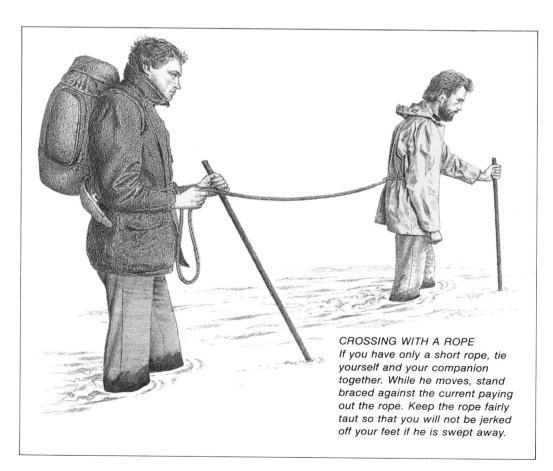

CROSSING WITH A ROPE
If you have only a short rope, tie yourself and your companion together. While he moves, stand braced against the current paying out the rope. Keep the rope fairly taut so that you will not be jerked off your feet if he is swept away.

Natural disasters

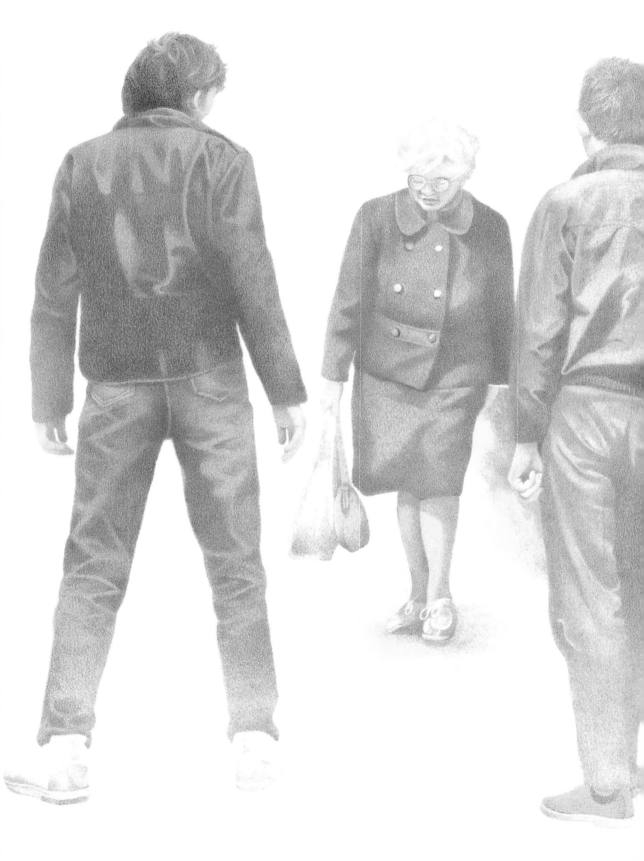

Crime

314   If you are attacked on the street

318   Threatened with sexual attack

319   Pestered by a drunk

320   When a crowd turns ugly

322   How to deal with an obscene telephone call

323   Caught up in a robbery

324   What to do if a bomb goes off

325   If your plane is hijacked

If you are attacked on the street

Escape if you can. Negotiate if possible. Fight only if you have no choice. These are the key rules for dealing with an attacker. Precisely what you do depends on your strength, confidence and willingness to fight back, and your assessment of the assailant.

Remember, an assailant who is drunk or on drugs acts impulsively. No one can predict what he might do if you try to defend yourself. In some cases, if you overreact or resist violently, you may increase your chances of being killed.

Faced with an armed mugger who wants your cash, it may be safer to hand it over rather than risk serious injury – or worse – in a fight.

On the other hand, faced with a potential killer and no escape, there may be nothing to lose by fighting. Nevertheless, try to negotiate or stall for time. Watch for a way of escape or rescue, or for a chance to disable your attacker. Fight only when you know there is no other option.

The techniques shown here need some practice, but not extensive training. All are danger-

THE STOMACH JAB

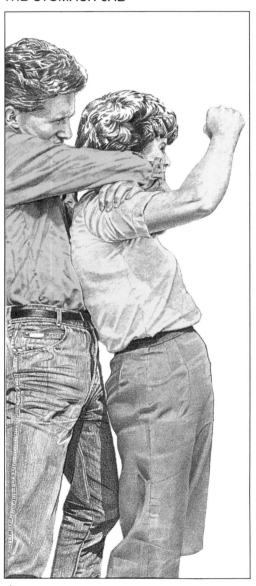

1 *If an assailant attacks you from behind, with his arms about your neck, the stomach jab is an effective deterrent. Twist your body slightly, clench your fist, and raise your arm. . . .*

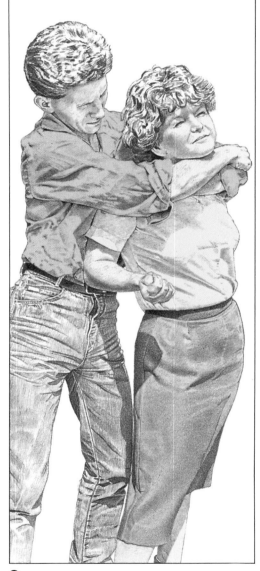

2 *Jab backward with your elbow into the attacker's stomach as hard as you can, aiming to wind him. This should force him to relax his grip enough for you to break free.*

THE SCRAPE AND STAMP

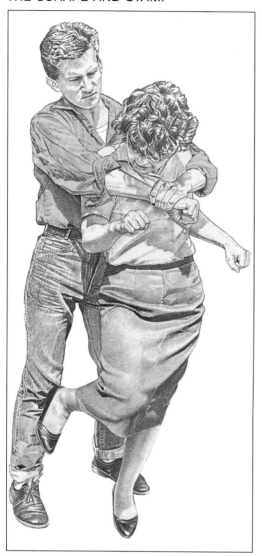

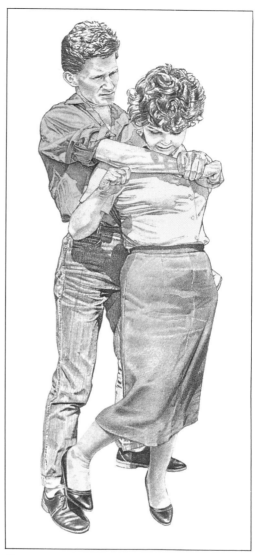

1 *If the stomach jab fails to break his grip, lift a foot and scrape the edge of your shoe down the front bony part of his shin. High-heeled shoes are particularly effective.*

2 *Stamp hard on the attacker's foot – a stiletto heel under the weight of a 110 lb. (50 kg) woman presses down with a force of more than 1,500 lb. (680 kg) per square inch.*

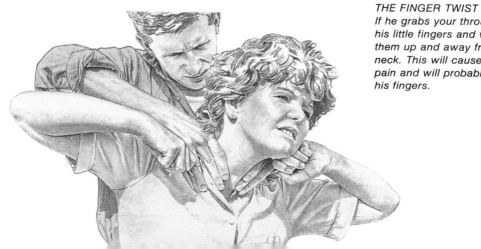

THE FINGER TWIST
If he grabs your throat, grasp his little fingers and wrench them up and away from your neck. This will cause extreme pain and will probably break his fingers.

Crime

315

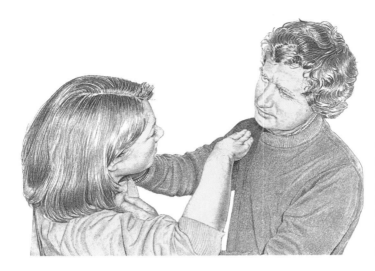

THE THROAT JAB
Hold the fingers of one hand rigidly straight and jab them into his throat, using either the ends of the fingers or the edge of your hand. Use this movement only in the worst situation.

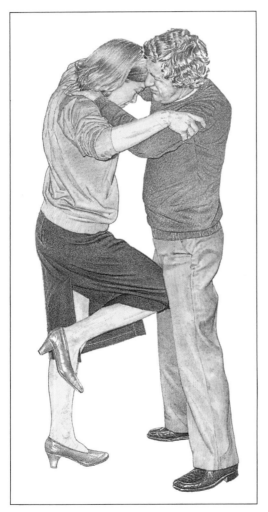

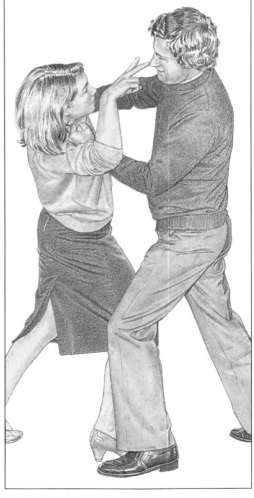

THE KNEE IN THE GROIN
Move in close and bring your knee up sharply into his groin. This will not work, though, if he is wearing a coat or if he twists away from you.

THE EYE JAB
Drop anything you are carrying to free your hands. Make a V with two fingers and poke them hard into the attacker's eyes.

ous – some are lethal. Never use them in earnest except in an emergency.

If you fight, never give a warning. Strike swiftly and as hard as you can. Be ready to repeat the blow or follow up with a different one. Scream for help as you fight. Keep on until you can escape or your assailant runs off or collapses.

How to escape

If you are approached by a suspicious-looking stranger, be wary – he may be armed. Act before he does. If you are on a busy street, scream as loudly as you can.

• If there are no other people about, run to the nearest occupied house and hammer on its door. Alternatively, run for the nearest well-lit street where other people are likely to be about.

HOW TO AVOID A MUGGER

• Walk with friends if possible, and ask them to stay with you all the way to your front door.
• If you are dropped off at home by a car, ask the driver to wait until you are inside.
• Stay on well-lit streets at night, and avoid lonely alleys or vacant lots.
• Walk on the street side of the sidewalk, or in the street if necessary, so that an attacker lurking in a doorway or alley has further to come to reach you.
• Walk with confidence, even if you do not feel it. An air of purposefulness is often enough to deter an attack.
• Carry a flashlight after dark. Flashed in an attacker's face, it could dazzle him and give you time to escape. It could also be used as a club.
• On a road, walk facing the traffic. That way, a car cannot pull up behind you unobserved. Do not hitchhike.
• If you have a bag, hold it in the hand or over the shoulder away from the road. Some muggers work on motorcycles, snatching handbags as they ride by.
• Carry a checkbook, credit cards, bills and cash in different pockets of your coat and handbag. If you have to hand over your cash, you will at least be able to keep other important items.
• Keep your keys in your pocket, not in a briefcase or handbag. Then, if a mugger steals the bag, you can still get home.
• Do not put your address on keys. If they are stolen, they could be passed on to a burglar. Instead, attach to the key ring a tag with your postal code. The code will be useless to a thief, but may help to identify the keys if they are stolen and are later handed in to the police.

USING AN UMBRELLA

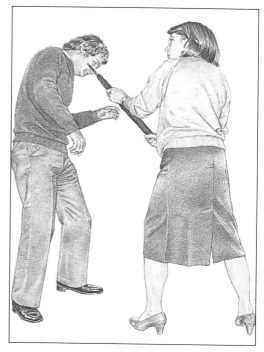

1 *An umbrella makes a powerful defense weapon. Hold it firmly in both hands and jab its end hard into the attacker's face . . .*

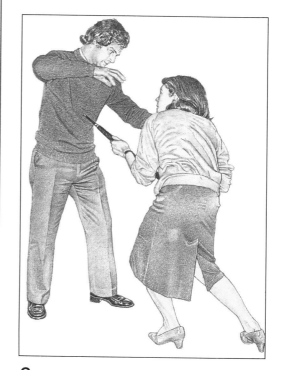

2 *. . . or stomach. If you have no weapon, feel for his testicles. Grasp and twist them violently. The pain can knock an attacker unconscious.*

Crime

Threatened with sexual attack

If you are threatened with attack — rape or, as Canadian law calls it, sexual assault — at home or on the street, police experts say that the best advice is to run away if you can. If no escape from the situation is possible, negotiate for your release or talk until you see an opportunity to get away. Some police experts recommend submission if the attacker is armed. Fight only if you have to (see *If you are attacked on the street*, page 314).

Police recommend that a woman at home who thinks she might be in danger from a would-be attacker should contact them, via a 911 call or through the operator, sooner rather than later (see *Intruders in your home*, page 178).

If you are followed on the street
• If you think you are being followed, cross the street to check your suspicions. Listen or glance back to see if the other person crosses the street after you.
• If you decide that you are being followed, go into any place where there are other people – a coffee shop, say, or a convenience store. Alternatively, knock at the first building or house that appears to be occupied.
• Tell the occupants you believe you are being followed and ask them to phone the police for you. Give the police a description of the person who was following you.
• Avoid using a phone booth on a quiet street to call for help. You could be trapped in the booth by an attacker.

If you are accosted
If you are approached by someone whose motives are plainly sinister, and you cannot get away at once, you can use any or all of a number of ways of dealing with him.

Which is best depends on the circumstances and on your own strength and confidence. None of the methods described here can guarantee your safety, but all have been used successfully by women to escape a would-be attacker.
• If you have time before the person accosts you, try to get some hard object in your hand – a comb, perhaps, or a bunch of keys – or a can of hair spray.
• If you pick keys, dangle them between your fingers and close your hand over them so that the jagged ends of the keys stick out from your fist.
• Keep your improvised weapon concealed until the attack starts. Then use the weapon – suddenly, without warning and as hard as you possibly can.
• Jab the end of the comb into his face or drag the teeth across underneath his nose. Scrape the keys across his face. Or spray into his eyes. At the same time, scream as loudly as you can.
• Keep using the weapon until the attacker lets go, then run to the nearest well-lit street or the nearest occupied building and get help.
• If you have no weapon, scream at the attacker to leave you alone. Use forceful language when you do this – as loud and vehement as possible. It may upset the fantasy a rapist often weaves

---

STAYING OUT OF DANGER

Most of the precautions you can take to avoid being attacked by a thief also apply to protecting yourself against the possibility of sexual attack (see *How to avoid a mugger*, page 317).

If you live alone, though, or if you have to go out alone – particularly after dark – consider taking some additional precautions.
• Consider, for instance, buying a hand-held screech alarm. Carry it in your hand, not in your handbag where it may be difficult to reach in an emergency.
• If you live in an apartment, use only your initials – not your full first name – on the tab beside your bell at the front door. That way, a stranger cannot tell whether a man or woman lives there.
• If you live alone, add another, fictitious name to the tab. An apartment that appears to be shared is far less likely to be picked out as a target by a rapist or a thief.
• Fit a heavy chain to the door, and a peep-hole viewer, and make a habit of using both

to check visitors. Do not use the chain alone.
• Do not open your door unless you are certain that it is safe.
• Arrange with your friends to use a special pattern of rings or knocks as a recognition signal, but even then make sure of your visitor's identity before opening the door. A thief or a rapist might have overheard the signal and could be copying it.
• If you are uncertain about the identity of a meter reader or serviceman, ask to see some form of identification or phone the company for confirmation. In an apartment, ask the janitor to accompany the meter reader or serviceman. In a house, read the meter yourself and inform the meter reader. Some companies permit users to fill in meter information on a form and to return it by mail.
• If you are on your own when someone comes to the door, pretend that you have company. As you approach the door, call out loudly to your fictitious companion something like: "Okay, Harry, I'll go."

around his intended victim, and make him abandon the attempt.

• At the same time as you shout, use a hand-held alarm if you have one, aimed into his face.

• If the attacker grabs you so that escape is impossible, and he is too strong for you to fight, pretend that you welcome the approach.

• Aim to buy time until an opportunity arises to escape. For instance, invite the attacker back to your apartment or house. Make the invitation sound convincing. Use earthy language to encourage him in the belief that once you get home you will be more than eager to do what he wants.

• Wherever you actually live, guide him toward a well-lit street with people in it. Then run toward the people yelling for help.

• Alternatively, try to persuade the attacker that you would love to spend the night with him, but in a few days' time. Give him a bogus telephone number to encourage him to believe you. Invent a plausible reason for the delay – tell him you have a heavy period, for example, or that you are suffering from a venereal disease.

• Once he hesitates, keep talking. Suggest, perhaps, going for a drink together in the mean-time. Again, once you are close enough to other people to call for help, break away and run toward them, shouting for help as loudly as you can.

• As soon as you get away from the attacker, dial 911, ask for the police and give them a detailed description of him (see *How to give a description to the police*, page 178).

If you are assaulted

• If you are attacked, get medical help as soon afterward as possible. Do not wash or tidy yourself up before doing this. A medical exami-nation will help to prove that you were forced to submit, and may be necessary to ensure that your attacker is convicted.

• Report the attack to the police and give them as detailed a description of the attacker as you can.

• Phone a rape crisis center for help and advice. The centers, which are staffed by women, exist in most large cities, and the phone number should be listed in the directory. If no number is listed, ask the police, a local women's center, or a hospital emergency department for the number.

• An internal examination, possibly by a male doctor, could be a traumatic experience if you are still suffering from shock. Later you might have to face your attacker in a police lineup and, if the case comes to a trial, give detailed evidence to a court in public. Many women find this an extremely painful experience. If you feel you cannot face the questioning, the medical examinations, or the subsequent legal processes, ask the rape crisis center to provide you with a companion – a woman trained to help you cope with these situations.

Pestered by a drunk

A drunken stranger is more likely to be a nuisance than a danger. Nevertheless, the un-predictability of his behavior and sudden switches in mood can be extremely frightening.

• Ignore a drunk, if possible, and keep out of his way. Do not invite his notice. On the subway, for example, get off and move to another car as soon as you can – ideally before he notices you. On the street, cross to the other side before you reach him.

• If you can't avoid him, assess his mood and character. If he seems harmless and merely wants to chat, humor him until he goes away or until you are able to leave. Try not to appear embarrassed, because this may encourage him.

• On the street, do not stop; just give a curt "Goodnight" in response to his opening con-versational gambit, and walk quickly by.

If he becomes aggressive

• Should he be either aggressive or maudlin, tell him firmly to go away, using language as forceful as you can make it. He is less likely to continue pestering someone fierce and firm than someone scared and submissive. If you make a fuss, you may get help from other people.

• If he is persistent and you are in a confined space such as a train, get up and sit next to another passenger. If you are on the subway, change cars at the next stop.

If he attacks you

• If he makes a grab for you, make as much noise as possible to attract other passengers.

• Some subways are equipped with a telephone for communicating with the operator in an emergency. Call the operator to inform him about the attack. There may be guards to deal with the attacker.

• Defend yourself if you have to. Hold him at bay by swinging something such as a handbag (see *If you are attacked on the street*, page 314).

Avoiding trouble on a subway or train

• To cut down the risk of being pestered by someone on a subway or train, always pick a car occupied by both sexes. Avoid a car where there is only one person – a man or a woman – or groups of unruly youths.

• At night on a train, try to sit in a car that will stop near the exit at your destination. Drunks sometimes seek out railroad stations, either in the hope of finding company or simply for shelter. Picking the right part of the train will save you a walk down what could be a lonely and shadowy platform.

• If you are not sure where the exit is on the platform at your destination, try to sit near the middle of the train. That way, you will at worst have to walk only half the length of the platform.

• If you feel insecure, arrange for someone to meet you at the station. You can also walk along with another passenger, or ask a train employee to accompany you through the station.

Crime

When a crowd turns ugly

Being part of a large, good-humored crowd – at a public occasion, say, such as the New Year's Eve celebration in Times Square, New York – can be exhilarating. But if the mood of the crowd turns sour for any reason, anyone caught in the crush, as a participant or simply as a bystander, can be seriously hurt or even killed.

Danger is most likely to arise in situations where people's feelings become inflamed for some reason – at or after hockey games, for instance, at protest meetings and demonstrations, and on picket lines. Panic, however, can turn any crowded place, such as a movie theater or discotheque, into a potential death trap.

If you are on foot
• If you find yourself in the path of an obviously unruly or frightened crowd, walk away from it and stay well out of its way.

• If you have no time to get right away from the scene before the crowd overtakes you, go into the nearest shop, knock at the door of the nearest house and ask for help, or tuck yourself into a convenient doorway.
• Stay put until the crowd has gone by.
• If you get caught up in the crowd, remember two overriding priorities: stay away from glass storefronts; and stay on your feet. If you get pushed through a plate-glass window or trampled by the crowd, you are unlikely to escape without serious injury.
• Hang onto something fixed, such as a lamp-post, if you can, and let the crowd surge on past you. Once the crowd clears, move calmly but briskly away from the scene.
• If you are swept along by the crush, create space for yourself by grasping one wrist in front of you with your other hand and bracing your elbows away from your sides. This will protect

IF YOU ARE SWEPT ALONG BY A CROWD

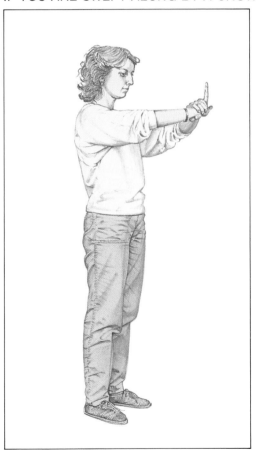

1 *In a crush you cannot escape from, create space for yourself around your chest so that you can breathe. Grip one wrist with the other hand and brace your arms in front of you with your elbows well out to the sides.*

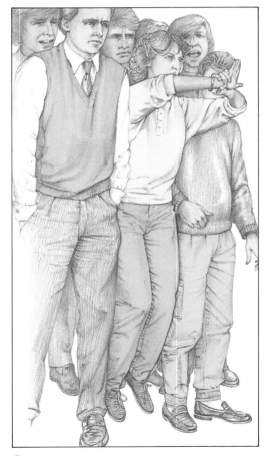

2 *Stay on your feet and stay away from glass storefronts for safety. If necessary, lift your feet off the ground so that your toes do not get trampled, allowing yourself to be supported by the people around you in the crowd.*

you from being squeezed by the people around you, and possibly fainting from sheer inability to breathe. Bend forward slightly at the waist at the same time to create extra room for your lungs to expand.

• Some experts suggest that you should bend your knees as well and lift your feet completely off the ground to avoid getting your toes trodden on. The crush of the people will support you.

• Be ready to put your feet down again as soon as the crowd begins to open up.

• If you are pushed to the ground, try to get against a wall.

• Roll yourself into a tight ball facing the wall with your hands clasped around the back of your neck. This will help to protect the most vulnerable parts of your body.

• Do not panic; a street crowd is likely to sweep on past you within a few seconds.

If you are in a car

• Never drive through a crowd, particularly if it is in an angry or hostile mood – or if it looks as though it could become hostile. You could be seriously injured if the mob turns on the car and breaks the windows or turns the car over.

• If you find yourself in the path of a crowd, do not stop to watch it. Turn into a side road, reverse or turn round, and drive away calmly.

• If you cannot get away from the approaching crowd altogether, park the car, lock it and leave it. Take shelter in a side street, a shop, a house or a doorway.

• If there is no time even to park the car, stop it – in the middle of the road if necessary – and turn the engine off.

• Lock all the doors and stay quiet inside the car until the crowd has gone by.

STAYING OUT OF TROUBLE

• At public events where there are large numbers of people, check the exits as you go in. But remember that the safest way out may not be the same as the way you came in. If a fire breaks out in a crowded place – in a baseball stadium, say, or a discotheque – look around for alternative escape routes. At a ball game, the safest place might be on the field, not pushing through narrow turnstiles.

• At a rock concert, try to avoid taking a seat at floor level. If fans rush the stage, you could be caught in the middle of a dangerous crowd.

• Every stadium has an evacuation plan. Follow the directions of security guards in your section. Keep pace with the flow of the crowd. Do not try to push ahead of other people.

• Stay behind at the end for 15 minutes to allow the main crowd to disperse.

IF YOU ARE PUSHED TO THE GROUND
Try to get beside a wall if you lose your balance and go down. Tuck yourself into a tight ball, facing the wall. Clamp your hands together around the back of your neck. Your fingers, back and legs may get hurt, but you will protect the most vulnerable parts of your body.

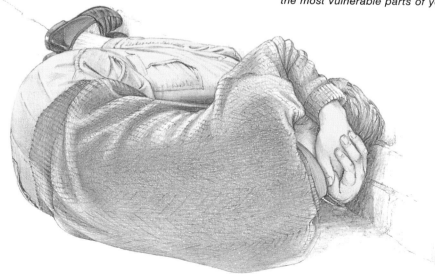

How to deal with an obscene telephone call

Obscene calls are unpleasant and may be upsetting, but they are extremely unlikely to lead to personal contact or a physical attack.

• Never give your number when answering the telephone, the police advise – just say "Hello." This is because, in many cases, nuisance callers do not bother to find specific numbers in a directory. They may dial a combination of numbers at random until a woman answers. As a result, they are unlikely to know your number, or to remember what they dialed, unless you remind them by saying it.

• If you have not had a similar call before, hang up without making any reply as soon as you realize the nature of the call. Do not say anything or betray any emotion. Check with everyone else in your home to find out if it has happened before.

• Do not try to dissuade the caller by blowing down the phone with a whistle, or using something that makes a screeching noise.

If nuisance calls continue

• If the calls persist, tell the phone company. Be prepared to supply a record of the calls, including dates and times. You can ask the phone company to put a trace on your calls. But it may be unwilling to trace sporadic nuisance calls, because it has more urgent cases and only limited equipment.

• If the nuisance calls continue, ask the police for help. The police may order the telephone company to put a trace on your calls. In this case, the phone company may want your assurance that you will press charges if the trace is successful. It may also ask to see a police report. It is unlikely that you will pay extra telephone charges if the police have ordered the trace on your telephone calls.

• Never try to keep a nuisance caller talking. With modern tracing equipment, it is unnecessary to keep him on the line. Try to listen for any distinctive background noise, such as machinery or traffic, in the few seconds before you hang up. Such clues might help the police track the caller down.

If you find the calls disturbing, or are afraid your child might answer an obscene call, you can do a number of things that might solve the problem while the police investigate the problem. The main options are listed below. To get detailed advice on any of them, contact your telephone company.

• Change your telephone number to reduce the chance of the same caller bothering you again. There may be no charge if the change is being made because of nuisance calls.

• If you have a plug and jack system, pull your phone out of the jack. When the phone is pulled out, the caller can hear it ringing but you cannot hear it at your end. The caller will think that you are out or have decided not to answer, and may give up dialing your number.

• Always use your phone in a professional way.

Let it ring twice. Answer in your usual way. If it is an obscene or nuisance call, hang up quickly and quietly. Do not ask repeatedly: "Who is it? Who is it?"

• Agree to a code with friends and relatives who are likely to phone you. Ask them, for instance, to let the phone ring three times, hang up and dial again. Then you will be sure that you are not answering an unwanted call.

AVOIDING UNWELCOME CALLS

Experts say that obscene callers are looking for an emotional reaction and, if you do not respond, they will probably look elsewhere. If you have a telephone answering service, never leave a message that could be construed as suggestive. Simply say something like this: "We are not available to come to the phone now. We will call back as soon as possible. Please leave your message." Do not give your name or your telephone number. Always use the plural "we" even if you live alone.

• If a caller asks you to confirm your number, do not do so; just ask what number is wanted. If it is not yours, do not give your number. Say: "Sorry, wrong number," and hang up. If it is your number, ask who wants to know.

• If your children are likely to answer the phone, tell them how to handle nuisance calls and make sure they do not give your phone number.

• If your teenagers are receiving nuisance calls, the cause may be a problem with friends at school. Discuss the problem with them.

• If you are uneasy about having your name and number published in the telephone directory, apply for an unlisted number. You can then expect calls only from people to whom you have given your number. This does not prevent a random obscene call, but as long as you do not mention the number when answering, a repeat call is unlikely.

• If you are having a new phone put in and you want an unlisted number, there will probably be an additional monthly fee. But if you want to change an existing number for an unlisted one, you may have to pay for the change as well.

• If you are a woman and want your name put in the directory, make sure that the entry gives only your surname and your initials – not your first name. Do not put Mrs., Miss or Ms. either.

Caught up in a robbery

Every day in the United States, there are more than 1,250 robberies – thefts involving violence or the threat of it – and in about one in three of them the robbers are armed. In Canada, there are about 30 robberies a day and in about one in eight cases the robbers are armed. Their targets are most commonly places where valuable goods, such as jewelry, or large amounts of cash are stored or handled: banks, for instance, armored cars, gas stations or convenience stores.

Burglary and housebreaking are far more common crimes. For details on how to cope with them, see *Intruders in your home*, page 178.

Most major robberies take place during the day, when the scene of the hold-up may be crowded with people. The thieves rely on speed and the terror they create to make an effective getaway.

If you are caught up in a robbery – at home, as a bystander when robbers burst in, as an employee of a firm that is being held up, or, in rare cases, as a hostage – police crime prevention experts recommend that you should not attempt to stop the raiders. Cash, they point out, can be replaced; life cannot.

What you can do, they say, is use your eyes and ears to help ensure that police catch the thieves afterward.

At home or in a shop
• If robbers – whether armed or not – burst into your house or into a shop where you are a customer, do not try to run away. By doing so, you make yourself the focus of the robbers' attention and could be killed or injured.
• Stay quiet. Do what you are told quickly and quietly. Do not argue.
• Make a mental note of everything you see and hear – including even the robbers' accents. Write details down as soon as possible, so that you do not forget anything in the confusion after the raiders leave.
• Dial 911 or call the operator and ask for the police as soon as you can after the robbery, and pass on your information to the police (see *How to give a description to the police*, page 178).
• If you are on the street and notice a robbery taking place – through a shop window, say – but you are not in danger yourself, do not go inside.
• Call the police at once. Do not put down the phone once you have raised the alarm. Keep talking. If you are close to the scene, you may well be able to pass on to the police an immediate description of the getaway car and the direction it heads in when the robbers leave.
• If you cannot get to a phone, make written notes of what you have seen as soon as possible.

In an office
If the office, store or factory where you work is raided by thieves, police recommend that you follow the same guidelines as those suggested for people who are caught up in a robbery at home or out shopping.
• Do not try to be a hero. Stay quiet and do what the robbers tell you. Observe, and make notes when the robbers have gone.
• Contact the police as soon as possible.

If you are taken hostage
The chance of your being taken hostage by robbers is very small. But it can happen.

The stress involved in being grabbed and threatened with death can be enough to drive every thought out of your head and create panic. But if you give way to panic, you only increase the danger you are in. Remember that anyone who takes a hostage does not intend to harm him or her. The intent is to use the *threat* of harm to force others to do what the robber wants.
• Do not struggle. Do not try to run away, unless you are certain you can make it.
• Do what you are told.
• Remember everything you can about your captor – his approximate age, build, type of voice, appearance, clothes and so on.
• As soon as possible after you are released, write down what you recall and dial 911.

GUARDING AN OFFICE

There are a number of precautions that can be taken in offices to prevent a robbery. In case of high-risk targets, for instance, a silent alarm can be connected directly to a security firm, which will call the police if the alarm is triggered. Reinforced doors and windows can make it difficult for thieves to get in.

Staff training can help as well. If, for instance, the cash-handling area is protected by a door that is kept locked from the inside, thieves may take a member of staff hostage to gain access. In this situation, a prearranged code – such as "George, can you let me in?" – could alert staff inside without arousing the thieves' suspicions. Police can then be contacted while other members of staff stall the thieves by, say, pretending that the mythical George has the key but he is not available for the moment.

Modern electronic locking systems can also have a code built in to warn staff of an attack.

A detailed security plan will depend on the size of the business being protected and the layout of the offices. Managers and staff can get free advice and help with training by contacting the crime prevention officer at the nearest police station.

Crime

What to do if a bomb goes off

A terrorist bombing is one of the least predictable and most terrifying emergencies anyone can be involved in. When traveling abroad in countries plagued by terrorism, be alert to the possibility of an attack. Busy public places – notably airports – are frequent terrorist targets. In these surroundings, look for the nearest exits and, if possible, try to stand away from the crowds. Always check in early at the airport to avoid the last-minute crush. Do not loiter in locker rooms or unattended luggage areas where bombs could be planted.

In the event of an explosion, you may feel helpless when faced with the sights and sounds of dozens, perhaps scores, of injured people. Nevertheless, your help could be invaluable.
- Give what help you can to the injured until the emergency services arrive and take over (see *Treatment priorities*, page 193).
- Do not, however, put your own safety at risk – from falling debris, say.
- If you feel you cannot help at the scene, leave the area quietly. Try not to run; you could start a panic and add to the casualty toll.
- If you have a camera, take photographs of the scene. Use a whole roll of film if possible. Concentrate on people leaving the scene after the explosion. The pictures could help identify a bomber.
- Make a note of everything you remember as soon after the incident as possible.
- Take your notes – and your film if you had a camera – to the police.

If you see a suspicious package
- Do not, under any circumstances, touch a package or container that you think might be a bomb. Many terrorist bombs contain anti-tampering devices which can trigger an explosion as soon as someone picks up or merely puts a finger on the package.
- Do not shout or do anything else that might cause panic.
- Move away from the package and encourage others to do the same.
- If you are in a crowded public place, find the nearest person in authority and tell him of your suspicions. If you are in an airport terminal, for instance, find the security guards; if you are standing on the platform of a railroad station, find a policeman or porter.
- If you see someone placing a suspicious package and making off, make a written note of what he looks like on anything handy (see *How to give a description to the police*, page 178).
- If you have a camera, take a photograph of him – if you can do so safely – and of the package. Even a fuzzy back view of the bomber may help to identify him. And if the package later explodes, knowledge of what it looked like to start with could give police experts clues in finding the terrorists who masterminded the operation.
- If you think the package might have been left

by accident, call to the person: "Is that yours?" If he denies it, act on the assumption that the package is a bomb.
- Get well clear of the package and make sure that others do so too.
- Alert the police at once.

HOW TO RECOGNIZE A LETTER BOMB

Letter bombs, like other types of terrorist bomb, are almost always disguised to look entirely harmless. Conversely, some hoax devices are deliberately designed to look like bombs in order to cause maximum panic. There is thus no reliable way of identifying a bomb.

Nevertheless, police experts do recommend looking for these warning signs among letters and parcels: any signs of wires or batteries; grease marks; or a smell of almonds.

More generally, they recommend that you look for the unusual. Is the package oddly bulky, for instance? Is it wrapped or sealed in an unusual way? If you are not expecting a package, do you know anyone living in the area where this one was postmarked?

If you find a suspicious letter
If you do come across a letter or package that arouses your suspicions, do not try to open it – letter bombs are designed to withstand postal handling and to explode on opening. Do not press, squeeze or prod it.
- Do not put it in another container. Do not put it in sand or water. Do not let anyone else do any of these things.
- Look for the name of the sender on the back. Phone the sender and check whether the package is genuine. If the package is not addressed to you, but to someone else in your home or office, ask the person to whom it is addressed if he or she is expecting a package.
- If these checks do not allay your suspicions, leave the package where you found it. Clear the room.
- If possible, lock the door and keep the key so that nobody can walk unknowingly into the danger zone.
- If there are windows in the room, tell colleagues and passersby outside to stay well clear of them to avoid being hit by flying glass if the bomb goes off.
- If you are at work, contact your firm's security officer, or the manager, or call the police at 911. At home dial 911.

If your plane is hijacked

Hijacking is not a common occurrence, but it does happen. In the 1980s, about 10 aircraft a year have been hijacked around the world. The planes affected have varied from light craft to huge jumbo jets.

At the start of any hijack, the hijackers, the crew and the passengers are all likely to be in a highly charged, emotional and excitable state which can lead to violence.

• Do not be aggressive. Try to melt into the background. Otherwise you may be singled out and put yourself and others at risk.

• Try to hide any possessions – such as military identification papers – which, if found, might arouse the hijackers' hostility.

• Keep a low profile – try not to call attention to yourself. Avoid eye contact with the hijackers.

• Never respond to hijackers unless you are questioned directly and then answer them briefly. Never show anger.

• As time passes, the situation will improve. Experience has shown that a rapport gradually builds up between passengers and hijackers. You may be asked to help with meals, clearing up and attending to the needs of others.

• Accept the more relaxed mood – but do not argue with your captors' political views.

• The hijack may last for days, and you may have to fly through a wearisome series of airports as the hijackers seek political sanctuary. Be alert for evidence of tension among fellow passengers, and reassure them where possible.

• Make allowances, too, for any symptoms of stress among hijackers and crew.

Surviving the ordeal

• If you are confined in a grounded aircraft, problems of heating and cooling may arise, especially if the aircraft has no ground power. Desert areas, for example, are hot by day and cold by night.

• At night, if the hijackers agree, distribute all available blankets and get everyone bedded down if possible.

• Be prepared for sanitation problems. The toilet arrangements on most aircraft are self-contained, chemical recirculation systems. They will quickly fill, become offensive, and may have to be drained by opening a valve outside the aircraft. Water for washing may be in short supply, or may not be available at all while the aircraft's engines are switched off.

• In the prolonged crisis of a hijacking, passengers may do unaccountable things. Some will become depressed and withdrawn. Others will become hyperactive, nervous and unpredictable. Children, however, may present fewer problems than anticipated – and can be a useful contact with your captors.

• If possible, try to keep your mind occupied with things other than the hijacking. Crossword puzzles, packs of cards, books and magazines will all help. It will also help if you can concentrate on small routines and maintain your self-control. A vacant mind, obsessed with the situation's dangers, tends to panic and take rash action.

• Try to keep fit – this is essential to maintain a healthy frame of mind. Opportunities for exercise may be limited, but take every opportunity to get sleep.

• Even catnapping is beneficial. If you are deprived of sleep, you will not be able to think straight.

• Take fluid whenever possible – it is more important than food. A healthy person can go without food for a month or more, but in high temperatures body fluid is lost quickly in the form of sweat and urine. While on the ground, an average individual not taking exercise needs at least a quart (about 1 liter) of water every day – at high altitudes 4-5 pints (2-3 liters) is needed daily. Do not drink alcohol, though, because it dehydrates the body.

• As any deadline given by the captors approaches, tension is bound to increase. Try to calm any passengers who are showing signs of hysteria.

• If the aircraft is attacked by rescuing forces, get down on the floor and stay there. Try to make yourself as small as possible; roll into a ball between the seats. There may be flashes of light, explosions, shooting and cries of terror. Do not stand up until the rescuers give the all clear.

• When this happens, leave the aircraft as quickly as possible.

• Outside the aircraft, the rescue services will meet all your needs, providing medical attention, clean clothing, washing facilities and – best of all – a bed. Accept their assistance. The press may be asking for interviews, but the airline staff will protect you from their approaches if you wish.

After the hijack

• Be prepared to face difficulties in the days that follow the ending of the hijack. You will feel completely drained physically and mentally. The experience may leave deep mental scars which may take weeks or months to heal.

• Be prepared especially for feelings of guilt. Some people may be disappointed with their own performance during the emergency. They may feel that they lacked bravery, panicked easily or behaved irrationally under stress. Others, however, may have surprised themselves by discovering unsuspected strengths of character.

• Under the Warsaw Convention, hijack victims can claim compensation for their ordeal from the airline they were flying with. However, it is more difficult to claim compensation from the country where the hijacking occurred. A claim must be substantiated by proof of damages, such as emotional upset, sleep disturbance and the like. A doctor's or psychiatrist's evaluation is necessary.

Crime

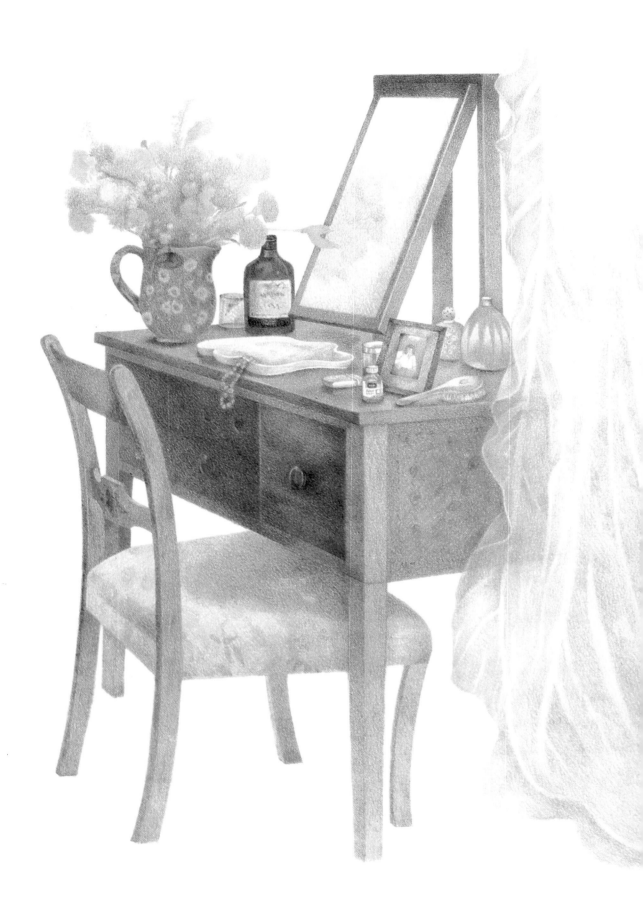

Alcohol and drugs

328   Spotting and coping with alcoholism
332   Staying on the wagon
333   Drug abuse: the risks
334   Drug identification and emergency treatment
335   Amphetamines
336   Amyl nitrite
336   Barbiturates
337   Cannabis
338   Cocaine
339   Glues, solvents, and lighter fuel
340   Heroin and morphine
341   LSD (and other hallucinogens)
342   Methadone
343   Opium
343   Tranquilizers

Spotting and coping with alcoholism

Though moderate and occasional drinking among friends is unlikely to prove harmful, alcohol *is* a drug.

Its damaging effects become more obvious when it is taken persistently or in excess.

Through abuse, alcohol can cause hallucinations as bad as those of LSD; like barbiturates, it can cause convulsions during withdrawal; and like heroin, it can induce coma and death.

Medically speaking, alcohol is a sedative with tranquilizing and hypnotic effects. Though a drinker may experience some initial elation, alcohol depresses rather than stimulates the central nervous system.

For this reason it belongs to the most dangerous category of abused drugs – those most likely to kill through overdose (see *Drug abuse: the risks*, page 333).

Alcohol as a drug

WHAT THE DRINKER FEELS Mild consumption of alcohol tends to free the drinker from inhibitions, reducing tension and anxiety. The drinker may feel relaxed, confident, euphoric or inspired. Large amounts induce excitement, agitation, nausea and vomiting. The drinker may *feel* alert both mentally and physically, but become confused, walk unsteadily and have difficulty in speaking clearly.

WHAT OTHERS SEE Alcohol reduces restraints and responsibility. These effects are often more evident to others than to the drinker. He or she may become impulsive and overtalkative, behaving in a grandiose, offensive or sometimes violent manner.

Judgment and concentration are affected progressively as more drink is consumed. The drinker may stagger and slur his or her speech. Accidents are a serious risk.

OVERDOSE SYMPTOMS After excessive drinking, the drinker may lapse into a stupefied state, leading to coma. In severe cases, he may stop breathing.

Do not automatically assume that because a person *appears* drunk, he is *drunk*. Other conditions – including diabetes – can produce similar symptoms, and so can numerous other drugs (see *Drug identification and emergency treatment*, page 334).

How to treat an overdose

• If the victim stops breathing, start artificial respiration at once (see page 50).
• If the victim is unconscious but still breathing, use your finger to clear any obstruction from the mouth and throat.
• Do not, however, try to induce him or her to vomit. Vomiting can kill an unconscious or comatose patient.
• Turn the victim onto his stomach, with his head facing sideways, in the recovery position (see page 136).
• Loosen his clothing and ensure that the airway

DRINKING – THE LONG-TERM EFFECTS

Besides the immediate risks associated with drunkenness, alcohol can also cause long-term damage. The liver and the central nervous system are especially vulnerable. Liver damage results from the poisonous action of the drug, while mental deterioration appears to result from organic changes which alcohol causes in the brain.

• Heavy drinkers tend to develop a fatty liver. Most will recover fully if they give up drink. A minority, however, develop more dangerous liver complications such as hepatitis (inflammation) and cirrhosis (replacement of healthy cells by fibrous tissue). With abstinence, the liver may recover from hepatitis, but the damage done by cirrhosis is irreversible. The condition can kill – but abstinence will at least check the progress of the disease.

• Other physical disorders include gastritis (inflammation of the stomach lining), pancreatitis (inflammation of the pancreas) and anemia (a reduction of the oxygen-carrying hemoglobin in the red blood cells).

• Damage to the central nervous system may lead to polyneuritis, which is also known as polyneuropathy. This is an inflammation of the nerves which may result in some degree of paralysis.

• The symptoms of brain damage may include loss of memory, pathological feelings of jealousy and persecution, delusions and hallucinations. Additionally, alcoholic dementia may occur. This is an irreversible deterioration of the intellect, with confusion, incoherence and numbed understanding resembling the symptoms of senile dementia. Heavy drinkers who escape these penalties are, however, no more likely than nondrinkers to lapse into senile dementia in old age.

• Women should not drink at all – or only moderately – during pregnancy. There are experts who claim that heavy drinking restricts growth and may also lead to mental retardation and physical defects. Some studies have shown that even moderate alcoholic intake – two drinks or more – is harmful to the unborn.

is still clear. Be sure to check that the tongue has not fallen back to block the windpipe.

• Call an ambulance if the victim is unconscious or if he cannot be roused. Other danger signs include an uneven or slow pulse rate, pale color and continued difficulty in breathing. If any of these occur, call an ambulance at once.

• Call an ambulance if the victim has sustained an injury, if he vomits persistently or if he remains in a state of excitement or agitation.

• Call an ambulance if the victim is a diabetic or if you suspect that any drugs have been taken in combination with the alcohol.

Withdrawal symptoms
Alcohol is an addictive drug, and with heavy drinking over a long period the body develops a tolerance for large doses.

The drinker may lose all pleasurable effects from drinking and may come to rely on alcohol simply to stay "normal" – to cope with the minor stresses and anxieties of life.

Often, a serious alcoholic problem is not detected until supplies are cut off or drastically reduced. When this happens, a serious withdrawal crisis may result. The symptoms resemble those experienced in withdrawal from barbiturates and tranquilizers.

• An alcoholic may exhibit anxiety, sweating and shaking before the onset of a withdrawal crisis. So-called "morning shakes," occasionally experienced by alcoholics, are in fact withdrawal symptoms which usually occur after sleep and are relieved by the first drink of the day.

• Delirium tremens (often known as the DTs) is a particularly severe, but rare, complication of alcohol withdrawal. Typically, it begins some two to four days after the last drink was taken and may follow a convulsion 12 to 36 hours after the last drink. A person suffering from delirium tremens begins trembling uncontrollably and becomes feverish and intensely agitated. Vividly realistic hallucinations may occur. These are usually visual and often terrifying.

• Whether or not delirium tremens develops, the withdrawal crisis may last for three days or longer before stopping, often abruptly.

• The withdrawal crisis may be so intense that there is a serious risk of accidental injury and of complications, such as pneumonia, setting in. For these reasons, a heavy drinker should not stop drinking suddenly without first seeking medical advice. Friends and relatives should encourage him or her to enter a hospital or specialist clinic for expert treatment.

How to deal with an alcoholic
There is no single cause of alcoholism. The disease may arise, for example, from a psychological problem.

But it can also arise from a particularly stressful occupation or simply from the company of hard-drinking friends who may themselves be dependent on alcohol. Similarly, alcoholism may appear in a variety of forms. Some people go for long periods without touching a drop – then go on prolonged binges in which they find it impossible to stop drinking.

Other people seldom get truly drunk, but they keep topping up with small quantities of alcohol from morning to night.

Whatever the cause or the pattern of drinking, remember that you cannot stop an alcoholic drinking. The drinker himself – or herself – must make the decision.

However, there are a number of things you can do to encourage positive thinking about the problem and assist the recovery process.

What not to do
• Do not start drinking yourself. Husbands and wives of chronic alcoholics are subject to the extra stress and tension of living with a drinker and sometimes they succumb to the same disease as their spouses.

• Do not put your own mental and physical well-being at risk. Make sure that you safeguard your health and constructive attitudes.

• Do not nag, lecture, preach or get involved in arguments. All hostile approaches tend to belittle the drinker. They may provoke violence or drive the drinker deeper into a sense of personal worthlessness for which drink has already become the remedy.

• Do not try to bargain with the drinker's emotions in an effort to make him or her stop drinking. Do not, for example, ask the drinker to demonstrate love for you by giving up alcohol. Similarly, do not threaten to leave – unless you are prepared to carry out your threat.

• Do not throw away any bottles you may find hidden about the house. You risk provoking violence and destroying such bonds of trust as still exist. An alcoholic will usually find some means of obtaining further supplies. And if he cannot find more drink, the enforced abstinence may only precipitate a withdrawal crisis with which you are unable to cope.

• Do not try to cover up for the drinker's habit by protecting him from its consequences. This mistake often takes the form of paying debts run up by the drinker. If money is owed, let the alcoholic face the problem. By smoothing the path, you act only as an "enabler," indirectly encouraging the drinking habit.

• Do not be misled by glib promises. If a resolution to give up drinking is made, make sure that it is backed up by definite action such as seeing the family doctor, joining Alcoholics Anonymous (see page 332), or both.

• Do not give up hope. Ultimately, most alcoholics who face up to their problem and accept qualified help do well. The addiction can be ended. About one out of every three alcoholics eventually recovers completely, and another can be greatly improved after treatment. So never be satisfied with doing nothing.

Alcohol and drugs

What you can do to help

• Recognize that alcoholism is a sickness. No good is served by considering it a sign of weak will or self-indulgence.

• Join Al-Anon (see page 332). This is a fellowship for the families and friends of drinkers. Learn as much as possible about the disease, and attend meetings regularly.

• Encourage the drinker to join Alcoholics Anonymous (AA). Make the suggestion with tact, and offer to go to open meetings with him – attendance carries no obligation, and he will not be asked for his full name.

• Leave literature such as AA pamphlets lying about the house. The drinker may resent lecturing but may nevertheless look at leaflets when you are not there.

• If the drinker shows any interest in giving up, encourage him to see the family doctor. In some cases, an alcoholic may not have acknowledged the scale of the problem to himself. Often, there will be reluctance to see a doctor but greater readiness to speak to an understanding clergyman, who may then persuade the drinker to seek medical advice.

• Strongly encourage any hobbies or activities which interest the drinker, so long as they keep him away from alcohol.

• If a serious problem occurs, for example through overdue debts, let the drinker face the problem. If he asks you for help, suggest that he contact Alcoholics Anonymous; the organization is skilled at advising on a wide variety of problems.

FOUR STAGES IN THE DEVELOPMENT OF AN ALCOHOLIC

Stage one –
the pre-alcoholic phase
Anyone who answers "yes" to any of these questions – particularly question 4 – should make an effort to control his drinking habits, as they could lead to serious problems.
1 Does he drink to feel at ease on social occasions?
2 Does he drink to forget worry or anxiety?
3 Does he feel more efficient or confident in his work when he is drinking?
4 Does he need to drink more than he used to in the past to obtain the same effect?

Stage two –
the warning phase
The answer "yes" to one or more of the following questions shows that the drinker is well on the road to alcoholism. He should cut down his intake sharply. Some people can manage to do this without outside help.
1 After a period of drinking during which he was not obviously drunk, does he find it difficult to remember things he said or did?
2 Does he drink surreptitiously or secretly?
3 If he thinks there will not be enough to drink at a party, does he "top up" with alcohol beforehand?
4 Does he arrange appointments so that they do not interfere with the opening hours of taverns and bars?
5 Does he gulp his drink?
6 Does he look for work in jobs where there is easy access to alcohol?
7 Does he ever drive after he has had several drinks?

Stage three –
the crucial phase
Every "yes" in answer to these questions is a warning that the drinker must cut down his intake drastically or in certain cases stop drinking altogether. He may need encouragement from his family or friends to do so or to seek medical advice. He is probably psychologically addicted to alcohol; he will become physically addicted unless he changes his habits immediately.
1 Does he continue to drink after initially deciding to have "just one or two"?
2 Does he frequently suffer from hangovers?
3 Does the idea of "a hair of the dog" as a remedy for a hangover appeal to him?
4 Does he suffer from morning shakes?
5 Does he have a drink first thing in the morning?
6 Does he neglect his meals because of his drinking?
7 Does he feel guilty about his drinking?
8 Does he prefer to drink alone?
9 Does he lose time from work because of drinking?
10 Does his drinking harm his family in any way?
11 Does he need to drink at a definite time each day?
12 Does he need to "top up" with a drink every few hours?
13 Does he carry drink with him, for example, in his car or briefcase?
14 Does his drinking make him irritable?

Where to go for help with an alcoholic problem
If you are trying to overcome an alcoholic problem of your own, keep in touch with your doctor. Remember, though, that a chronic alcoholic should not try to give up drinking suddenly without taking medical advice.

In a specialized treatment center, you may be given vitamins and possibly anticonvulsants (to guard against seizures).

Additionally, the family doctor may prescribe pills to cope with a drink problem. Keep strictly to the prescribed doses. As an alcoholic, you may be prone to excess and to the dangerous belief that four pills are better than one.

• Remember that no pills can "cure" alcoholism. They offer only a temporary aid, not an alternative, to the help which organizations such as Alcoholics Anonymous can provide (see page 332). Social service agencies also provide help for alcoholics.

• Under certain conditions, the doctor may recommend alcohol-sensitizing tablets, such as Antabuse or Temposil. These are deterrent drugs which, combined with alcohol, induce unpleasant effects such as headache, nausea, vomiting and breathing difficulties. They are available only on prescription.

• Psychotropic drugs (which alter the taker's mood) are occasionally recommended. They should, however, be avoided unless your doctor strongly advises them. Psychotropic drugs can themselves be addictive and they may prove harmful, by weakening your determination to stay off drink.

---

15 Has he become jealous of his wife since he started heavy drinking?

16 Does his drinking cause physical symptoms, such as stomach pains?

17 Does drinking make him restless, or prevent him from sleeping?

18 Does he need a drink to be able to sleep?

19 Does he lose self-control after drinking?

20 Does he show less initiative, ambition, concentration or efficiency than before?

21 Has his sexual desire decreased?

22 Is he particularly moody?

23 Has he become more isolated and lost friends?

24 Have his wife and children had to change their way of life – for example, by not going out, or not inviting guests – because of his drinking?

25 Has drinking made him harder to get on with, or otherwise changed his personality?

26 Does he tend to drink with people of a different background to his own or in places where he hopes he will not meet friends and acquaintances?

27 Does drinking affect his peace of mind?

28 Does he feel resentful, self-pitying or that everyone is treating him unfairly?

29 Is drinking jeopardizing his job or damaging his reputation?

Stage four –
the chronic phase
The answer "yes" to any one of the first three questions means that there is a strong likelihood that the drinker is an alcoholic. The answer "yes" to any one of the last five questions means that he is an alcoholic. He needs help *now* or he may do himself irreversible mental or physical harm.

1 Has he ever seriously considered suicide when drinking?

2 Does he feel incapable of coping with life, whether or not he has been drinking?

3 Does he suffer from any of the following conditions, all of which (in the absence of any other cause) are complications of heavy drinking? Vomiting blood; passing blood in the stools; severe abdominal pains; unsteadiness of gait when not drinking; pain in the calves; epileptic-like seizures; hallucinations (delirium tremens, or DTs); or severe tremors or sweating at night.

4 Does he go on alcoholic binges, drinking for several days in succession?

5 Does he get obviously drunk on much less than in the past?

6 Is he unable to take any action unless he has fortified himself with a drink beforehand?

7 Does he feel unable to give up drinking, even though he has been warned it is going to kill him?

8 Does he return to uncontrolled, excessive drinking again and again, even though he has tried to cut it down or give it up altogether?

Alcohol and drugs

Staying on the wagon

If you discover yourself to be heavily dependent on drink, you may need specialist care to cope with withdrawal symptoms. Afterward, friends, relatives and advisers can help you to stay off drink. But remember that, ultimately, the responsibility for recovery is yours.

• At all costs, stay away from the *first* drink. If you allow yourself one, others will almost certainly follow.

• Stay in close touch with the local branch of a specialist organization (see box, this page).

• Build up your own network of nondrinking friends whom you can contact whenever you feel the need for support.

• Keep in close touch with your doctor.

• Do not let the prospect of keeping off drink for the rest of your life become an obsession. Tackle the problem a day at a time: the days will mount to weeks, months and years. In time, abstinence will become part of your daily life.

• Do not be discouraged if, for some time after giving up drink, you still experience occasional cravings. Feeling like a drink is not the same as having one. The longer you stay sober, the less you will be troubled by cravings.

• Try to fill the gap created by giving up drink.

Keep busy, exploring any activities which interest you.

• Examine your own emotional makeup. Certain attitudes may have led you into alcoholism, such as feelings of guilt, inadequacy or self-destructive urges. If you can acknowledge and overcome them, the urge to drink may diminish. Professionals who have been trained to help addicts may be useful in this context.

• Do not give up hope. Alcoholics who *really* want to get better usually do so.

Things to avoid

• Keep away from bars and other drinking places. If you have drunk heavily for long, you most likely have particular haunts and drinking companions – avoid them at all costs.

• Avoid keeping drink in your home. Only when you are certain that you have conquered your problem should you risk keeping alcohol.

• Avoid stressful situations which have encouraged drinking in the past. Learn when to call "*HALT.*" The letters of the word are a simple reminder of the states in which you are most vulnerable – when you are *Hungry, Angry, Lonely, Tired* or *Thirsty.*

ORGANIZATIONS THAT CAN HELP

IN THE UNITED STATES

Alcoholics Anonymous World Services Inc.
P.O. Box 459
Grand Central Station, New York, NY 10163
(212) 686-1100

Al-Anon Family Group (includes ALATEEN)
P.O. Box 862, Midtown Station
New York, NY 10018-0862
(212) 302-7240

National Clearinghouse for Alcohol Information
P.O. Box 2345, Rockville, MD 20852
Federal government agency that supplies information and printed material.

National Council on Alcoholism
12 West 21st Street, Suite 700
New York, NY 10010
(212) 206-6770
or 1-800 NCA-CALL (24-hour service)

IN CANADA

Addiction Research Foundation
33 Russell Street
Toronto, Ont. M5S 2S1
(416) 595-6000 (9 a.m.-9 p.m. service)
or (416) 595-6111

Alcoholics Anonymous
234 Eglinton Avenue East, Suite 502
Toronto, Ont. M4P 1K5
(416) 487-5591

Al-Anon Family Group (includes ALATEEN)
P.O. Box 161, Station S
Toronto, Ont. M5M 4L7
(416) 366-4072

PUBLICATIONS

National Directory of Alcoholism and Drug Abuse Programs
U.S. Journal Inc.
1721 Blount Road, Suite 1
Pompono Beach
FL 33069
(305) 979-5408 or
1-800-851-9100

The Annual National Directory of Alcoholism and Addiction Treatment Programs Quantum Publishing
23860 Miles Road
Cleveland, OH 44128
(216) 475-9010 or
1-800-342-6237

Drug abuse: the risks

Drug abuse may warp behavior patterns, increase the risk of accidents and cause distress among the user's friends and relatives. Most drug-related emergencies are caused by overdose, and in this area the greatest risks arise from strong sedatives.

Sedatives induce sleep and reduce muscle activity. When taken in excess, they may slow bodily reactions to the point where the user goes into a coma. In extreme cases, they can kill by stopping the victim's breathing. Even if a patient who is in a coma goes on breathing, he may choke to death on vomit or suffocate because the tongue falls back and blocks the windpipe.

The drugs most likely to induce coma are: heroin; morphine; strong tranquilizers; barbiturates; alcohol; and the vapor from solvents, glues and similar volatile fluids. Death through coma is less likely to result from stimulants such as cocaine and amphetamines; hallucinogens such as LSD; cannabis; and mild tranquilizers.

The risk of accidents

Whatever the risk of overdose and coma, all drugs are more or less intoxicating, depending on their strength and the dose taken. They can impair judgment and behavior, creating risks of dangerous accidents. An LSD user, for example, might imagine that he can fly – and might jump to his death from a window in that belief. Large doses of amphetamines may cause the user to lose his grip on reality and to commit crimes without regard for the consequences.

The risks from injection

If an addict injects any drug, he courts risks to himself, in addition to the risks of the drug itself. Unskilled injection may result in ulcers on the skin, collapsed veins or a potentially lethal internal blood clot (a thrombosis). Addicts also often become victims of infectious diseases such as AIDS and hepatitis. The diseases are caused by handling hypodermics carelessly, sharing syringes or needles, or by using impure water to dilute the drug in the syringe.

In general, injection into a vein is the most dangerous way of taking a drug, because the whole dose acts immediately on the body. Amphetamines, for example, are only moderately harmful if swallowed, because digestion spreads the effect of the dose over several hours. If the same dose of an amphetamine is injected, the intensity of the resulting "hit" makes the drug as dangerous as heroin.

The risk of impure drugs

The dangers of taking pure drugs are multiplied because those on the streets have often been mixed with other substances. The additives may be poisonous or contaminated with disease organisms, or they may be quite unsuitable for the use to which the drug is put. For example, an addict may inject impure heroin (suitable only for smoking) with unpredictable toxic effects.

Other drug risks

Users may mix drugs with disastrous consequences. For example, a sedative may be taken to offset a stimulant. But drugs – even those with opposite effects when taken singly – do not necessarily counteract each other when they are taken in succession. In some cases, they can combine with tragic results.

Different drugs affect the body's chemistry in different ways. LSD, for example, rarely produces an overdose. Taking more than the normal dose may not alter the user's experience. With glues and solvents, however, there is a narrow margin of safety between the dose the user needs to achieve a "high" and a dose that could threaten his life. While a single dose may only intoxicate, a double dose could kill.

TEENAGERS ON DRUGS

A teenager may succumb to drugs simply to be "one of the gang." In this case, explaining the dangers may be enough to stop him using drugs. Often, a drug problem stems from mental or emotional stress. For some teenagers, drugs appear to offer a solution to the problems of growing up.

A teenager's drug problem may come to light before an emergency arises. Your suspicions may be aroused by an unexpected change in behavior or by poor performance at school. Faced with evidence of drug-taking, it is best not to overdramatize the situation. But there are some steps you can take:

• Try to keep on good terms with the teenager and discuss his problems sympathetically.

• Try to establish some facts about the drug or drugs being used. Are they smoked, swallowed, injected or inhaled? For how long and how often have they been taken?

• Ask your doctor for advice on coping with the problem. He can refer you to a drug clinic or hospital where specialist treatment is available.

• If possible, direct the teenager's attention toward making friends away from the drug scene and toward activities that will help to boost his or her confidence.

In cases of long-term addiction, expert help may be needed. But the support of friends and family is essential. The majority of addicts return to drugs after treatment, and more die than achieve lasting cures. Few among the survivors can kick the habit for good without the support of those closest to them.

Alcohol and drugs

Drug identification and emergency treatment

The ten-page section that begins here covers, in alphabetical order, all the drugs which are most commonly abused in North America.

Each entry describes what an individual drug looks like and illustrates its most common forms – this may be a form in which it is usually prescribed by doctors or the form in which it is most often sold on the streets. The entry goes on to explain what it is commonly called by users (since a parent's first knowledge of a drug problem in the family may be a teenager's chance remark).

Each entry also explains what a user feels when he or she is "high," what someone else might notice, and tells you how to recognize and treat an overdose. For first aid details on how to treat an overdose of an unknown drug, see page 92.

The size of a dose is no guarantee of immunity from an overdose because drugs do not always act on different individuals in the same way. A single aspirin may cause acute stomach pain in some people. Others are hypersensitive to cocaine and may collapse in life-threatening shock immediately after sniffing the powder. There is, therefore, no amount of any of these drugs that can be taken in complete safety.

Age, weight and general health also play a part in determining what effect a given dose will have. Other factors being equal, an older or less healthy person runs a greater risk of suffering from an overdose than a fit person in his late teens or early twenties.

Similarly, the bigger the user, the more diluted the dose becomes in his body. So someone who is physically large and heavy is likely to be less affected by a given dose (again, other things being equal) than someone who is small and slight.

How the drug is taken makes a difference, too. A dose that is injected has a far more dramatic effect – and thus carries a greater risk of overdose – than the same quantity sniffed, smoked or eaten.

Moreover, a user who buys drugs on the black market has no reliable way of knowing what he is getting, or how strong it is. The drug is likely to have been "cut" – in other words, adulterated – to an unknown degree in order to boost the pusher's profit.

The additive may itself be poisonous, or it may be a cheaper drug whose effects may magnify the effects of the drug it has been mixed with, affecting in an unpredictable way the chances of an overdose (see *Drug abuse: the risks*, page 333).

EMERGENCY SYMPTOM SORTER

A person who has taken a drug overdose may be in no condition to identify the drug involved or may be unwilling to admit to taking a drug at all. This list shows the major overdose symptoms and the drugs that are most likely to cause them. For more details and for how to treat the overdose, look under the entry for the appropriate drug. For the details on alcohol and on how to treat an alcohol overdose, see page 328.

Symptom	Possible causes	Symptom	Possible causes
Apparent drunkenness	Amyl nitrite barbiturates glues tranquilizers	**Fast pulse and fever**	Amphetamines cocaine
Coma	Barbiturates glues heroin morphine methadone opium tranquilizers	**Flushed skin**	Amyl nitrite
		Hallucinations	Cannabis, cocaine, glues, LSD
		Hysterical outbursts	Amphetamines cocaine, LSD
		Severe headache	Amyl nitrite
Drowsiness	Barbiturates cannabis tranquilizers	**Terror**	LSD
		Twitching and seizures	Amphetamines cocaine
Extreme restlessness	Amphetamines cocaine	**Violence**	Amphetamines, LSD

Amphetamines (and other stimulants)

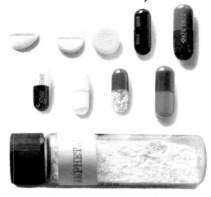

Amphetamine sulphate powder.
Pills and powder, all about actual size

WHAT THEY LOOK LIKE When prescribed by doctors, amphetamines and other stimulants come in the form of tablets or capsules. Shapes and colors vary greatly. Many of these legally issued drugs – which may be prescribed for slimming, for depression and fatigue during pregnancy, or for epilepsy, hyperactivity and other conditions – find their way onto the streets.

A white powder, amphetamine sulphate, is also sold by drug dealers. Often, the powder is adulterated with chalk or talcum, and it is sometimes passed off as cocaine.

TRADE NAMES Benzedrine, Dexedrine, Ritalin, Tenuate, Preludin, Methedrine.

WHAT THEY ARE CALLED Speed, pep pills and uppers are among the slang terms loosely used by drug-takers to cover the whole range of stimulant drugs.

Black bombers, blues, and hundreds and thousands take their names from the appearance of specific capsules and pills. Bennies and dexies are slang contractions of trade names.

HOW THEY ARE TAKEN Tablets and capsules are swallowed.

WHAT THE TAKER FEELS The short-term effects include heightened mental and physical activity. Users may feel no need for sleep, and may lose their normal inhibitions.

The drugs cause dryness in the mouth, so users often feel a strong thirst.

Excessive or repeated doses result in a sense of detachment from reality, sometimes accompanied by delusions. As the stimulation wears off, a depressed reaction sets in. The hangover may be severe and persistent, leading to craving for another dose. The drugs become habit-forming, and addicts often experience acute craving, depression and anxiety when supplies are cut off.

WHAT OTHERS SEE Moderate stimulation produces talkative, erratic and restless behavior. The user may sound hoarse and may drink much more than normal.

Larger doses block an awareness of reality. The user may stop communicating with other people and may become accident-prone. Users also lose awareness of the consequences of their actions and may commit crimes or become violent.

With the craving for renewed supplies, an addict may plead for money, and there may be evidence of pilfering at home.

OVERDOSE SYMPTOMS In an overstimulated or "blocked out" state, there may be extreme restlessness, irrational acts, outbursts of frustration, hysteria and delusions.

Physical symptoms can include a faster-than-usual pulse rate, fast breathing, twitching and even seizures. If symptoms persist, the whole body temperature may rise.

How to treat an overdose
• Make sure that no more stimulants – or any other drugs – are taken.
• Keep the patient away from bright lights, loud noise and fast movement – all will intensify the crisis.
• Try to calm the patient and keep a constant watch on him or her to prevent accidents. With a violent patient, some physical restraint may be necessary.
• Seek medical advice by telephoning your doctor or a hospital. If the patient is taken to hospital, doctors may administer a stomach washout to remove any drugs not yet absorbed. In severe cases, the overdose takes several hours to wear off, and the doctor may give a sedative or tranquilizer.

Alcohol and drugs

335

Amyl nitrite

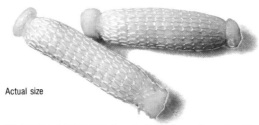

Actual size

WHAT IT LOOKS LIKE Amyl nitrite is a clear liquid contained in a small glass ampoule. The container is usually sheathed in a cotton cocoon. The drug is used medically to treat angina, a heart condition.

TRADE NAMES None.

WHAT IT IS CALLED Ammies, poppers, sniffers, snappers, amps and nitrite amps are the commonest names.

HOW IT IS TAKEN The glass ampoule is crushed so that the volatile liquid soaks into the cotton covering. The vapor is then inhaled.

WHAT THE TAKER FEELS Users experience an intoxicated "high." However, the state often requires several ampoules to attain, and it is often accompanied by a pounding headache.
    Large doses produce hallucinations.

WHAT OTHERS SEE Users appear drunk, elated or confused. The skin is often flushed, and the user may complain of a headache. The liquid also has a distinctive ether-like smell which may linger about the user.

OVERDOSE SYMPTOMS An excessive dose results in intensified symptoms. The headache may cause anguish and the skin can appear brightly flushed.
    Staggering, incoherence and other symptoms of intoxication all become worse.
    In a very severe case, the user may suffer temporary collapse and may have difficulty in breathing.

How to treat an overdose
• Apply artificial respiration at once if the patient stops breathing (see page 50).
• If artificial respiration is necessary, get medical help at once by dialing 911.
• Otherwise, stay with the patient to prevent accidents happening while he is intoxicated.
• Wait for the drug's effects to wear off. They should do so within about 30 minutes, provided no other drugs are involved.

Barbiturates

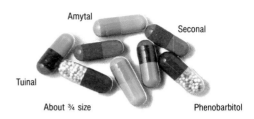

Amytal

Seconal

Tuinal

About ¾ size

Phenobarbitol

WHAT THEY LOOK LIKE Most barbiturates take the form of tablets or colored capsules containing white powder. Phenobarbitol, one of the most commonly prescribed barbiturates, comes in the form of a white tablet or a half blue, half clear slow-release capsule called a Spansule. Occasionally, barbiturates reach the black market as loose white powder.

TRADE NAMES Nembutal (yellow capsules), Amytal (blue), Seconal (orange-red), Tuinal (half red, half blue). Luminal and Gardenal (white tablets) contain phenobarbitol. Ampoules of white powder are usually Pentothal, which is used by doctors as an anesthetic.

WHAT THEY ARE CALLED Users refer to barbs, downers, goofballs and sleepers.
    Specific capsules often get their names from their appearance: blues, bluebirds, yellows and yellowjackets, for instance. Slang terms (phenobarb, ammies) come from chemicals.

HOW THEY ARE TAKEN Capsules and tablets are usually swallowed. Users often take them with alcohol – a combination which can prove fatal. Pentothal is injected.
    Attempts are also made to inject powders extracted from capsules and tablets and dissolved in water, but most barbiturates are dangerously unsuitable for this use. The powder is caustic, only partially dissolves and may burn or cause serious ulcers.

WHAT THE TAKER FEELS The sensations felt by users who take even mild doses of barbiturates resemble drunkenness, but users are more prone to accidents and they progress more easily into drowsiness. Barbiturates are addictive, and withdrawal symptoms include acute anxiety, headache, abdominal cramps, pains in the limbs and convulsions.

WHAT OTHERS SEE Users exhibit the typical symptoms of drunkenness, including talkativeness, slurred speech, stumbling, confusion and drowsiness.

OVERDOSE SYMPTOMS Heavy doses produce drowsiness deepening into semiconsciousness and coma. Breathing may stop, especially after the injection of a large dose.

How to treat an overdose

• Dial 911 and ask for an ambulance at once, stating clearly that you believe the emergency has been caused by an overdose of barbiturates.
• Provided the patient is conscious and cooperative, induce vomiting by putting your fingers down his or her throat.
• If the patient is not conscious or if he or she is not cooperative, however, do not try to make him or her vomit.
• Prevent any more drugs or alcohol being taken, and keep a close watch to prevent accidents.
• If the patient is comatose or unconscious but breathing, clear any obstruction from the mouth and put the patient in the recovery position (see page 136).
• If breathing has stopped, start artificial respiration immediately (see page 50).
• When medical help arrives, a stomach washout will be urgently needed to remove any unabsorbed drugs from the patient's body. The patient will need to be admitted to hospital.

Cannabis

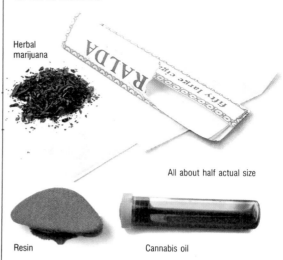

Herbal marijuana

All about half actual size

Resin   Cannabis oil

WHAT IT LOOKS LIKE In herbal form, cannabis – which comes from the hemp plant, *Cannabis sativa* – resembles a coarse tobacco. The dried leaves are greenish brown, often chopped up with stems, seeds and flower parts.

The sap of the plant is also dried to extract cannabis resin, which takes the form of a greenish, brownish or blackish block, stick or lump, or a coarse brown powder.

Very occasionally, the drug appears in liquid form, either as yellowish brown cannabis oil, or as cannabis tincture (a practically obsolete medical preparation).

TRADE NAMES None.

WHAT IT IS CALLED The herbal form is often known as grass, pot, marijuana, Mary Jane, weed, kef, bhang, dagga or ghanja. Resin is commonly referred to as hash, hashish, dope or resin. Other slang terms – such as Thai sticks, Moroccan gold, Lebanese gold and Nepalese black – derive from the drug's place of origin and its color.

Cannabis cigarettes are described as joints, spliffs or reefers. The butt of a used joint is often referred to as the roach.

HOW IT IS TAKEN Cannabis is usually smoked in joints (often made with larger-than-usual cigarette papers) or in pipes to produce an immediate effect. In herbal form, it may be smoked on its own. Alternatively, in any form, it may be mixed with tobacco.

Sometimes, powdered resin is added to cake mixtures, which are cooked and eaten. The drug's effects are then more delayed.

WHAT THE TAKER FEELS The drug is unpredictable. A user, especially one who is already depressed or worried, may become withdrawn and experience deepening anxiety.

Alcohol and drugs

337

Large or repeated doses may produce deep drowsiness or provoke delusions or hallucinations resembling those of an LSD trip. The skin is especially prone to imaginary creeping or crawling sensations.

WHAT OTHERS SEE Evidence of cannabis smoking may be present in the form of discarded butts, cigarette papers or torn strips of cardboard (used to make improvised cigarette filters).

Additionally, cannabis smoke has a distinctive smell, resembling that of burned grass or a garden bonfire.

The eyes of a user are often red. He or she may appear unusually relaxed and distant, mildly confused or prone to senseless laughter.

Judgment is impaired, and users may appear clumsy and accident-prone.

Cannabis rarely produces a hangover, but habitual users may become anxious and urgent in their search for more drugs when supplies are cut off.

OVERDOSE SYMPTOMS Large doses produce intensified symptoms of drowsiness, disorientation or hallucinations. The symptoms may cause distress, but are not normally life-threatening. Nevertheless, intoxication may create serious accident risks, especially if the user is driving or operating machinery. Large or repeated doses can also produce "cannabis psychosis" – a state of mental disorder and delusion which may take several days to pass.

How to treat an overdose
• Restrain the user from taking any more cannabis. Try to calm and reassure him. Take care to prevent accidents, remembering that, in severe cases, his judgment may be impaired for several days.
• If the user has persistent delusions or his behavior becomes severely disordered, seek medical or psychiatric advice.

Cocaine

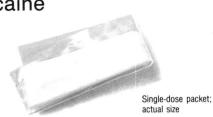

Single-dose packet; actual size

WHAT IT LOOKS LIKE Cocaine is a fine white powder. On the streets it is often sold in individual doses, folded in small pieces of paper or plastic. Because pure cocaine is extremely expensive, most doses are heavily adulterated with inactive powders such as chalk or talc. Some doses may contain no cocaine at all, but consist of cheaper amphetamine, often mixed with lidocaine or procaine (an anesthetic and a stimulant).

"Crack," a more powerful and addictive form of cocaine, is made by "cooking" it with water and baking soda.

TRADE NAMES None.

WHAT IT IS CALLED It's known as coke, crack, snow, lady snow, C, big C, princess, snuff, flake, leaf, nose candy, speedball (when mixed with heroin), and bombita (when mixed with amphetamine). Individual doses are referred to as snorts.

HOW IT IS TAKEN The powder is most commonly sniffed ("snorted"). Alternatively, it may be dissolved in water and injected into a vein, a practice known as "mainlining." The drug may also be mixed with tobacco and smoked, a practice known as "freebasing." Wads of coca leaves – whose effects are much weaker than the powder's – are chewed. "Crack" is usually smoked.

WHAT THE TAKER FEELS The user feels energetic and euphoric. The drug counters drowsiness and prevents sleep. Large doses may give rise to hallucinations.

A depressed reaction sets in as the effects of the drug wear off. Depression is relieved by a further dose, and so the drug becomes habit-forming.

WHAT OTHERS SEE The user's mood may visibly brighten and his behavior may become more uninhibited. He may seem mildly intoxicated or become accident-prone. Behavior can also become erratic and may extend to violent outbursts if the user is frustrated.

Physically, cocaine tends to dry out the lining of the nose, and some users develop sniffing as a nervous tic.

An intensely depressed hangover is often experienced on the morning after taking the drug. Cocaine addicts develop powerful cravings with severe withdrawal symptoms if supplies are cut off. Frantic drug-seeking behavior may result, often leading to crime to raise money.

OVERDOSE SYMPTOMS A few individuals are hypersensitive to cocaine; even a small dose may cause sudden collapse through an allergic reaction known as anaphylactic shock.

In any individual, an overdose may produce hysteria, delusions, physical tremors, muscle twitching and convulsions. Pulse, breathing rate and body temperature may also rise.

How to treat an overdose
• If a user collapses suddenly, call a doctor or ambulance immediately. Urgent medical care will be needed to treat anaphylactic shock (see *Dealing with an allergic reaction*, page 110).
• Otherwise, an overdose is rarely life-threatening. Prevent any more drugs being taken and try to calm and reassure the patient. Keep him or her away from bright lights, loud noise or fast movement, and keep watch to prevent accidents.
• The effects decline spontaneously over a few hours. A stomach washout is not necessary unless other drugs have been taken. If the overdose symptoms persist for longer than a few hours, however, or if they are very severe, get medical help.

Glues, solvents, and lighter fuel

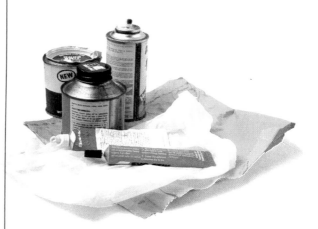

WHAT THEY LOOK LIKE Many household and industrial products are based on solvents that give off intoxicating vapors that are poisonous and sometimes fatal.

These freely available products include a wide range of glues, thinners, varnishes, paint strippers, dry-cleaning fluids, nail polishes and nail-polish removers. Gasoline, lighter fluid, and some aerosol products have similar properties.

WHAT THEY ARE CALLED Users refer to glue, thinner, sniffer and contractions of familiar trade names.

HOW THEY ARE TAKEN Glues and solvents are either sniffed or inhaled by the mouth. Sometimes the vapors are obtained directly from the tube, tin or aerosol spray.

More often the vapors are inhaled from a plastic or paper bag into which the glue has been poured, or from a cloth which has been soaked in the fluid.

WHAT THE TAKER FEELS Users experience a rapid intoxication that relaxes and sedates like alcohol, and that may include hallucinations. Drowsiness or drunken stupor may follow.

WHAT OTHERS SEE Inhaling produces mild intoxication resembling drunkenness, with staggering and slurred speech. However, the use of solvents is often readily identified by the pervasive smell of the vapor inhaled.

Spilled glue, impregnated cloth or discarded plastic bags are all signs that a product may have been abused.

OVERDOSE SYMPTOMS Severe intoxication may lead rapidly to coma. In severe cases, breathing may stop. This is a particular risk if the patient falls forward and continues to inhale vapor while unconscious. Abuse of these products can also

Alcohol and drugs

cause serious weight loss, lead poisoning, and brain and liver damage. The user may sometimes be injured when these products explode or catch fire.

How to treat an overdose
• Remove the source of the vapor at once.
• In a room, open doors and windows.
• Clear any obstruction from the patient's mouth and apply artificial respiration if breathing stops (see page 50).
• If the patient is unconscious or comatose, put him or her in the recovery position immediately (see page 136).
• Then dial 911 and call an ambulance.
• If the patient is conscious but disorientated, watch him closely. If his condition deteriorates or fails to improve within five minutes, call an ambulance.
• Keep watch to prevent accidents while the patient remains under the influence.
• Take special care to avoid fire risks. Many glues and solvents are flammable – or even explosive – as well as intoxicating. This is a special risk where gasoline or lighter fuel have been used: even a sparking light switch could ignite the vapor.

Heroin and morphine

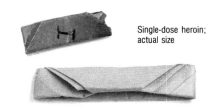

Single-dose heroin; actual size

WHAT THEY LOOK LIKE Heroin and morphine are usually sold in powdered form. Both are prepared from opium, and although the refined powder is white, it often appears brownish yellow because of impurities. Heroin (a derivative of morphine) is the stronger of the two and probably the most dangerous drug in illegal use. Both drugs are usually adulterated with an inactive powder for sale on the streets.

TRADE NAMES None in general use.

WHAT THEY ARE CALLED Horse, H, smack and shit are among the slang terms for heroin. Morphine is usually known as M or morph. An individual dose is referred to as a fix or a hit.

HOW THEY ARE TAKEN Heroin and morphine are usually taken by injection, with the powder dissolved in water. Addicts generally inject directly into a vein, a practice known as "mainlining." Alternatively, the drugs may be injected under the skin, a practice known as "skin popping." Addicts occasionally "snort" – that is, sniff – heroin powder.

WHAT THE TAKER FEELS Users of either drug lose touch with reality and feel drowsy. Some people, however, experience only unpleasant effects after taking heroin.
  Heroin and morphine are both addictive, and habitual users tend to stop feeling any pleasurable effects. The drugs become necessary simply to remain "normal" or to escape from harrowing withdrawal symptoms.

WHAT OTHERS SEE Signs of intoxication are often slight. The user may seem merely withdrawn into a private world and have tiny, pinpoint pupils. Larger doses produce more marked drowsiness. Scars of injection, known as "tracks," may be visible on the user. These are commonly found on the inside of the forearms and the front of the elbows. There may also be ulcers or the scars of healed ulcers.
  Discarded syringes and needles, or foil and tube (used for sniffing the smoke from the drug), may indicate that the drugs are being used. If supplies are threatened, the user is likely to exhibit acute withdrawal symptoms and to become frantic and violent. He or she may turn to crime in the search for more.

OVERDOSE SYMPTOMS The patient is in a deep coma and is breathing but cannot be wakened. The pupils of the eyes are reduced to mere pinpoints. Breathing may also stop.

An overdose is a particular risk when an addict has been off drugs for some time – in hospital, for example, or in prison. A single injection within days of discharge can kill, because the body can no longer tolerate doses to which it was previously accustomed.

How to treat an overdose
• Dial 911 and call an ambulance at once.
• If breathing stops, immediately clear any obstruction from the mouth and throat and apply artificial respiration (see page 50).
• Continue until breathing restarts or until medical help arrives.
• If the patient is breathing but unconscious, check that the airway is clear and place him or her in the recovery position (see page 136).

LSD (and other hallucinogens)

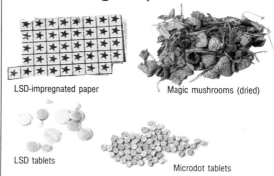

LSD-impregnated paper   Magic mushrooms (dried)

LSD tablets   Microdot tablets

All about actual size

WHAT THEY LOOK LIKE Lysergic acid diethylamide (LSD) and other chemical hallucinogens usually come in the form of tablets or capsules. Shapes, sizes and colors vary greatly, and include tiny microdot tablets (each about the size of this letter "o," or even smaller) and squares of transparent plastic.

More rarely, LSD may be sold in the form of a colorless liquid, which is dropped onto sugar cubes, cookies, paper or blotting paper for consumption.

In the picture above, for instance, each star on the sheet of yellow paper contains enough LSD for one "trip."

Mescaline, obtained from the Mexican peyote cactus, is sold in small, dried, brown portions of the plant.

Some fungi – often sold in dried form – contain hallucinogens, as do the seeds of some varieties of the morning glory plant.

TRADE NAMES None.

WHAT THEY ARE CALLED Acid is the common term for LSD. Doses are referred to as tabs (from tablets). Other chemical hallucinogens are known by their abbreviated names, such as STP, DMT and PCP (also known as angel dust).

Portions of the mescaline cactus are known as buttons, or mescal buttons. Hallucinogenic fungi are known as magic mushrooms.

HOW THEY ARE TAKEN Almost all hallucinogens are swallowed. Very rarely, LSD is injected. PCP may be swallowed, inhaled, or injected.

WHAT THE TAKER FEELS Users experience a hallucinated "trip," or sequence of disordered sensations. It starts about 30 minutes after the drug has been taken and may last for four or more hours, depending on the dose.

Sense impressions become distorted, and users may experience highly colored dream sequences. Sometimes, these are nightmarish and include terrifying imagery and visions.

Alcohol and drugs

341

Users may also experience a loss of self-awareness.

WHAT OTHERS SEE Few physical symptoms are visible. The user appears to be in a daydream or trance but may describe his or her experience more or less coherently.

The user may be prone to accidents through being detached from reality. Some imagine that they have acquired the power to fly or to walk on water – with obvious dangers.

On a so-called "bad trip," the user may cower from illusory terrors or try hysterically to escape them. Violent behavior may result from imagined threats.

OVERDOSE SYMPTOMS True overdoses are very rare. However, excessive quantities of any hallucinogen will intensify or prolong an experience. The most common emergency results from the persistent terrors of a bad trip.

Some hallucinogens can be poisonous. They include magic mushrooms, PCP and impure LSD. The user's behavior may become grossly disordered, and there may be symptoms of poisoning such as nausea, vomiting or physical collapse.

How to treat an overdose
• If poisoning is suspected, call an ambulance immediately.
• If the patient is unconscious, clear any obstruction from the mouth and put him or her in the recovery position (see page 136).
• If the patient is experiencing the horrors of a bad trip and remains conscious, there is no immediate need for medical help.
• Stay with the patient to prevent accidents and to stop him or her taking any further drugs. Some physical restraint may be necessary if the patient is violent.
• Keep him or her away from bright lights, loud noises and fast movement. Where possible, keep him in dim lighting and try to talk him down, calming and reassuring him until the worst is over.
• If the crisis lasts longer than four hours, seek medical help. Call the doctor to the patient. Do not take the patient to the doctor, or you risk stirring up the horrors again.

Methadone

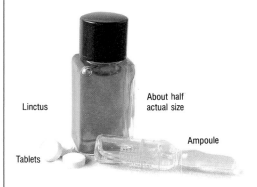

Linctus

About half actual size

Ampoule

Tablets

WHAT IT LOOKS LIKE Methadone can be a clear solution in a small ampoule. The drug may also be sold as a linctus or colored syrup, as wafers that are mixed with juice, or in the form of small white tablets.

TRADE NAME Physeptone, Dolophine and Amidon.

WHAT IT IS CALLED Meth, phy or linctus.

HOW IT IS TAKEN The drug may be injected, either in a vein or under the skin. In drug clinics, it is widely used to treat heroin addiction since it may reduce heavy craving and dependence.

Linctus and tablets are swallowed. In clinics they are used to try to break the heroin-injection habit.

WHAT THE TAKER FEELS Methadone has effects similar to those of heroin and morphine. The effects last somewhat longer, however. Methadone itself is addictive and may produce withdrawal symptoms.

WHAT OTHERS SEE The observable effects and signs of methadone abuse are the same as those of heroin and morphine abuse.

OVERDOSE SYMPTOMS The same as those of heroin and morphine.

How to treat an overdose
• Treat as for an overdose of heroin or morphine (see page 340).

Opium

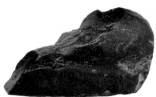

Actual size

WHAT IT LOOKS LIKE Raw opium (pictured above) appears in the form of blackish or brownish dried sap from the opium poppy. Refined opium is much paler in color and often powdered. It was once widely used in medical preparations such as tinctures and cough linctus. But most have been phased out because of the dangers of creating dependency.

TRADE NAMES None.

WHAT IT IS CALLED Poppy.

HOW IT IS TAKEN Raw opium is usually smoked, in an opium pipe. It may also be swallowed. Refined opium may be smoked, swallowed or (in some forms) injected. All forms are addictive.

WHAT THE TAKER FEELS The effects are similar to those of heroin and morphine, which are both derived from opium. The sensations are generally milder, though.

WHAT OTHERS SEE Dreaminess, drowsiness and detachment may be evident, though less marked than in heroin or morphine users. Injection scars will not necessarily be present.

There may be evidence of smoking in the form of an opium pipe with a sweet, heady smell. Some experts, however, say that the smoke smells like burning cloth.

OVERDOSE SYMPTOMS An excessive dose may produce effects similar to those of heroin and morphine, but there is less risk that the patient will fall into a coma or stop breathing.

How to treat an overdose
• If the patient appears comatose – breathing, but incapable of being woken – treat as for heroin and morphine (see page 340).
• In milder cases, the patient can be allowed to recover on his own.
• Keep him under observation to ensure complete recovery, and to prevent any other drugs from being taken.

Tranquilizers

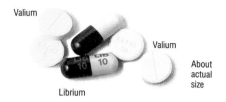

Valium

Valium

Librium

About actual size

WHAT THEY LOOK LIKE   Tablets and capsules of various shapes and colors. Some are also sold as syrup or in ampoules.

TRADE NAMES   Librium, Valium and Xanax are known as "mild" tranquilizers. In normal doses they tend to relieve stress without inducing sleep. Mandrex, Largactil, Quaaludes and Sparine are stronger tranquilizers, and are sometimes prescribed for mental disorders. They have a sedative effect, and may induce drowsiness even in a normal dose. Quaaludes are no longer legally prescribed but are available on the streets.

WHAT THEY ARE CALLED Like the stronger sedatives (see *Barbiturates*, page 336), tranquilizers are known as downers because they tend to relax rather than stimulate.

Mandrax tablets and capsules are known as mandies and blues. Quaaludes are also known as ludes.

HOW THEY ARE TAKEN Tranquilizers are usually swallowed.

Drug users often take them in dangerous combinations with alcohol, or in order to counteract the effect of stimulants. Occasionally, the drugs are injected.

WHAT THE TAKER FEELS   An easing of mental agitation and emotional stress. The drugs are mildly intoxicating, but more strongly so – sometimes much more strongly so – when they are taken with alcohol.

WHAT OTHERS SEE   Users display the characteristic symptoms of mild drunkenness, which may include staggering and clumsiness. Large doses, or smaller ones taken with alcohol, lead to greater confusion, drowsiness, slurred speech and uncoordinated movements.

Habitual use of tranquilizers may create a dependency, so that users exhibit anxiety when supplies are cut off.

OVERDOSE SYMPTOMS   Excessive doses may lead to coma, though this is less common than with barbiturates.

How to treat an overdose
• Treat as for an overdose of barbiturates (see page 336).

Alcohol and drugs

Index

Page numbers in **bold** type indicate a major treatment of a subject. Page numbers in *italic* indicate that the information is wholly or mainly explained in illustrations.

A

AA (Alcoholics Anonymous) 330, 332
abdominal injuries................ **46-7**
abdominal pain, recurrent in childhood........................... 81
abdominal thrusts
  relieving choking by......... *82-5*
abrasions
  sports injuries..................... 131
accelerator, jammed........ 213-14
accidents
  in inland waters
    avoiding........................... 220
  road accidents **192-5**
ACTA (Alliance of Canadian Travel Associations) 272
air sickness
  prevention.................. 270, 275
  treating............................ 270-1
air travel
  discomfort in the ears 275
  hijacked plane..................... **325**
  missing the plane.............. 272
  plane crash.......................... **274**
  staying comfortable in flight.................................. 275
airlines, collapse of 272
Al-Anon............................. 330, 332
alcohol poisoning 92
  first aid summary 18
Alcoholics Anonymous (AA) 330, 332
alcoholism **328-32**
allergic reactions
  to drugs............................. 333
  to insect stings and bites... 110
Alliance of Canadian Travel Associations (ACTA) 272
alphabet, phonetic
  in radio messages 259
American Society of Travel Agents (ASTA) 272
amphetamines **335**
amputation 48
amyl nitrite............................. 336
Amytal 336
anaphylactic shock................ 110
anchors, improvising *258*
animals
  accidents involving............. **198**
    avoiding...................... 197
  bites from.............................. 48
    cleaning and dressing *48*
    and rabies...................... **119**
    snakes.......................... **125**
  sick and injured.............. **181-9**
  threatened by bears ... **299-301**
ankle injuries **49**
  sprains *132, 133*
    moving the victim............ 112
ant stings................................ *110*
appendicitis **49**
  symptoms in children 81

arm
  bruised *65*
  fractured 99
    recovery position for........ *33*
    securing *127*
    sling for *121*
  jerky movements of in children 78-9
  severe bleeding from **60-2**
    first aid summary................. 4
  severed................................. 48
artificial respiration **50-3**
  and effects of cold water 239
  external chest compression................. **52-3**
  mouth-to-mouth resuscitation.................. **50-1**
    first aid summary................. 2
asphyxiation **54**
ASTA (American Society of Travel Agents)................. 272
asthma
  attacks **54-5**
  symptoms in children 79
athlete's foot 131
attacks
  on the street................. **314-17**
  sexual............................ **318-19**
attics
  safety measures 167
avalanches.............................. **304**

B

babies
  artificial respiration
    external chest compression..................... 53
    mouth-to-mouth resuscitation............... 50, *51*
  childbirth **72-5**
  choking 82-3
    first aid summary.............. 14
  crying **88-9**
  diaper rash 80
  hypothermia **108**
  newborn
    breathing difficulties.......... 75
  safety measures
    in the kitchen *163*
  suffocation risks................. *166*
  thrush 81
back injuries 55
  slipped disc **124**
bad weather, signs of.... 254, *255*
badminton, injuries from 130
bandages and bandaging.... **56-9**
  abdominal wounds *47*
  in first aid kit *44-5*
  fractured leg *98-9*, 128
  improvised 45, 56
  scalp injuries *102-3*
barbed objects
  removing from paws.. 186, *187*
barbed wire
  horse caught on............. 188-9
barbiturates **336-7**
barometers, reading 254
basketball, injuries from........ 130
bathrooms
  blocked toilet..................... 161

danger points 164-5
toilet flush failure................ 161
toilet tank dripping............. 160
baths
  water leaking under........... 160
Beaufort wind scale........... 256-7
bedrooms
  danger points 167
beer stains, removal of 176
bees
  stings............................... *110*
  to cats and dogs.... 186, 188
  swarms of 188
bicycles
  safety measures 217
birds
  treatment of injured 188
bites
  by animals **48**
    and rabies...................... **119**
  on cats and dogs.............. 186
  by insects 110
  by snakes 125
black eye **59**, 131
blanket splints
  fractured leg *129*
bleach
  child swallowing................ **117**
  first aid summary........... 27-8
bleeding................................ **60-3**
  detecting in the dark 60
  ear 62, *63*
  face *104*
  first aid summary 3-6
  injured cat or dog...... 182-3
    applying a tourniquet..... *182*
  mouth............................ 62, *63*
  nose 62, 116, 117
  stopping severe bleeding *60-1*
  pressure points *62*
  scalp.................................. 102-4
blindness **63**
blisters **64**
blocked drains *160*, 161
blocked toilets........................ 161
blood stains, removal of 176
blowouts **203**
board sailing............................. **240**
boats
  abandoning ship **260-2**
  avoiding a collision **242-3**
  canoeing **263**
  caught in a storm............. **258-9**
  dealing with a leak........... **248-9**
  falling overboard............. **236-7**
  fire on a boat **250-1**
  kayaking **264-5**
  plugging a hole **248-9**
  righting a capsized dinghy.......................... **240-1**
  rough seas....................... **252-3**
  running aground............... **244-7**
  wind and weather **254-7**
body splinting....................... *127-9*
bodysurfing.............................. *224*
bogs, trapped in..................... **280**
boils....................................... **64**
bomb going off....................... **324**
bones, broken....................... **98-9**
  ankle 49
  arm 99
    recovery position for........ *33*
    securing *127*
    sling for *121*

elbow
  splinting............................ 128
jaw... 104
leg... 98-9
  blanket splint for 129
  cats and dogs.................. 183
  recovery position for......... 33
  securing 128
  when skiing....................... 288
nose 116
rib cage........................... 69, 70
skull 102-3
sports injuries...................... 131
bottled gas
  safe use of........................ 152
bowline knot.................... 238, 239
brachial pressure point 62
brain damage
  and alcohol abuse 328
brake failure in cars................ 202
braking distances 201
  in fog.................................. 203
  on ice................................. 206
  on a motorcycle................. 216
breath tests
  law on 217
breathing
  abnormal breathing in
    children 78
  checking unconscious
    person for 136
  difficulties
    asthma attacks.................. 54
    choking 82-5
      first aid summary..... 13-16
    in newborn babies 75
    painful breathing 71
  rate.............................. 118-19
breech births 75
broken bones.......................... 98-9
  ankle 49
  arm 99
    recovery position for......... 33
    securing 127
    sling for 121
  elbow
    splinting............................ 128
  jaw... 104
  leg... 98-9
    blanket splint for 129
    cats and dogs.................. 183
    recovery
      position for 33
    securing 128
    when skiing....................... 288
  nose 116
  rib cage........................... 69, 70
  skull............................. 92, 102-3
  sports injuries...................... 131
broken fan belt......................... 211
bronchitis
  symptoms in children 79
bruises 65
bullet wounds........................... 102
burglaries
  dealing with 178-9
  protection against.............. 180
burns.................................... 66-7
  blisters caused by................ 64
  chemical burns
    to the eye...................... 94-5
  electrical 93
  first aid summary 7-10
burst water pipe...................... 159
  action summary 11-12

C

calf (leg)
  cramp in........................... 86-7
camping.............................. 276-7
cannabis 337-8
canoeing.............................. 263
capsized dinghy................. 240-1
carotid pulse 52, 119
cars
  accidents 192-5
    abroad........................... 195
    and animals.................. 198

helping victims of........ 192-3
avoiding a collision 195
batteries
  lighting a fire with........ 293-4
blowouts 203
brake failure 202
caught in a thunderstorm... 278
controlling a skid............. 200-1
defensive driving............. 196-7
driving in fog....................... 203
driving in snow and ice 206
driving through
  floodwater...................... 210
emergency repairs........ 211-15

All about CHILDREN

Babies and toddlers
  Giving artificial respiration to a baby
    external chest compression.......................... 53
    mouth-to-mouth resuscitation.................50, 51
  Dealing with an emergency childbirth...........72-5
  Dealing with diaper rash.................................. 80
  If a baby has thrush.. 81
  If a baby is choking.....................................82-3
    first aid summary....................................... 14
  If a baby is crying..88-9
  Recognizing symptoms of hypothermia 108
  Safety measures in the kitchen...................... 163
  Avoiding suffocation by pillows....................... 166

First aid for children
  Giving artificial respiration to a small child
    external chest compression.......................... 53
    mouth-to-mouth resuscitation...................... 50
  If a child is burned or scalded 67
  Diagnosing childhood illnesses....................76-81
    if a child has a runny nose and raised
      temperature 76-7
    if a child has diarrhea................................. 77
    if a child has jerky movements of the
      limbs 78-9
    if a child has abnormal breathing..............78-9
    if a child has stomach pain 80-1
    if a child has a rash for more than
      a week..80-1
  If a child is choking.......................................82-3
    first aid summary....................................... 14
  If a child eats a poisonous plant.................... 117
    first aid summary....................................... 28
  If a child swallows a household chemical
    first aid summary....................................27-8
    prevention 165

Child safety
  Avoiding accidental poisoning 117
  Making the kitchen safe................................162-4
  Making the bathroom safe.............................164-5
  Making the stairs safe 168
  Avoiding drowning accidents 164, 165
  If a child gets lost...284-5

car *continued*
  escaping from a car
    underwater.................. **208-9**
  fatigue during journeys....... **204**
  fire in **205**
  fitting a fire extinguisher..... 205
  sickness during journeys ... 270
  stopped by the police........ **217**
  stopping from 60 mph........ 201
  stuck on a rail crossing..... **205**
  stuck in snow **206-7**
  survival kit in........................ 300
cats
  accidents involving............ 198
  barbed objects in paws...... 186
  bee stings................... 186, 188
  broken leg 183
  choking 185
    avoiding risk of............... 185
  injured 181-3
    handling 181-3
  stopping bleeding 182
  fights between..................... 186
    treatment of injuries....... 186
  fits.. 184
  giving ear drops/ointment
    to 184
  giving medicine to...... 183, *184*
  giving pills to *183*
  and the law.......................... 198
  limping............................. 185-6
  wasp stings 186, 188
caves **290-1**
  lost in 290
  safety in 290
  stuck in passage................. *290*
  without lights in................... 291
ceiling, water leaking through
  burst pipes................. *158*, 159
    action summary........... 11-12
  leaking roof...................... 170-1
central heating repairs
  leaking pipe 160
  leaking radiator 159
chain saws
  safe use of.......................... *175*
chemicals
  burns from 66
  to the eye....................... 94, 95
  poisoning by household
    chemicals........................ **117**
    first aid summary........... 27-8
chest
  external chest
    compression................. **52-3**
  injuries............................ **68-70**
    asphyxiation caused by.... 54
    bleeding from 62
    rib fracture 120
  pain 71
chewing gum on clothing
  removal of 177
chicken pox **71**
  symptoms in children 77
childbirth................................. **72-5**
childhood illnesses............. **76-81**
children
  artificial respiration
    external chest
    compression................. *52-3*
    mouth-to-mouth
    resuscitation 50-1
  choking **82-3**
    first aid summary.............. 14
  lost................................... 284-5

poisoning **117**
  first aid summary........... 27-8
safety with
  in the bathroom........... 164-5
  in the kitchen.............. 162-4
  on stairways 168
chimney pots
  blown off during storm........ 171
chocolate stains 176
choking **82-5**
  cats and dogs 185
  first aid summary 13-16
cholera vaccination 268
circuit breakers 175
circulation problems
  in the eye............................. 63
cirrhosis of the liver.............. 328
clothing
  for cyclists 217
  on fire.......................... 67, 146
    first aid summary.............. 23
  for hot climates................... 270
  for motorcyclists **217**
  removing burned clothing *66*
  when struck by lightning 278
cocaine **338-9**
coffee stains.......................... 176
cold, common
  symptoms in children 77

cold water
  effect on swimmers 222-3
  perils of, for swimmers....... 239
cold weather, coping with...... 171
colic
  in children...................... 79, 81
  in horses............................ 189
collapse in the street............. 199
collision mats
  (for boats).................. 248, *249*
collisions, avoiding
  cars 195
  at sea **242-3**
common cold
  symptoms in children 77
compass
  using with a map............. **286-7**
compression
  head injuries......................... 86
computer on fire 148
concussion............................... **86**
contact lenses
  eye injuries caused by......... 94
convulsions
  symptoms in children 78
cooking equipment
  fires caused by.................... 147
  safe use of........................... *21*
cosmetics stains.................... 176

All about DRIVING

Road accidents
At the scene of an accident **192-5**
Warning other traffic.. 192
Sending for the police 192
Immobilizing the crashed vehicles 192
Helping the injured.. 192
Causes of road accidents 193
If you are involved in an accident **194-5**
Making a sketch of the accident..................... *194*
What to do after an accident....................... 194-5
If you have an accident abroad....................... 195
How to avoid a head-on collision.................... 195
If you hit an animal **198**

Defensive driving
Watching other road users........................... 196-7
Approaching a parked car............................ 196-7
Watching road signs.. 197
Watching approaching animals 197
Driving safely in fog...................................... **203**
Driving safely on snow and ice...................... **206**
Safety on a motorcycle or bicycle................. **216**

Problems on the move
Controlling a skid **200-1**
How to avoid skidding 201
How tires and weather affect braking............. 202
If your brakes fail 202
Why brakes fail.. 202
How to double-clutch 202
Blowouts **203**
How to drive through fog **203**

countryside, the
  camping **276-7**
  lost in the
    countryside **282-5**
  survival **292-301**
  using a map **286-7**
cramp
  attacks while
    swimming 222, *223*
  helping a swimmer with *230*
  treatment for **86-7**
credit cards
  safeguarding when
    traveling abroad 269-70
crime
  attacked on the street .. **314-17**
  bomb explosion **324**
  hijacked plane **325**
  intruders in your home ... **178-9**
  obscene phone calls **322**
  pestered by a drunk **319**
  robberies **323**
  threatened by a crowd ... **320-1**
  threatened with sexual
    assault **318-19**
crop spraying
  poisoning by **285**
croup
  symptoms in children 79

crowds
  avoiding dangers from ... **320-1**
crush injuries **87**
  chest 69-70
crying baby **88-9**
currency regulations 270
current
  swimmer caught in 222
cuts **89**
  bleeding from **60-3**
  first aid summary 3
  sports injuries 131
cycling
  injuries from 130
  safety measures 217
cyclones 306

delayed journeys
  compensation claims for 272
delirium tremens (DTs) 329
deserts
  survival in **298-9**
detached retina 63
dew trap, making
  in the desert *298*, 299
diabetes
  eye damage caused by 63
diabetic coma **90**
diaper rash 80
diarrhea
  in children 77
  traveler's 269
dinghy, capsized **240-1**
dining rooms
  danger points 165-6
dislocated joints **90**
distress signals
  heliographs 282-3
  lost in the countryside 282-3
  at sea 259
  while swimming *223*
  while windsurfing 240
distributor cap, cracked *214*
doctors
  seeing a doctor overseas .. **273**
dog bites
  treatment *48*
dogs
  accidents involving 198
  barbed objects in
    paws 186, *187*
  bee stings 186, 188
  broken leg 183
  choking 185
  fights between 186
    treatment of injuries 186
  fits 184
  giving ear drops/ointment
    to 184
  giving medicine
    to 183, 184, *185*
  giving pills to *183*
  heat stroke 186
  injured 181-3
    handling 181-2
    moving *181*
    stopping bleeding *182*
  and the law 198
  limping 185-6
  poisoning 184
  wasp stings 186, 188
doors
  frozen car-door lock 215
  opening during a fire *142-3*
  preventing toddlers from
    opening *165*
  safety measures 168
    glass doors 168
drains, blocked *160*, 161
dressings for wounds 56, *57*
  improvising 45
driving
  blowouts **203**
  brake failure **202**
  braking distances 201
    in fog 203
    on ice 206
    on a motorcycle 216
  burst tire **203**
  controlling a skid **200-1**
  defensive **196-7**
  fatigue during journeys **204**

D

deep fat fryer **148**
  action summary 21
  preventing fire in 162-3
defensive driving **196-7**
dehydration
  symptoms in
    children 77, 79, 80

If you feel drowsy at the wheel **204**
Staying awake during car journeys 204
If the car catches fire **205**
Getting out of deep snow 207
How to drive through floodwater **210**
If you are threatened by a hitchhiker **216**
If you are stopped by the police **217**
If you suffer from car sickness 270-71

Stranded in a car
  If you are stuck on a rail crossing 205
  If you are stuck in snow **206-7**
  If you are in a snowbound car 207
  Trapped in a car underwater **208-9**
  If you are caught in a thunderstorm 278
  Lighting a fire with a car battery *293*, 293-4
  Motorist's survival kit 300
  If you are caught in an earthquake 307
  If you are caught in a forest fire 308
  If you encounter a hostile crowd 321

Emergency repairs
  If the fan belt breaks 211
  If the gas gets low 211-12
  If the windshield wipers fail 212
  If you lose the wheel nuts 212-13
  If the engine is flooded with gasoline 213
  If the engine fades out because of
    vapor lock 213
  If the accelerator jams 213-14
  If the distributor cap is cracked 214
  If a fuse blows 214-15
  Thawing a frozen door lock 215
  Spare parts for everyday motoring 215

driving *continued*
  through floodwater............. **210**
  in fog.................................... **203**
  in snow and ice................ 206
  stopping from 60 mph........ 201
  in a thunderstorm 278
drowning
  and effects of cold
    water 222-3, 239
  rescuing a drowning
    person **228-31**
    from river or lake............. *221*
  reviving a drowning person . *91*
drownproofing technique **237**
drugs
  identification and emergency
    treatment **334-43**
  overdose........................... **92**
    first aid summary........ 17-18
  risks of drug abuse............. **333**
drunken strangers
  pestered by **319**
drunkenness **328-32**
  alcohol poisoning................. 92
  first aid summary.............. 18
DTs (delirium tremens)........... 329
dysentery................................ 269

E

ear
  bleeding from 62, *63*
    first aid summary.............. 5-6
  discomfort during
    air travel........................... 275
  infection in children 76, 77
  injuries.................................. **92**
ear drops
  administering to a pet 184
earthquakes **307**
egg stains, removal of........... 176
elbow
  fractured
    splinting........................... *128*
  sprained.............................. 133
elderly people
  coping with cold weather... **171**
  safety for
    in the bathroom.............. 164
    in the bedroom................ 167
    on the stairs.................... *168*
  treatment for
    hypothermia................. **108-9**
electric blankets
  on fire................................. 148
  safety with *167*
electric shock........................... **93**
  first aid summary 19-20
electric wiring
  water touching 161
electrical appliances
  in the bathroom
    safety with 165
  on fire
    action summary................ 21
electricity
  safe use of...................... 153-4
elevation slings........... 121-2, *123*
elevators, trapped in 177
engine, car
  emergency repairs........ **211-15**
  flooded with gasoline 213

vapor lock............................ 213
epiglottitis
  symptoms in children 78, 79
epileptic seizure...................... **94**
  helping victims on the
    street................................ 199
exposure................................. **281**
extended ladders
  raising *172*
extension cords
  safe use of...................... 153-4
    with power tools.......... 174-5
external chest
  compression................... **52-3**
eye
  black eye **59**, 131
  blindness **63**
  injuries............................. **94-5**
eye drops
  administering to a pet 184
eye jab
  for dealing with an
    attacker............................ *316*
eye ointment
  administering to a pet 184

F

face injuries........................ **102-3**
  bleeding *104*
  on the sports field.............. 131
fainting................................... **96**
  helping a victim on the
    street................................ 199
falls, treatment of injuries
  abdominal injuries............. **46-7**
  ankle injuries **49**
  back injuries **55**
  fractures.............................. **98-9**
  head injuries................... **102-3**
  neck injuries **55**
fan belt, broken....................... 211
febrile convulsion 78
feet, care of............................ 131
femoral pressure point............ *62*
fever fit.................................... 79
finger
  applying a tubular bandage
    to *59*
  severed................................. 48
finger twist
  for dealing with an
    attacker............................ *315*
fire
  on a boat **250-1**
  burns caused by **66-7**
  in a car............................... **205**
  causes of, in the home 147
  fighting **148**
    action summary............ 21-4
  forest fires **308**
  making in the wild........... 292-4
  prevention
    on a boat 250-1
    in the home **150**
  rescuing someone
    from............................ **148-9**
  in a tent............................. 276
  trapped in a blazing
    house **142-7**
fire extinguishers
  in cars 205

in the home **150**
fire screens.......................... *166*
fire-fighting equipment
  on a boat 251
fireman's lift *148-9*
first aid kits *44-5*
fits in animals 184
floats, improvising
  for survival in water ... 236, *237*
flooded house 309
flooded river
  crossing *310-11*
flooded tent 277
floodwater
  driving through **210**
flu... **97**
  symptoms in children 77
foam furniture on fire............. 148
fog
  driving through **203**
  lost in 284
  safe sailing in 248
food
  finding in the wild
    cooking 295
    edibility test.................... 296
  safeguards when eating
    abroad.............................. 271
food poisoning **97**
  avoiding abroad 271
foot
  care of feet 131
  cramp in.............................. 86-7
  frostbitten *99*
  severed................................. 48
football, injuries from.............. 130
football games
  avoiding trouble at.............. 321
foreign bodies
  in bleeding wounds........ 60, *61*
    first aid summary................. *4*
    making a ring-pad for *58*
  in the ear 92
  in the eye.......................... **94-5**
  in the nose..................... 116-17
forest fires 308
four-wheel skid 200-1
fractures **98-9**
  ankle 49
  arm 99
    recovery position for........ *33*
    securing *127*
    sling for *121*
  elbow
    splinting........................... *128*
  jaw...................................... *104*
  leg....................................... *98-9*
    blanket splint for *129*
    cats and dogs.................. 183
    recovery position for........ *33*
    securing *128*
    when skiing...................... 288
  nose 116
  rib cage 69, 70
  skull............................ 92, 102-3
  sports injuries...................... 131
freezers
  and power cuts 156
front-wheel skid 200
frostbite.................................. **99**
  see also exposure **281**
frozen car-door lock 215
frozen water pipes.................. 159
fruit juice stains, removal of .. 176
frying pan fire **148**

All about FIRE

In the home
If an electrical appliance catches fire 21
If an oil heater catches fire 22
If you smell burning at night 23-4
If a person's clothes catch fire 67, **146**
action summary 23
If your clothes catch fire.................. 67, *145,* 146
Fighting a fire... **148**
If a frying pan or deep fryer flares up 21, 148
If a computer catches fire 22, 148
If a television catches fire 22, 148
If foam furniture catches fire 22-3, 148
If an electric blanket catches fire 148

Outdoors
If fire breaks out in a stable 189
If your car catches fire.................................... **205**
Fire on a boat... **250-1**
If your tent catches fire 276
If someone is struck by lightning..................... 278
Forest fires... **308**

Escaping from a fire
If you are trapped on an upper floor 145
action summary.. 24
How to rescue a victim of smoke
inhalation... *124*
If a house is on fire **142-7**
Getting out of a blazing house *142-5*
If the exit is blocked *144-6*
Escaping from a high-rise building................. 146
Using a rope ladder.................................... 146-7
Rescuing someone from a fire **148-9**
How to do a fireman's lift **148-9**
Escaping from a sleeping bag....................... *276*
Escaping from a forest fire........................... **308**

Fire prevention
The causes of house fires 147
How to protect your home against fire 150
Choosing a fire extinguisher 150
Choosing a fire detector................................ 150
Preventing fires in a frying pan or a deep
fryer 162-3
How to use fire screens 166
Guarding against fire on a boat.................... 262-3

First aid for fire victims
How to treat burns...................................... **66-7**
first aid summary... 7-10
Treating blisters caused by burns 64
Removing burned clothing.............................. *66*
Treating chemical burns................................. 66
Treating burns or scalds in the mouth............. 67
Treating electrical burns................................. 93

action summary **21**
fungal infections
thrush in children 80, 81
furniture on fire 148
action summary 22-3
fuses
blown fuse in a car 214-15
in the home 154

G

gardens
safety measures 168-9
gas
appliances
safety with 151-2
asphyxiation by **54**
bottled
safety with 152
leak...................................... **151**
first aid summary........... 25-6
poisoning **100**
gasoline
car low on..................... 211-12
vapor lock..................... 213
gastroenteritis **97**
in children 77, 79, 80
German measles **101**
symptoms in children 77
glass doors
safety measures 168
glaucoma.................................. 63
glue-sniffing **339-40**
glue stains, removal of.......... 176
grand mal (epilepsy)................ **94**
helping victim on the
street........................... 199
gravy stains, removal of......... 176
grazes...................................... **101**
grease stains, removal of 176
grit in the eye *94-5*
gunshot wounds **102**
gymnastics, injuries from 130

H

hand
cramp in................................. 86
severed................................ 48
hand tools
safe use of........................ 174-5
hand brake failure
on a steep hill 202
head injuries........................ **102-3**
bleeding from 62
concussion **86**
fainting 96
head-on collision, avoiding.... **195**
heart attack............................. **105**
first aid summary 29-30
heart failure
giving external chest
compression.................. **52-3**
Heat Escape Lessening
Position............................... *262*
heat exhaustion **106**
prevention........................... 271
heatstroke **107**
in dogs 186

heatstroke *continued*
prevention............................ 271
hedge trimmers
safe use of.......................... 175
heights, working at **172-3**
heliographs, homemade 282-3
HELP position *262*
hepatitis vaccination.............. 268
herbal marijuana 337
heroin.................................... **340-1**
hiccups **108**
high blood pressure
eye damage caused by........ 63
hijacked plane........................ **325**
hikers
bad weather signs
for 254, *255*
exposure........................... **281**
first aid kit for 45
lost in the countryside.... **282-5**
survival in the wild **292-301**
hitchhikers
dealing with threats from ... 216
hockey, injuries from 130
horses
caught on barbed wire ... 188-9
colic................................... 189
lame 188
and motorists 197
sick or injured................. 188-9
handling 188, *189*
stable fires........................... 189
hostages
taken hostage by
hijackers.......................... 325
taken hostage by
robbers............................. 323
house
break-ins.......................... 178-9
protection against 180
danger points **162-9**
fires
action summary............. 21-4
causes of **147**
escaping from **142-7**
fighting **148**
rescuing someone
from **148-9**
smoke inhalation............. 124
floods *309*
storm damage................. 170-1
strangers calling at............. 178
hurricanes.............................. **306**
hypothermia **108-9, 281**
hysteria **109**

I

ice
driving in icy conditions...... 206
falling through **232-3**
rescuing someone fallen
through.......................... **234-5**
melting for water................. 295
ice cream stains, removal
of 176
immunization against disease
when traveling abroad.... 268-9
impetigo
symptoms in children 77
infantile paralysis (polio)
vaccination 269

influenza **97**
symptoms in children 77
injured person moving...... **112-15**
ink stains, removal of 176
insecticides
child swallowing................. **117**
first aid summary........... 27-8
insects
in the ear 92
stings and bites
to cats and dogs.... 186, 188
prevention........................ 301
treatment **110**
swarms of 188
insurance
accidents abroad 195
cash lost or stolen on
vacation 269
medical 273
plane hijacked.................... 325
vacation firm going out of
business........................... 272
internal injuries
abdominal............................. 47
head and chest.................... 62
International Association for
Medical Assistance to
Travelers (IAMAT)........... 273
intruders in the home........ **178-9**

J/K

jam stains, removal of............ 176
jaundice (hepatitis)
vaccination 268-9
jaw, broken.............................. **104**
joints
dislocated **90**
sprained.............................. **130**
journeys, delayed 272
jump start 215
jungles
survival in.......................... 295-6
kayaking **264-5**
kitchens
blocked sinks *160*, 161
danger points 162-6
knots
bowline....................... 238, *239*

L

ladders
carrying *172*
for rescuing someone fallen
through ice...................... 235
rope ladders 146-7
steadying *173*
stepladders......................... *168*
lakes
falling into **220**
rescuing someone from **221**
lameness
cats and dogs 185-6
horses 188
landings
safety measures 168
Largactil................................. 343
lawn mowers, electric ... *174*, 175

leak under bath...................... 160
leak through ceiling
burst pipes.................. *158,* 159
action summary........... 11-12
leaking boat......................... **248-9**
leaking radiator 159
leaking roof **170-1**
leg
cramp in........................... 86-7
fractured *98-9*
blanket splint for *129*
cats and dogs................. 183
recovery position for........ *33*
securing *128*
when skiing..................... 288
jerky movements of
in children 78-9
severe bleeding **60-2**
first aid summary................ **5**
severed................................ 48
letter bombs........................... 324
Librium 343
life jackets
choosing 260
staying afloat with.............. *262*
life preserver rings
in rivers 221
in the sea 236
life rafts.............................. 260-1
adrift in................................ 262
lightning storms **278**
lightning strikes...................... 278
treatment of victim...... 66-7, **93**
limbs
jerky movements of
in children **78-9**
severed................................ 48
lipstick stains
removal of 176
living rooms
danger points 165-6
locks, frozen car door 215
lost child 284-5
lost in the countryside........ **282-5**
LSD **341-2**
lung injuries 62, **68-70**

M

magic mushrooms......... 341, 342
malaria
preventive measures......... 269
man overboard **238-9**
maps
using in the
countryside.................. **286-7**
if you are lost 282
marijuana (cannabis).......... 337-8
Mayday calls 259
measles **111**
symptoms in children 76
medical insurance 273
medical treatment
on vacation........................ **273**
paying for........................... 273
medicines, administering
to a cat................... 183, *184*
to a dog.................. 183, *185*
taking abroad 269
meningitis
symptoms in
children 76, 77, 78, 80

mescaline 341
methadone **342**
microwave ovens
  safety with 162
migraine 63
milk stains
  removal of 176
mine workings
  hazards of............................ 290
miscarriage............................... **111**
mist, lost in 284
money
  when traveling abroad.. 269-70
morphine **340-1**
motion sickness................... 270-1
motor boats
  caught in a storm............. 258-9
  in rough seas **252-3**
  plugging a hole **248-9**
motorcycles..................... **216-17**
  braking techniques 216-17
  protective clothing 217
  safety measures 216-17
mountains
  avalanches **304**
  exposure on **281**
  survival in 297
  volcanic eruptions.............. **305**
mouth
  bleeding from 62, *63*
    first aid summary............... 5-6
  burns and scalds in 67
  insect stings in 110
  tooth injuries...................... 135
  toothache........................... 135
mouth-to-mouth
  resuscitation..................... **50-1**
    first aid summary................. 2
mouth-to-nose
  resuscitation..................... **50-1**
moving the injured........... **112-15**
mowers, electric,
  safe use *174*, 175
muggers, dealing with **314-17**
mumps................................... **116**
  in children............................ 77
muscles
  pulled 130
  stiff.......................... 130, 131
  strained..................... *132*, 133

N/O

neck injuries.............................. **55**
Neighborhood Watch
  schemes 180
nicotine stains, removal of 176
north, finding
  by the stars...................... *284*
  with a watch *283*
nose
  bleeding from 62, *63*
  injuries........................... **116-17**
  runny nose in children...... 76-7
  sports injuries.................... 131
  treating a nosebleed *117*
  first aid summary 5-6
object impaled in the eye 95
obscene telephone calls....... **322**
offices
  dealing with suspicious
    letters 324

robberies............................. **323**
  security precautions
    against........................ **323**
oil heater on fire
  action summary 22
oil stains, removal of 176
old people
  safety for................. 164, 167-8
  treatment for
    hypothermia................. **108-9**
opium....................................... **343**
otitis media............................... 76
overboard
  if someone falls **238-9**
  if you fall **236-7**

P/Q

packages, suspicious............. 324
  and letter bombs................. 324
paint stains, removal of.......... 176
paint stripper
  child swallowing.................. **117**
    first aid summary........... 27-8
parked cars
  approaching while
    driving........................... 196-7
passports
  safeguarding....................... 268
  and visas 268
perspiration stains, removal
  of 176
petit mal (epilepsy) 94
pets
  and rabies........................... 119
  sick or injured................. **181-9**
phone calls, obscene............. **322**
pills, giving of
  to a cat............................. *183*
  to a dog *183*
pipes, central heating
  leaking 160
pipes, water
  blocked 160-1
  burst *158*, 159
    action summary........... 11-12
  frozen pipes....................... 159
  layout *157*
  leaking joints 159
planes (aircraft)
  hijacked plane.................... **325**
  missing the plane................ 272
  plane crashes.................. **274-5**
  staying comfortable in
    flight.............................. 275
plants, poisonous 117
  first aid summary 28
  identifying in the wild......... 296
plugs, electric......................... 153
plumbing
  emergency repairs........ **157-61**
pneumonia
  symptoms in children **78, 79**
poisoning **117**
  cats 184-5
  by a crop sprayer............... **285**
  dogs 184-5
  drinking water as
    antidote............................ 117
  risks of 164
  first aid summary 27-8
  food poisoning **97**

poisonous plants 117
  first aid summary 28
  identifying in the wild......... 296
poisonous substances
  storage of *169*
police
  giving a description to 178
  and motorists **217**
    accidents 194, 195
  reporting road accidents
    to 192
poliomyelitis vaccination........ 269
polyneuritis
  (polyneuropathy)............. 328
power boats
  avoiding a collision
    in............................ 242, *243*
power cuts............................... **156**
power tools
  safe use of.......................... 174
pregnancy
  and alcohol 328
  miscarriage........................ 111
pressure points
  stopping blood flow at......... *62*
prickly heat............................. 107
psychotropic drugs and
  alcoholism 331
pulled muscles....................... 130
pulse, checking....................... *52*
  with breathing.................... 118
  at the throat...................... *119*
  at the wrist...................... *119*
pulse rates..................... 118, 119
quicksands, trapped in.......... **280**

R

rabies **119**
radiator leaks 159
rail crossings
  car stuck on........................ **205**
rain
  damage caused by 170-1
rain forests
  surviving in....................... 295-6
rape.................................. **318-19**
rape crisis center................... 319
rash in children
  prolonged 80-1
rear-wheel skids *200*
recovery position *136-7*
  and broken limbs *33*
  first aid summary *31-2*
reef knot *57*
retina, detached....................... 63
rib cage fracture 69, *70*
rib fracture............................... **120**
  symptoms 62, 120
ring-pad bandages *58*
rivers
  capsized canoe.................. 263
  caught in a current 222
  caught in waterweeds 222
  crossing flooded *310-11*
  falling into **220**
  kayak caught in rapids ... 264-5
  rescuing someone from..... **221**
road accidents **192-5**
  abroad.............................. 195
  and animals........................ **198**
  avoiding............................ 197

road accidents *continued*
avoiding a head-on
collision.............................. 195
causes of................................ 193
helping victims of........... **192-3**
prevention braking
distances 201, 203, 206
defensive driving......... **196-7**
keeping your
distance...... 203, 206, 216
roadside signs
approaching............ *196,* 197
robberies **323**
roofs
storm damage to 170-1
room on fire.......................... 148-9
action summary 23-4
smoke inhalation................. **124**
rope ladders........................ 146-7
ropes
crossing a river with 310-11
for rescues
from ice........................... *235*
from river or lake............. *221*
rubella (German measles)..... 101
symptoms in children 77
rust stains, removal of 176

S

sailing boats
avoiding a collision *242*
capsized dinghy.............. **240-1**
caught in a storm........... **258-9**
fire on board.................... **250-1**
heavy weather................ **252-3**
plugging a hole **248-9**
windsurfing **240**
sauce stains, removal of........ 176
scabies 81
scalds.................................... **66-7**
first aid summary 7-10
scalp injuries 103-4
bandaging........................ *102-3*
scorch marks, removal of...... 176
scrape and stamp.................. *315*
sea
avoiding collisions **242-3**
falling into **236-7**
heavy weather................ **252-3**
lifesaving....................... **228-31**
shark attacks..................... **227**
snorkeling **226**
storms at........................ **258-9**
survival at 262
swimming difficulties...... **222-3**
wind and weather at....... **254-7**
windsurfing **240**
seasickness 270
Seconal................................... 336
sedatives 333
septicemia, symptoms in
children 76, 77, 80
sexual assault **318-19**
shark attacks........................ **227**
shingles blown off
during storm 170
shipwreck **260-9**
shock **120**
shoulder, sprained.................. 133
sink, blocked.............. *160,* 160-1
overflowing 160

skidding car......................... **200-1**
skiing accidents **288-9**
avoiding an avalanche 304
injuries from 130
tobogganing on skis........... *289*
skull, fractured 102-3
symptoms of.................. 62, 92
sleeping bag
escaping from *276*
slings.................................. **121-3**
slipped disc **124**
smoke inhalation **124**
snakes 279
treatment of bites **125**
snorkeling.............................. **226**
snow
avalanches **304**
car stuck in..................... **206-7**
caught in a whiteout........... 282
making a shelter in *297,* 298
melting for water................ 295
skiing accidents **288-9**
snow blindness 63
snowshoes
improvising *289*
solar still, making
in the desert *299,* 299
solvent abuse.................. **339-40**
Sparine 343
splinters, removal of............. **126**
splints, making............ **127-9, 288**
sports injuries........................ 130-1
sprained ankle 49
moving someone with 112
treatment of................ *132, 133*
sprained joints........................ 130
sprains **132-3**
squash, injuries from............. 130
stab wounds............................ **133**
abdominal injuries caused
by.................................. **46-7**
chest injuries caused by **68-70**
stables on fire 189
stain removal **176-7**
stairs, safety measures.......... 168
stars
finding your way by.... *284,* 284
status epilepticus (epilepsy) **94**
stepladders *169*
stomach
injuries.............................. **46-7**
pain in children................. 80-1
upsets
gastroenteritis **97**
symptoms in
children 77, 79, 80
in the wild 295
stomach jab
for dealing with an
attacker............................ *314*
storms
damage to the home...... **170-1**
hurricanes.......................... **306**
lightning storms.................. **278**
at sea **258-9**
strained muscles *132,* 133
strangers
calling at your house 178
drunken
pestered by..................... **319**
stretchers
improvising 114, *115*
putting a person on *115*
supporting an unconscious
person on *138*

stroke..................................... **134**
first aid summary 29-30
symptoms of................. 29, 134
'sucking' wounds in chest ... 68-9
suffocation................................ **54**
sun
finding your way by............ 283
sunburn........................... 135, 271
surf
kayaking through 264
swimming in..................... **224-5**
survival
on a life raft 262
in the water 261-6
in the wild **292-301**
survival kits
for hikers 301
for life rafts 261
for motorists 300
in snowy weather............... 207
swimming
bodysurfing........................ *224*
cold water hazards 239
cramp attacks 222, *223*
difficulties **222-3**
drowning 91
exhaustion 222
injuries from....................... 130
lifesaving....................... **228-31**
safety measures 222
snorkeling **226**
in turbulent waves **224-5**

T

tar stains, removal of 176
tea stains, removal of 176
teenagers
drug abuse 333
telephone calls, obscene....... **322**
television on fire 148
temperature, raised
in children 76-7
tennis, injuries from............... 130
tents
blown down *277*
burning............................... 276
collapsed *277*
flooded *277*
leaking 276-7
pitching *277*
terrorist bombs...................... **324**
tetanus................................... **126**
antitetanus injections .. 131,269
thigh, cramp in 87
throat
insect stings to................... 110
taking pulse at................... *119*
throat jab
for dealing with an
attacker............................ *316*
thrush
symptoms in children 80, 81
thunderstorms
safety during...................... 278
tick bites 110
tiles
blown off during storm........ 170
tiredness
during car journeys............ **204**
tires
blowouts **203**

All about TRAVELING

Traveling abroad
How to obtain a visa 268
How to obtain immunization 268
How to prevent malaria 269
How to safeguard money and
valuables 269-70
How to cope with traveler's diarrhea 269
How to obtain the best rate of
exchange 270
Clothing for hot and humid climates 270
How to deal with motion sickness 270-1
Preventing motion sickness 270
How to avoid infected food
and drink 271
How to treat altitude sickness 271
How to avoid sunburn 271
If your vacation firm goes out of
business **272**
If your journey is delayed 272
How to obtain medical treatment
abroad 273
How to have a comfortable flight 275
How to clear your ears 275

Crises away from home
If you have a car accident abroad 195
If your train crashes 274
If your plane crashes 274

toddlers
safety measures
in the home **162-9**
on stairways 168
toe, severed 48
toilet-paper dressings............... *45*
toilets
blocked 161
dripping tank........................ 160
flush failure 161
tonsillitis
symptoms in children 77
tools
safe use of........................ **174-5**
tooth injuries 135
toothache 135
tornadoes 306
tourniquets
applying to animals............. *182*
trains
avoiding trouble on 319
crash.................................... 274
drunken strangers on 319
tranquilizers............................ **343**
trap, blocked *160, 161*
travel firms
collapse of........................... 272
travel sickness **270**
traveler's cheques
changing......................... 269-70
safeguarding.................. 269-70
traveler's diarrhea.................. 269
traveling abroad............. **268-71**
on airplanes........................ 275

triangular bandages........ 56, 57-8
in first aid kits *44*
improvising with *58*
for slings 121
tubular bandages............... 58, *59*
Tuinal 336
tunnels
exploring 290-1
safety in 290
typhoid vaccination 269
typhoons................................. 306

U/V

umbrellas
use as a weapon *317*
unconscious person........... **136-8**
checking for breathing *136*
choking *84-5*
first aid summary......... 15-16
collapse in the street.......... **199**
concussion 86
drowning.................... 229, *230*
epileptic seizure **94**
fainting **96**
first aid summary 31-3
gas poisoning..................... **100**
moving *113*
poisoned by a
crop sprayer **285**
recovery position for....... *136-7*

rescued from icy river......... 235
sports injuries...................... 131
suffering from exposure 281
supporting on a stretcher... *138*
turning.................................. *138*
underground
exploring **290-1**
safety 290
urine stains, removal
of 176, 177
vacation firms
collapse of........................ **272**
vacations abroad............. **268-71**
Valium 343
vapor lock................................ 213
varicose veins, burst 62
varnish stains, removal of...... 176
vertigo..................................... **139**
visas....................................... 268
volcanic eruptions **305**
vomit stains, removal of........ 176

W/Y

wasps..................... **110**, 186, 188
water
as antidote to poison.......... 164
car underwater.............. **208-9**
falling into a river or lake ... **220**
falling through ice **232-3**
filtering contaminated........ 295
leaking under baths 160
leaking through ceiling ... 170-1
leaking roof...................... 170-1
treading............................. *220*
water pipes
burst........................... *158,* 159
action summary........... 11-12
layout *157*
leaking joints 159
noisy................................ 161
waves, swimming through .. **224-5**
wheel nuts, loss of 212-13
wheelchair
carrying disabled person
in................................ 112-13
whiteout
lost in 284
whooping cough **139**
symptoms in children 79
wild animals
and the law......................... 198
treatment of injured 188
wind damage to houses..... 170-1
windows
blown in by storm 170
windshield wipers, failure of .. 212
windsurfing **240**
wine stains 176, 177
wounds
abdominal...................... **46-7**
applying bandages to....... *56-7*
bleeding....................... **60-3**
first aid summary.............. 3
chest **68-9**
gunshot 102
'sucking' wounds in chest *68-9*
stab wounds 133
wrist
sprained 133
taking the pulse at............. *119*
yellow fever vaccination 269

Credits

The publishers wish to acknowledge their indebtedness to the following books, which were consulted for reference:

Action Manual: How to Conduct a Small Boat Safety Campaign (National Safe Boating Council, Inc., Seattle, 1988); *AMA Family Medical Guide*, ed. Jeffrey R.M. Kunz and Asher J. Finkel (Random House, New York, 1987); *America's Camping Book,* Paul Cardwell, Jr. (Charles Scribner's Sons, New York, 1976); *Be Expert with Map and Compass*, Bjorn Kjellstrom (Charles Scribner's Sons, New York, 1976); *Canadian Aids to the Navigation System* (Canadian Coast Guard, Ottawa, 1986); *Canoe Travel Handbook* (Canadian Recreational Canoeing Association); *Canoeing Instruction and Leadership in Canoeing*, Kurt Wipper (Canadian Recreational Canoeing Association); *Childhood Symptoms*, Edward R. Brace and John P. Paconowski (Harper and Row, New York, 1985); *Don't Drink the Water: The Complete Traveler's Guide to Staying Healthy in Warm Climates*, Stanley Seah (Canadian Public Health Association and Grosvenor House Press, Inc., Toronto, 1983); *Down But Not Out*, RCAF Survival Training School Staff (Canadian Government Publishing Centre, Ottawa, 1978); *Drug Abuse and Drug Abuse Research*, The Second Triennial Report to the Congress from the Secretary, U.S. Department of Health and Human Sciences, Rockville, Md., 1987; *Everyday Law: A Survivor's Guide for Canadians*, Jack Batten and Majorie Harris (Key Porter Books, Toronto, 1987); *Federal Requirements for Recreational Boats* (United States Coast Guard); *First Aid* (Canadian Red Cross, Ontario Branch, 16th edition, 1984); *First Aid Guide* (American Medical Association, Chicago, 1987); *First Aid Safety Oriented* (St. John Ambulance, Ottawa, 1983); *Forbidden Highs: The Nature, Treatment and Prevention of Illicit Drug Abuse*, Reginald Smart (Addiction Research Foundation, Toronto, 1983); *A Guide to Immunization for Canadians* (Laboratory Center of Disease Control, Health and Welfare Canada, Ottawa, 1984); *Injuries Associated with Selected Consumer Products* (National Electronic Injury Surveillance System, U.S. Consumer Product Safety Commission, Washington, 1985); *Modern Survival*, Dwight R. Schuh (Hurtig Publishers, Edmonton, 1979); *National Drug Intelligence Estimate 1986/87*, The Royal Canadian Mounted Police (Public Relations Branch of the RCMP for the Drug Enforcement Directorate, Ottawa, 1987); *Northern Survival*, Employment and Related Services Division of the Department of Northern Affairs, Ottawa (Fitzhenry and Whiteside, Don Mills, Ont., 1979); *Outdoorsman's Emergency Manual (The)*, Anthony J. Acerrano (Winchester Press, New York, 1973); *Practical Law: A Layman's Handbook*, Chester S. Weinerman (Prentice-Hall, New Jersey, 1978); *Safe Boating Guide* (Canadian Coast Guard, Ottawa, 1987); *Standard Tests of Achievements in Canoeing* (Canadian Recreational Canoeing Association); *Survival in the Bush*, Bernard Assiniwi (Copp Clark Publishing Company, Toronto, 1972); *Surviving the Unexpected Wilderness Emergency*, Gene Fear (Survival Education Association, Tacoma, Wash., 1972); *Travel and Health Guide: A Guide for Canadian Travelers* (Health and Welfare Canada); *Things Your Travel Agent Never Told You: The Traveler's Survival Guide to Health, Fitness and Worry-Free Travel*, Gordon W. Stewart (Canadian Public Health Association and Grosvenor House Press, Inc., Toronto, 1983); *Travel and Health Guide: A Guide for Canadian Travelers* (Health and Welfare Canada, Ottawa, 1986); *Visual Distress Signals for Recreational Boaters* (U.S. Coast Guard, U.S. Department of Transportation, Washington, 1976); *Wilderness Survival* (British Columbia Forest Service); *Your Teens and Drugs*, Norman Panzica (McGraw-Hill Ryerson, Toronto, 1983).

Picture credits

The photographs in this book were provided by the following photographers and agencies. Work commissioned by Reader's Digest is shown in *italics*.

Page 254 *Johan du Plessis/ Reader's Digest, South Africa;* **251** *all* Professor R. Scorer; **256** *all* John Lythgoe/Planet Earth Pictures; **257** Jonathan T. Wright/ Bruce Coleman Ltd.; **305** S. Jonasson/Frank Lane Picture Agency Ltd.; **307** S. McCutcheon/Frank Lane Picture Agency Ltd.

Typesetting: MGM Typographers, Inc., Montreal; **Film work**: R.P.J. Litho, Inc., Montreal; **Printing and Binding**: Fabrieken Brepols N.V., Belgium